Total Knee Replacement and Rehabilitation

Dedication

We would like to dedicate this labor of love to our families for all their support and caring during this project. And we would also like to thank all our patients over the years who have taught us so much about life and TKA.

Ordering

Trade bookstores in the U.S. and Canada please contact:

Publishers Group West
1700 Fourth Street, Berkeley CA 94710
Phone: (800) 788-3123 Fax: (510) 528-3444

Hunter House books are available at bulk discounts for textbook course adoptions; to qualifying community, health-care, and government organizations; and for special promotions and fund-raising. For details please contact:

Special Sales Department
Hunter House Inc., PO Box 2914, Alameda CA 94501-0914
Phone: (510) 865-5282 Fax: (510) 865-4295
E-mail: sales@hunterhouse.com

Individuals can order our books from most bookstores, by calling **(800) 266-5592,** or from our website at **www.hunterhouse.com**

Total Knee Replacement & Rehabilitation

The Knee Owner's Manual

Daniel J. Brugioni, M.D., and Jeff Falkel, Ph.D., P.T., CSCS

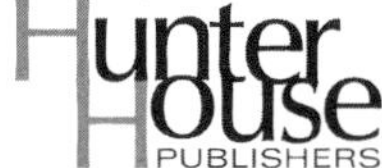

Hunter House Inc., Publishers
PO Box 2914
Alameda CA 94501-0914

Library of Congress Cataloging-in-Publication Data

Brugioni, Daniel J.
Total knee replacement and rehabilitation : the knee owner's manual / Daniel J. Brugioni and Jeff Falkel.
p. cm.
Includes bibliographical references and index.
ISBN 0-89793-439-3 (pbk.)
1. Total knee replacement—Popular works. I. Falkel, Jeff. II. Title.
RD561.B786 2004 617.5'810592—dc22
2004002785

Project Credits

Photographer: Andy Boudreau
Cover Design: Jinni Fontana Graphic Design
Book Production: Jinni Fontana Graphic Design
Developmental and Copy Editor: Kelley Blewster
Proofreader: Lee Rappold
Indexers: Robert and Cynthia Swanson
Acquisitions Editor: Jeanne Brondino
Editor: Alexandra Mummery
Publicist: Lisa E. Lee
Foreign Rights Assistant: Elisabeth Wohofsky
Customer Service Manager: Christina Sverdrup
Order Fulfillment: Washul Lakdhon
Administrator: Theresa Nelson
Computer Support: Peter Eichelberger
Publisher: Kiran S. Rana

Printed and Bound by Bang Printing, Brainerd, Minnesota

Manufactured in the United States of America

9 8 7 6 5 4 3 2 1 First Edition 04 05 06 07 08

Contents

Contents

Important Note

The material in this book is intended to provide a review of information regarding knee-replacement surgery. Every effort has been made to provide accurate and dependable information. The contents of the book have been compiled through professional research and in consultation with medical professionals. However, health-care professionals have differing opinions, and advances in medical and scientific research are made very quickly, so some of the information may become outdated.

Therefore, the publisher, authors, and editors, as well as the professionals quoted in the book, cannot be held responsible for any error, omission, or dated material. The authors and publisher assume no responsibility for any outcome of applying the information in this book in a program of self-care or under the care of a licensed practitioner. If you have questions concerning the application of the information described in this book, consult a qualified health-care professional.

Acknowledgments

A book like this would not be possible without the time, talents, and commitment of many people. First of all, we would like to thank our colleagues, particularly Dr. Cynthia Kelly; Dr. Douglas Dennis; Don Duntsch, PT; and Julia Juliusson, PT, for their expertise and professionalism in getting Dr. Falkel back on his feet. We would also like to thank our models, Sonny, Violet, Dianne, and Jerry for lending their time, talent, and knees to our photos. Andy Boudreau is our friend and photographic guru, and he made our ideas come to life. Finally, we would like to thank the staff at Hunter House for saying "yes" to this book and then for making this project a very positive experience; our acquisitions editor Jeanne Brondino for recognizing our potential; the always available and extremely brilliant Alex Mummery, who made our questions seem intelligent; and Kelley Blewster, whose attention to detail and command of the English language is pure poetry.

Please address all correspondence to:

Daniel J. Brugioni, M.D.
E-mail: dbrug@aol.com

General Statement about Scars in Figures

In order to more clearly illustrate which leg in a photo is the TKA leg, we have enhanced the surgical scar on the front of the knee with a marker.

Introduction

Orthopedic surgeons in the United States perform approximately 250,000 total knee replacements each year.[1] Total joint replacement is a relatively new technique that has improved dramatically over the past twenty-five years. It is considered one of the most reliable and cost-effective surgical procedures in medicine today. With the aging of the baby boomers, there has been an exponential increase in the number of people who require total knee replacement (more formally known as total knee arthroplasty, or TKA). Arthritis is the most common knee-joint disorder, especially in an aging population. As people demand a more active lifestyle, knee arthritis can be a source of daily and disabling pain. Although several treatment options are available for these patients, the end-stage treatment of knee arthritis is total knee replacement. The number of knee arthroplasties is predicted to rise significantly in the next decade due to the growth of the senior population, the increase in the incidence of arthritis, and wider acceptance of joint replacement.[2] With the improved surgical and anesthetic techniques available today, more patients than ever before are becoming safe candidates for total knee replacement.

The Need for a Book on TKA

The practice of medicine in this country has changed dramatically in the past twenty years due to the introduction of managed care. Within managed care, demands of the health-care system conflict with the demands of the patient. Health-care professionals—whether physicians or physical therapists—are reimbursed less for each patient, forcing them to see more patients. Therefore, they have less time to spend with each individual. Total joint replacement requires a great deal of time and attention to detail to enable the patient to experience the best possible result. A patient facing total knee replacement requires a significant amount of preparation and education to assist with the decision-making process and treatment. Once the surgery has been performed, the patient faces a long and arduous road to recovery. However, the length of supervised postoperative rehabilitation following total knee replacement is most often dictated by a case manager for an insurance company and is not always in accordance with an individual patient's needs. It is becoming increasingly difficult to provide quality care within the present health-care system because there is less direct contact between patients and their health-care providers. Therefore, it has become necessary for patients who need a total knee replacement to assume more responsibility for their own education and rehabilitation.

Because of the conflict between what the TKA patient needs and unfortunately fails to receive in our current health-care system, we felt an overpowering need to write this book. Its purpose is to assist patients in receiving the greatest benefit from their total knee replacement and rehabilitation. The book's early chapters discuss knee arthritis and its various treatments, making the decision to undergo TKA surgery, preparing for the operation, the surgical procedure itself, and the hospital experience. The remaining chapters concentrate on postoperative rehabilitation. They provide daily and weekly exercise suggestions and progressions that any patient can perform with or without a physical therapist. The book is unique in that it is organized chronologically along the timeline of total knee rehabilitation, starting with preoperative decisions and progressing through the days and weeks that follow. Appendix A describes potential complications following TKA surgery, and Appendix B provides a convenient index to all the exercises included in the book. Our goal is to provide patients with valuable, detailed information for each step of the journey, allowing them to get answers to their questions and concerns.

Let us note that if you are reading this book before undergoing TKA surgery, some of the exercises we've included may seem elementary. However, after surgery you will understand why this is the case. Rehabilitation following total joint replacement involves breaking down and isolating the mechanics behind the simplest of our everyday movements. Only then can we progress to more complicated activities.

The Authors' Personal and Professional Experience

It has been common practice for many surgeons to recommend that their patients with arthritis wait as long as possible to have their knee replaced. This is because the average life expectancy for a TKA is only ten to fifteen years. However, most surgeons fail to realize how the pain and discomfort of arthritis totally change their patients' lives. Jeff Falkel was one of those patients. For twenty years both of his knees gave him a hard time. For several years he was unable to do anything, even walk, without indescribable pain. The pain intruded upon every aspect of his life, including his job as a homecare physical therapist in Denver. He had to give up many activities that he truly enjoyed because the pain was prohibitive.

On October 19, 2000, Dr. Falkel underwent bilateral total knee arthroplasties, performed simultaneously by two surgeons. (*Bilateral* means the surgery was performed on both knees at the same time.) Over the course of twenty-five years as a physical therapist he had treated hundreds of patients with total knee replacements, and now he himself was one of those patients. Although the daily pain he had experienced was gone, he was faced with the challenge of getting his new knees to function properly. Even with all his clinical experience treating TKA patients, he was unprepared for the rigors of the twelve months following his own surgery.

Following an extensive rehabilitation program Dr. Falkel now has no pain, and his overall function has improved dramatically. He can walk up or down any surface without *any* pain or assistive device. He feels as if he can do anything he wants, and because the pain is gone he enjoys life much more than he ever thought he could.

Dr. Falkel's role as a patient with bilateral TKAs has changed his professional approach to the treatment of his TKA patients. With a new perspective, he is able to share his thoughts, questions, gains, disappointments, and unique experiences as both a patient and as a medical professional with those who need to consider this life-changing surgery. And it *is* life-changing...for the better.

Coauthor Daniel J. Brugioni also brings a perspective to this book as both surgeon and patient. He is a board-certified orthopedic surgeon in private practice in the Denver area. He performed over four hundred surgical procedures each year, with special expertise in total joint replacement. After practicing orthopedic surgery since 1982, a painful lumbar spine condition made it impossible for him to continue to perform surgery. On May 19, 2001, he underwent an extensive lumbar spine fusion, changing his perspective as a surgeon.

Dr. Brugioni will explain the surgical options, describe the preparation for surgery, and outline in detail what takes place during and after total knee arthroplasty. He will also discuss the decision-making process for both patient and surgeon, outlining the important factors to consider for each decision. His recent experience as a surgical patient provides valuable insight from the patient's side of the scalpel.

Why This Book, and Why Now?

The answers to these questions are simple: because every day, more and more people in this country are undergoing TKA surgery, and they need to know what to expect and how to get the most out of their rehabilitation. Many surgeons offer preoperative classes, but they are typically taught by health-care professionals who have not personally experienced the TKA procedure as a patient. Many surgeons provide booklets or pamphlets about total knee rehabilitation, but they are not comprehensive, and many times they leave the patient with more questions than answers. Between them, Dr. Brugioni and Dr. Falkel have over forty-five years of clinical experience in the medical field and have treated thousands of patients. A significant percentage of those patients suffered arthritic knees and underwent total knee replacements. The authors are able to share their thoughts on the full spectrum of total knee replacement and rehabilitation from the viewpoint of surgeon, physical therapist, and patient.

Our aim is to provide a comprehensive overview of total knee arthroplasty for the prospective patient and his or her family and friends. We have recorded our thoughts in an organized and chronological order to provide readers with a quick and easy guide to specific information they will need before, during, and after surgery. However, the book in no way attempts to be a substitute for the information provided to the patient by her or his surgeon and physical therapist. Rather, it is designed to supplement the information given to the patient, allowing him or her to ask more informed questions of the health-care professionals. Our goal as authors is to empower prospective patients to make informed decisions concerning their treatment. We intend to give the patient a better understanding of what to expect, when to expect it, and how to deal with the trials and tribulations of total knee rehabilitation. Being prepared for surgery and getting the most out of rehabilitation are critical factors in increasing the chance of each patient obtaining an excellent result. It is our pleasure to share with you our expertise and experience with total knee replacement and rehabilitation.

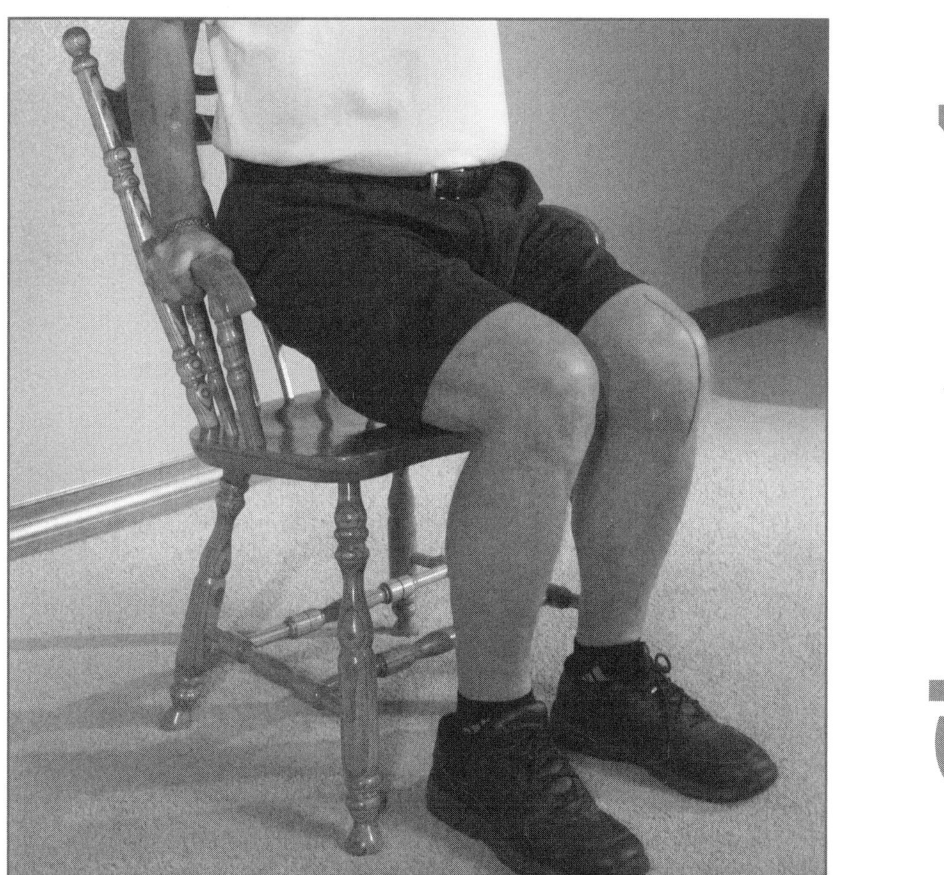

Chapter 1

Knee Arthritis

Why Do My Knees Hurt So Much?

The medical definition of arthritis relates to the breakdown, or wearing away, of the cartilage surfaces on the ends of the bones inside the joint. Arthritis is the most common cause of joint pain today.[3] Many problems cause knee pain; however, as with other types of joint pain, the most prevalent cause of knee pain is arthritis, particularly in our aging population.

The biomechanics of the knee are such that a person's full weight is distributed with each step through the knee over a small area of bone and joint surface. This results in an extremely high mechanical force through the knee joint. The knee must handle the stresses caused by gravity and muscle contractions, as well as those caused by the actual design of the joint. The ends of the bones in the knee joint are coated with a low-friction surface called *articular cartilage*. It is this cartilage layer that allows the bones to smoothly glide across each other. The next time you eat a piece of chicken, notice the white glistening cartilage at the end of the bone. This is similar to human articular cartilage. Stress transfer and joint motion both occur between adjacent surfaces of articular cartilage, thus making joint failure synonymous with cartilage failure.

The articular cartilage layer in the joint provides a smooth, low-friction, shock-absorbing surface between the bones of the knee. As mentioned above, arthritis involves a breakdown, or destruction, of a joint's articular cartilage.[4] When arthritis destroys the cartilage layer, the bone ends eventually rub together, causing joint pain. Joint failure due to arthritis can be caused by abnormal mechanical stresses, insufficient cartilage, inflammation (swelling), or infectious disorders. A good analogy is the wearing away of the rubber tread on a tire, eventually exposing the steel belts deep within the tire. When cartilage wears away in the human knee, the result is a painful and dysfunctional joint.

Symptoms associated with knee-joint arthritis include swelling, stiffness, loss of motion, limping, increased pain with weight-bearing activities, and pain that increases at night. The symptoms can be successfully treated; however, the arthritic disease process is irreversible and there is no known cure. Although the disease can be quite disabling, it is usually not life threatening. Many theories exist as to the cause of the various forms of arthritis, but no definitive cause has been found. Without an identifiable cause, the disease is more difficult to treat.

A detailed description of arthritis is beyond the scope of this book. Several texts have already been written on the subject. For more information we suggest contacting the Arthritis Foundation branch office in your area.

Over a hundred types of arthritis have been identified. The most common types are *osteoarthritis* (also known as *degenerative arthritis), traumatic arthritis*, and *rheumatoid arthritis*. The next three sections provide a brief description of these major forms of arthritis.

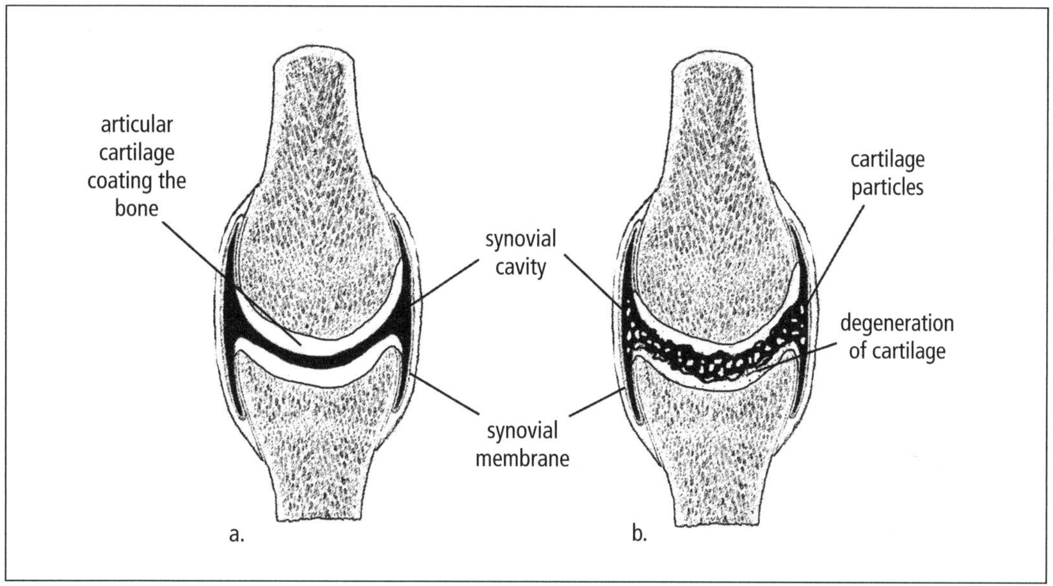

Figure 1.1. Figure 1.1a is an illustration of a normal, generic joint. Figure 1.1b shows the degenerative changes that occur with osteoarthritis. Note the cartilage breakdown and loose cartilage particles in the joint.

Osteoarthritis

Osteoarthritis (OA), or degenerative arthritis, is the most common form of arthritis (Figure 1.1). Millions of people in the United States have symptomatic or asymptomatic osteoarthritis. It is recognized as the most prevalent joint disorder in humans and as the most frequent cause of long-term disability in people over age sixty-five. More than one-third of people over age forty-five suffer joint symptoms that vary from occasional stiffness and aching after activity to permanent loss of motion and constant pain in at least one joint, usually the knee.[5] The prevalence of OA produces a significant impact on the national economy. The cost of medical care, combined with nonmedical costs such as lost wages and limited employment opportunities, creates a large burden on our society.[6]

Although the cause of osteoarthritis is unknown, we do understand a great deal about the disease process. Mechanical factors associated with wear and tear on the joint may be linked with osteoarthritis.[7] Repetitive and excessive stresses that occur during sports and recreational activities, as well as during the activities of daily living, may compromise normal joint mechanics and lead to osteoarthritis over a long period of time.[8] This sequence of events is common in the aging athlete—more affectionately referred to as the "weekend warrior."[9]

Genetics may also predispose a person to osteoarthritis. The condition is not passed on to offspring in a single gene like those for eye color or hair color, but it does tend to run in families. The lifestyle of certain families may contribute in a way that is not well understood. One of the major contributing risk factors for osteoarthritis is obesity or being overweight. Because the knee must bear a person's full weight with each step, excessive weight causes the cumulative wear and tear on the knee to be a problem sooner rather than later in life.

Traumatic Arthritis

Traumatic arthritis is sometimes considered a secondary osteoarthritis. Trauma to the joint can cause damage to the articular cartilage. With continued use of the joint, the damaged cartilage is weakened and cannot withstand the stress. The articular cartilage layer begins to break down prematurely. Fracture of the bone that results in improper alignment of the cartilage layer after healing places abnormal stress on the joint surface. Congenital malformation of the bone can also have this effect. The abnormal stress leads to early cartilage destruction. Significant cartilage damage can also result from ligament injuries that occur during sports or during a traumatic event such as a fall or a motor vehicle accident. It can also result from multiple minor traumatic episodes over time. The classic example is the athlete who sustains several minor knee injuries over the length of his or her career.

Although trauma is the cause of this form of arthritis, once the cartilage begins to degenerate, the condition looks very similar to osteoarthritis.

Rheumatoid Arthritis

Rheumatoid arthritis is an inflammatory disease of the soft sling membrane lining the joint cavity, called the *synovium* (Figure 1.2). The synovial tissue becomes swollen and inflamed, which eventually leads to cartilage breakdown and joint destruction. In this country, rheumatoid arthritis has a prevalence estimated at between 0.3 percent and 1.5 percent of the population, depending on the diagnostic criteria.[10] It affects women more than twice as often as men. Rheumatoid arthritis is considered an autoimmune disease, meaning the body begins to attack a portion of its own tissue, in this case destroying the joint cartilage. The body erroneously recognizes the joint as being "foreign tissue," and as a result it "attacks" these structures, which eventually results in joint damage. The cause of rheumatoid arthritis is unknown, although some researchers have theorized that it may be related to a viral infection or to environmental factors that have yet to be determined.

Other Forms of Arthritis

As mentioned earlier, osteoarthritis, traumatic arthritis, and rheumatoid arthritis are

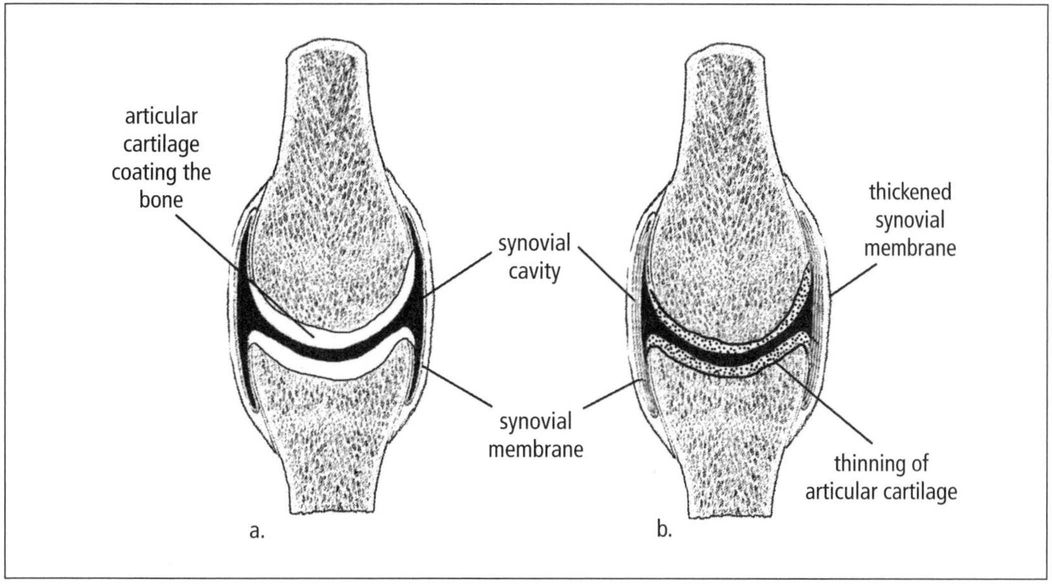

Figure 1.2a/b. Figure 1.2a is an illustration of a normal, generic joint. Figure 1.2b shows the changes that occur with rheumatoid arthritis. Note the thickening of the synovial membrane and the thinning of the articular cartilage.

the most common types of arthritis, and the knee is one of the most common joints where arthritis may occur.

Less frequent forms of arthritis include gout, psoriatic arthritis, systemic lupus erythematosus, ankylosing spondylitis, juvenile arthritis, Reiter's syndrome, Lyme disease, and septic arthritis. Other conditions also exist that affect the bone adjacent to the joint surface and that can lead to arthritis. These include trauma (as discussed above), avascular necrosis (the dying off of blood vessels), and tumors. Conditions such as these weaken the structural integrity of the bone underneath the cartilage layer. The articular cartilage loses its underlying support and starts to degenerate. A detailed discussion of the uncommon forms of arthritis is outside the focus of this book; however, more information on these conditions is available at any library.

Diagnosing Arthritis

A primary-care physician, rheumatologist, or orthopedic surgeon usually makes the initial diagnosis of arthritis. An experienced physician can frequently diagnose arthritic conditions by medical history alone. However, a physical examination of the joint is very important in gathering information.[11] The examining physician must check for any swelling, warmth, loss of motion, tenderness, muscle weakness, or ligament instability. X rays are strongly recommended to aid in the diagnosis of arthritis and,

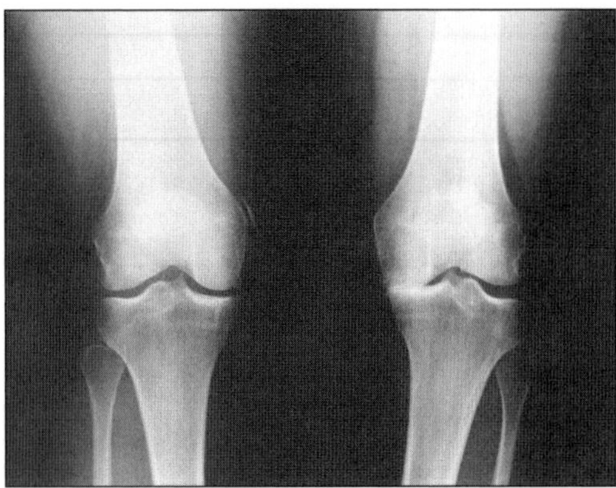

Figure 1.3. This is an X ray that shows a normal knee (on the left) and an osteoarthritic knee (on the right). Note the joint space narrowing (bone-on-bone) on the inner part of the knee with osteoarthritis.

especially, to help quantify the severity of the disease. In an arthritic knee, the X ray will show narrowing of the space between the bone surfaces. Because arthritis causes the cartilage layer in the knee to wear away and become thinner, there is less space between the bones. Although we cannot see cartilage on an X ray, if the bones appear closer together, this implies a loss of cartilage. The significant narrowing of the joint space on an X ray is an indication of severe arthritis (Figure 1.3). Sometimes blood tests are needed, particularly to help diagnose rheumatoid arthritis or gout. For the case that is difficult to diagnose, arthroscopic surgery is occasionally utilized to look into the knee joint and perhaps biopsy the joint lining and/or cartilage.

Regardless of which type of arthritis the patient may have, they all result in the breakdown of the low-friction cartilage surface of the knee joint. It is this breakdown that causes all the symptoms and pain that the patient experiences. Each of the treatment forms available to the patient, whether medical or surgical, is designed around the fact that the cartilage in the knee is damaged. The common thread in all arthritic conditions is the degenerative cartilage. Therefore, the treatment options available to the patient will be similar, regardless of which form of arthritis is present. The next chapter addresses the different treatment options available for arthritis.

? Common Questions and Some Answers

Our experience over the years has proven that different patients tend to ask the same questions about knee arthritis and TKA surgery. We have listed these most frequently asked questions at the end of each appropriate chapter. Most of the questions are related to issues discussed in the respective chapters, but they do not summarize the material covered in the chapter. The questions and their answers are meant to supplement the chapter rather than to replace it.

What causes my knee to swell?

All arthritic conditions are associated with inflammation. Inflammation is a chemical process that releases certain by-products into the knee joint, which results in swelling. Swelling is the result of an overproduction of normal joint fluid, which is triggered by this chemical process.

What causes pain in my arthritic knee?

Many factors can cause pain in the knee. Swelling, or overproduction of joint fluid, in the closed confines of the knee joint can cause the synovial lining of the joint to be put under tension, which can result in pain. Due to the degenerative changes in the cartilage around the bones in the knee, there is little or no shock absorption or protection of the bone. When an exposed bony surface comes in contact with another joint surface, the result is pain. Pain sensors are located in the ends of the bones in the knee, and when there is no cartilage present to help distribute the pressure of the body weight, these pain sensors are stimulated.

Why are my knees stiff?

There are several reasons for knee stiffness. The excess fluid in the arthritic knee joint occupies space, causing tension in the soft tissues surrounding the joint, which makes movement more difficult. As the cartilage surfaces break down in the knee, they resemble the surface of the moon or a cobblestone street. The smooth, low-friction surface of the cartilage is lost, and the resulting rough surfaces rub together and contribute to stiffness. Another reason for knee stiffness is because the body naturally reacts to a painful joint by limiting its movement. If this "protective" stiffness lasts for an extended period of time, the lack of movement of the joint results in more stiffness, creating a vicious cycle.

What causes bone spurs, and do they cause pain?

Bone spurs, also known as *osteophytes*, accompany the changes in articular cartilage and bone that are caused by arthritis. They are a response to abnormal stress and inflammation of the cartilage surface. Bone spurs are not the primary cause of joint pain, but rather the by-product of arthritic changes in the joint. However, once bone spurs grow large enough, they can limit motion and result in a grinding sensation in the knee, which is also very painful.

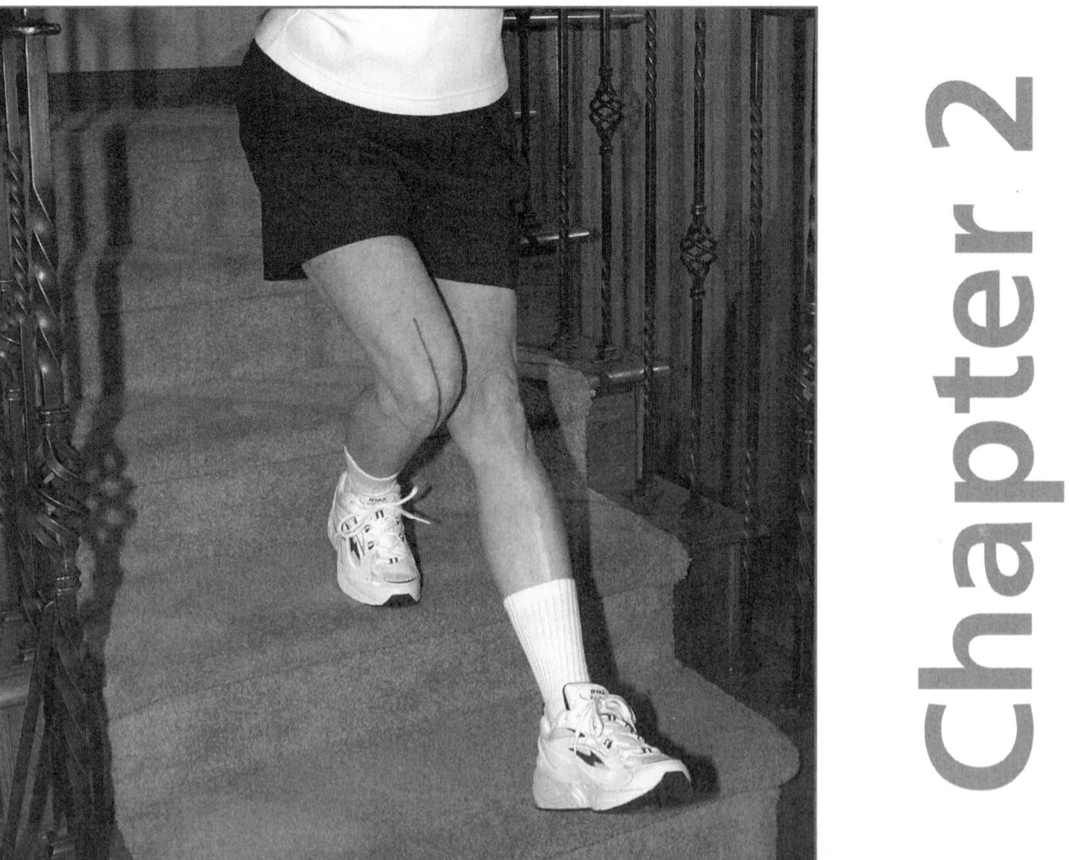

Chapter 2

Treatment Options

What Can I Do to Get Rid of the Pain?

The early symptoms of knee arthritis include occasional pain, swelling, and warmth in the joint. As the disease progresses, the symptoms become more consistent and more severe. Signs of progressing disease include decreased range of knee motion, tenderness, crepitation (crunching sensation), bone enlargement, and deformity. The treatment of advancing arthritis is multifaceted and is focused on controlling pain and maintaining function. There is no cure for arthritis; therefore the treatment is symptomatic—that is, it focuses on easing the symptoms. Mild forms of the disease are treated with the easiest and most conservative modalities. As the disease progresses, more involved treatments are utilized, depending on the severity of pain and dysfunction.

Lifestyle Changes

The initial treatment, which is also the most conservative, is a change in lifestyle. The relationship between diet and arthritis is poorly understood; however, evidence suggests that diet may affect the progression of the disease. It is thought that a change in diet may be helpful in decreasing arthritis pain. Foods high in fat and cholesterol may worsen arthritis. Increasing one's dietary intake of fibers such as fruits and vegetables may help alleviate symptoms. Decreasing salt, sugar, and alcohol intake may also be beneficial.

Weight loss generally alleviates pain in weight-bearing joints such as the knees. In the early stages of arthritis, weight loss can often relieve the symptoms completely! Even if surgical treatment is inevitable, losing weight will make the postoperative rehabilitation much easier.

Certain recreational activities have been shown to worsen the symptoms of arthritis. Sports that involve a great deal of stopping, starting, and lateral movement can make knee pain worse. Examples of these sports include tennis, jogging, racquetball, skiing, soccer, and basketball. It is helpful to identify these activities and to cut back or stop participation altogether. Doing so may cause symptoms to improve dramatically. However, at the same time it is important to continue to exercise, as discussed in the subsection below.

Certain types of work may also aggravate knee pain. We can often identify a specific activity or activities that are hard on the knees. This mostly applies to very physical jobs. An example of a harmful job activity is jumping off a truck bed or a loading platform repetitively over time. It is worthwhile to discuss any potentially harmful duties with your doctor and employer if you think a change in job activity could be helpful.

Let's take a closer look at two lifestyle factors that are commonly addressed when treating arthritis: exercise and nutritional supplements.

Exercise

Probably the most important lifestyle change in the treatment of the arthritic knee is exercise. Regular exercise offers the very beneficial effects of minimizing joint stiffness, increasing the tone and strength of the muscles surrounding the joint, and helping with weight management. The added strength around the knee provides the equivalent of a "built-in" brace for the patient.

Exercises frequently need to be modified so the knee is able to tolerate the stress applied to it during the exercise activity. For example, high-impact exercises, such as jogging or high-impact aerobics, often aggravate an arthritic joint. Substitution of medium- or low-impact exercises is usually better tolerated. Examples of lower-impact activities include swimming, cycling, walking on soft surfaces, rowing, Nordic track, elliptical trainer, or low-impact aerobic classes. One or two days of rest between periods of exercise is helpful in allowing the joint to recover. Applying ice to the knee for ten to fifteen minutes following exercise will often reduce joint pain and inflammation.

Levels of exercise may need to be modified on a daily or weekly basis in order to optimize the health of the joint. A general rule of thumb is to monitor how much exercise you can tolerate by thinking back about the pain you experienced during or after exercise. A certain amount of pain during or immediately after exercise is a normal response. However, if the pain persists after stopping exercise and continues through the night or into the next day, this is a sign that the joint was overstressed. Appropriate modification of the amount and/or duration of exercise may be needed in the future.

It is important for you to do as much exercise as possible within your comfort zone. Stopping all exercise should definitely be avoided, because doing so deconditions the muscles and increases the possibility of weight gain. At the same time, however, advanced stages of knee arthritis involve a paradox. Because of the increased pain in the knee with any or all exercise, many patients find it difficult or impossible to exercise. Therefore, they gain weight because of the reduction in their physical activity. As they gain weight their knee pain increases, which further limits their physical activity. In most cases the solution to this vicious cycle of pain is surgery.

Nutritional Supplements

The next step in conservative treatment is to try nutritional supplements, specifically *glucosamine* and *chondroitin sulfate*. These "cartilage-protecting" agents can be purchased over the counter without a prescription and are not regulated by the Food and Drug Administration. Glucosamine and chondroitin sulfate help with joint pain by aiding articular cartilage metabolism, protecting against articular cartilage breakdown, and providing a mild anti-inflammatory effect. Over thirty clinical studies have been performed in humans and animals using these substances, with five double-blind trials performed in the 1980s.[12] All studies showed consistent results with improvement in symptoms.

Glucosamine and chondroitin sulfate are usually taken orally, with the dose dependent on the patient's weight. As recommended in the book *The Arthritis Cure*, patients weighing less than 120 pounds should take 1,000 mg (milligrams) of glucosamine and 800 mg of chondroitin sulfate daily. Those weighing between 120 and 200 pounds should take 1,500 mg of glucosamine and 1,200 mg of chondroitin sulfate daily. Those weighing more than 200 pounds should take 2,000 mg of glucosamine and 1,600 mg of chondroitin sulfate daily. If the supplements are going to be effective in reducing symptoms, most people will see results after a three-month trial.[13]

Researchers also note that symptom relief does not occur equally in all joints. Some patients may experience profound pain relief in specific joints, while other joints are unaffected. To provide continued relief of pain, it is important to take these supplements indefinitely.

Side effects with these "cartilage-protecting" agents are quite rare in humans. However, chondroitin sulfate has a molecular structure similar to the "blood thinner" heparin, and, therefore, patients who are taking anticoagulation medication should use it only under a doctor's supervision. Gastrointestinal side effects occurred in less than 3 percent of people, and drowsiness in less than 1 percent of the patients tested, according to Tapadinhas et al.[14] Glucosamine and chondroitin sulfate are indicated only for the treatment of osteoarthritis. They should not be used by children or pregnant women. For diabetic patients, blood glucose should be monitored carefully by a physician because glucosamine contains sugar.

Although many other products on the market claim to aid in joint health, they have not withstood the rigors of scientific testing that glucosamine and chondroitin have. Nutritional supplements are not always benign, and they may interact with various types of prescription medications. Therefore, prior to taking any form of nutritional supplement, it is recommended that you consult your physician.

Nutritional supplements as a form of alternative medicine have been slow to gain acceptance by physicians in the United States. This may be due to the system in this country whereby the pharmaceutical industry controls much of the information on drug treatment given to physicians. Since glucosamine is a natural agent and cannot be patented, there is limited opportunity for profit by drug companies. Only after the discovery of glucosamine and chondroitin sulfate by the American consumer has the information about their effectiveness become more readily available.[15]

Medications

Traditional medications are effective in relieving the symptoms of arthritis. These can be obtained with or without a prescription. The most common over-the-counter pain relievers include acetaminophen, ibuprofen, naproxen sodium, and aspirin. Acetaminophen (Tylenol) has analgesic effects, but minimal anti-inflammatory properties. It has a low incidence of gastrointestinal side effects, but may cause liver toxicity in large doses. Ibuprofen (Advil, Motrin), naproxen sodium (Aleve), and aspirin offer better anti-inflammatory properties. However, gastrointestinal side effects and bleeding may occur with these drugs. Even though these medications may be purchased without a prescription, one must be careful of their possible side effects. They may be taken quite safely with occasional use, however. If such medications are to be used for long-term pain relief, it is advisable to first discuss the matter with your physician.

Prescription medications for arthritis include nonsteroidal anti-inflammatory drugs (NSAIDs). Some of the common brand names are Motrin (ibuprofen), Naprosyn (naproxen sodium), Clinoril, Feldene, Voltaren, Arthrotec, Lodine, Celebrex, and Vioxx. These medications have passed the test of time and have proven to be effective against the symptoms of arthritis. The most common side effects include gastrointestinal upset, bleeding, allergic reactions, and liver and kidney toxicity. A blood test should be performed every three to six months to monitor liver and kidney function in patients requiring long-term use of NSAIDs.

The newest of the NSAIDs are the cox-2 inhibitors, Celebrex and Vioxx. They are typically taken once a day and have minimal side effects. The cox-2 inhibitors are the only NSAIDs that may be used in conjunction with anticoagulants (blood thinners) under doctor supervision.

Usually it is prudent to try over-the-counter medications first. If they fail, ask your doctor for a prescription NSAID. Finding the right medicine for you may take several trials. The best drug for one patient may not work for another, and several changes may be needed.

Steroids are agents with more potent anti-inflammatory capabilities. Steroids are given orally, as an intramuscular injection, or intravenously. The most common is oral prednisone. Steroids are usually reserved for short-term use with severe flare-ups of symptoms, or long-term use for difficult cases that fail to respond to other treatments. They are most commonly used for the treatment of rheumatoid arthritis. Because of the potentially serious side effects, steroids should only be prescribed by physicians who have experience with them. Gold salts and methotrexate are two more powerful medications used in the treatment of resistant cases of rheumatoid arthritis. Usually these are prescribed under the supervision of a rheumatologist.

Injections

The next treatment option for knee arthritis is somewhat more invasive. It is a shot in the joint, or an *intra-articular injection.* For years steroid medications have been injected into the knee joint to help with severe pain or flare-ups of pain. Instead of the patient taking the steroid orally, it is placed directly in the joint to decrease inflammation. The most common steroids injected are dexamethasone, Depomedrol, and Celestone. These agents may potentially give quick, impressive, and long-lasting relief of symptoms. Unfortunately, obtaining relief requires a needle stick, and the duration of relief sometimes lasts only a few days. Repeated injections in the knee may produce destructive side effects in the joint. The connective tissue around the joint may be weakened, or the articular cartilage in the joint may degenerate further, making the treatment counterproductive. We recommend a maximum of four to five injections total in a single joint. Any more than this should be discussed thoroughly with your doctor. When successful, the injections may reduce or eliminate some of the pain of the arthritic joint. However, the injection does not cure the joint or prevent progression of the disease. Therefore, if multiple injections are required (more than three per year), perhaps an alternative treatment should be considered.

Another type of treatment using intra-articular injections in the knee is *viscosupplementation.* This process involves a series of injections using a substance called *hyaluronate.* Viscosupplementation has been approved by the Food and Drug Administration only for the treatment of osteoarthritis of the knee. Hyaluronate is not considered a drug, but rather a fluid prosthesis. In osteoarthritis the joint fluid becomes thinner than normal, losing some of its lubricating and shock-absorbing properties. Hyaluronate increases a joint's fluid viscosity—in other words, makes it thicker. Thicker joint fluid provides better joint lubrication and shock absorption between the cartilage surfaces. Hyaluronate has also been shown to slow the deterioration of cartilage surfaces and promote the health and restoration of damaged cartilage. Additionally, it provides an anti-inflammatory effect on the joint.[16] The only two commercial products of hyaluronate currently available for knee-joint injections are Hyalgan and Synvisc. The choice of product is usually based on the physician's experience and preference.

Viscosupplementation is usually performed by an orthopedic surgeon or other appropriately trained physician. The series of injections involves a minimum of three and a maximum of five, performed at one-week intervals. Symptomatic relief is usually noted within a month after the last injection. Duration of relief can vary from a few months to a year. Beneficial results are achieved in greater than 70 percent of patients.[17] If symptomatic relief is achieved for six to twelve months or longer, it is possible and advisable to repeat the series of injections. There is some evidence to support the finding that hyaluronate is more effective when more than one series of injections are given. If symptomatic relief is obtained for only a few weeks or not at all, a repeat series of injections should be considered with caution.

Hyaluronate has not been shown to have any adverse interactions with other medications. Side effects predominantly consist of inflammation at the injection site or inside the joint. A retrospective analysis of fifteen hundred patients reported an incidence of adverse events of 7 percent per joint.[18] Joint infection is also a concern because of the invasive and repetitive nature of the procedure. This complication is minimized in the hands of an experienced physician.

Viscosupplementation is most useful for patients who cannot tolerate NSAIDs, who have failed conservative treatment, or who are considered a poor surgical risk due to medical problems or old age. Viscosupplementation is not a cure for osteoarthritis, but it may be effective in reducing the pain and dysfunction associated with the disease. It may be used to "buy time" before more aggressive surgical procedures are needed.

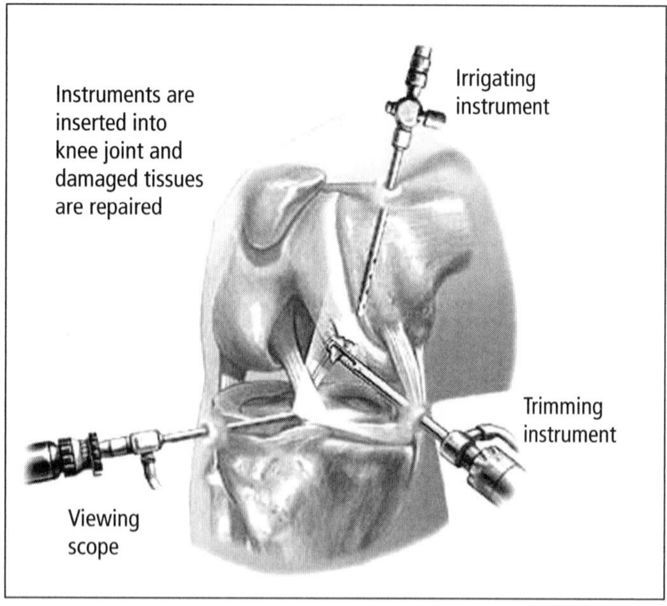

Figure 2.1. Arthroscopy of the knee. (Illustration courtesy of Stryker Endoscopy)

Arthroscopy

If conservative treatment fails to relieve the symptoms of knee arthritis, surgery is the next step. The least invasive surgical procedure is *arthroscopy of the knee joint*, or "knee scope" for short (Figure 2.1). Knee arthroscopy involves receiving an anesthetic—usually a brief general anesthetic less than an hour long. Other alternatives include regional (spinal or epidural) or local anesthetics. Barring any health risks, most patients choose a general anesthetic due to the short length of the procedure.

The arthroscopic procedure consists of three or more small slitlike (¼ inch) incisions on the front of the knee to insert instruments that are approximately the diameter of a pencil. With a small fiber-optic camera, the surgeon explores the joint to make a definitive diagnosis. The surgery is then performed with small instruments that cut, shave, trim, and vacuum inside the joint. Arthroscopic procedures for an arthritic knee typically include debridement (removal of loose tissue), chondroplasty (smoothing of cartilage), synovectomy (trimming of joint lining), meniscectomy (removing torn portions of meniscal cartilage), and drilling of the bone (to promote cartilage growth). In essence this accomplishes a "housecleaning" of the joint, and it often relieves the pain. A joint cleaning does not always provide symptomatic relief of arthritis, as it does not alter the natural course of the disease. However, if the patient experiences two or three years of improvement it is considered a successful surgery.

Knee arthroscopy is usually performed as an outpatient procedure. This means the patient is in and out of the hospital on the same day. The surgery may be performed in a hospital operating room, a freestanding day-surgery center, or an orthopedic surgeon's office that is properly equipped. Crutches are usually required for one to three days after surgery, depending on the patient's symptoms and the procedure performed. The knee may get wet in the shower two days after surgery. Exercise is required to overcome joint weakness and stiffness. For the most part, formal physical therapy is not needed because most patients are able to manage their own exercise program. Rehabilitative exercises such as those that are utilized after knee arthroscopy are discussed in more detail later in the book.

Cartilage Replacement

The technique of cartilage replacement in the knee has been gaining popularity since the mid-1990s. It is used when there are full-thickness defects in the articular cartilage layer of the knee, usually resulting from trauma. The procedure is not intended as a treatment for diffuse arthritis of the joint. Results vary depending on the location and size of the defect in the joint. The technique requires proper joint alignment, stability of the ligaments, and good range of motion in the knee. Cartilage replacement is also called *autologous chondrocyte implantation* (ACI).

The first step of the technique involves a knee arthroscopy for diagnosis of the cartilage defect, cartilage debridement, and cartilage biopsy. The biopsied cartilage cells are grown in a lab for approximately three weeks to increase the number of cells. The cells are then transplanted back into the knee through an open incision during a second surgery. The transplanted cells are contained within the cartilage defect using a periosteal cover, which is a patch of membrane taken from the upper tibia (lower leg bone). The entire technique involves two surgical procedures. It is quite expensive and may not be covered by insurance. Only certain patients are properly suited for the procedure, depending on the exact condition of their knee, and selecting them properly is critical for the surgery's success. Only orthopedic surgeons who are specially trained in ACI are capable of performing it.

Postoperative rehabilitation following ACI includes walking with crutches without putting any weight on the knee for approximately two weeks, with a gradual increase to walking while bearing full weight on the knee at six weeks after surgery. A continuous passive motion machine (CPM) is used for two to three weeks (Figure 2.2). The CPM is a cradle that very slowly flexes and extends the knee to begin early motion. A locked-hinge knee brace is also used to control joint movement. The goals of rehabilitation are to protect the cartilage tissue from excessive load and shear forces while controlling stress transfer to promote cartilage cell growth and healing.

Clinical results of ACI on 219 knees with an average of four years follow-up were reported by the surgeon L. Peterson.

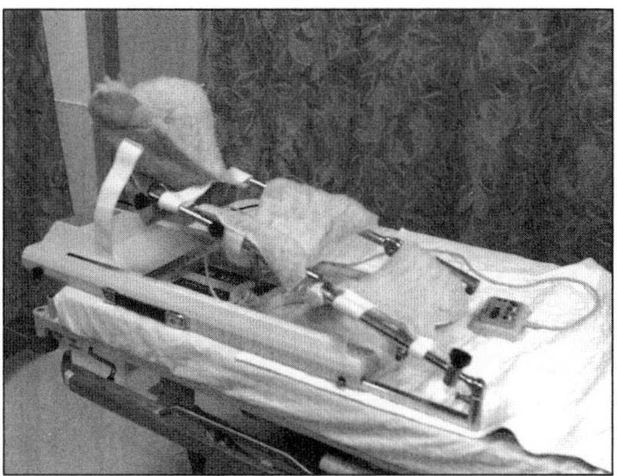

Figure 2.2. Continuous passive motion (CPM) machine, used to improve range of motion following surgery

He reported 80 to 90 percent good to excellent results, depending on the location of the cartilage defect.[19] Most of these patients had failed previous arthroscopic procedures. Unfortunately, most people are not candidates for ACI, due to the diffuse nature of their arthritis. The procedure is reserved for knees with focal cartilage defects in a well-defined area.

Cartilage replacement involves a great deal of time and many resources in order to obtain a good result. Therefore, as mentioned earlier, patient selection is critical. It is a relatively new technology. As surgeons gain more experience with the technique, they will be able to perform the surgery more efficiently, with better results, for less cost.

Osteotomy

For a select group of patients, an osteotomy may help alleviate the pain associated with knee arthritis. *Osteotomy* means cutting the bone. This surgical procedure is used in patients who have arthritis that affects only half of the knee joint, while the other half remains relatively normal. When only half of the joint is affected by arthritis, the knee is usually out of alignment, causing a bow-legged or knock-kneed deformity. In an osteotomy, depending on the deformity, the bone of the upper tibia or lower femur (thigh bone) is cut, creating a controlled fracture. The leg is realigned, and the osteotomy site is fixed with either internal fixation (plate and screws) or external fixator (screws into the connecting bone with rods outside of the skin). In principle, the leg is realigned to shift the weight-bearing forces away from the arthritic portion of the joint to the joint's better half—that is, to the part of the joint that still has a normal cartilage surface. By doing this, the weight-bearing forces of the knee are decreased across the arthritic portion of the knee joint and increased across the normal cartilage layer.

Although this can be a successful surgery when chosen for the proper patient, there are drawbacks. The procedure is lengthy, essentially creating and then fixing a fracture. Bone healing may take three months or more. Stiffness and weakness in the knee joint are a problem. Because the arthritic portion of the joint still exists, residual joint pain is common. An osteotomy is usually performed for osteoarthritis or traumatic arthritis in a patient who has the strength to remain non-weight bearing for a prolonged period using a walker or crutches. It is typically reserved for younger patients who are trying to "buy time" before their inevitable knee replacement.

It takes a great deal of time for the patient to heal from an osteotomy, and the procedure requires an experienced surgeon. Over the years, total knee replacement has become a surgery with increasingly reliable and reproducible results. Therefore, osteotomy procedures are performed with less frequency as more and more patients choose the option of a total knee replacement.

Total Knee Replacement

We have now arrived at the focus of our book, total knee replacement, more appropriately called *total knee arthroplasty* (TKA). *Arthroplasty* is defined as the plastic surgery of a joint or joints, or the formation of movable joints.[20] Total knee arthroplasty is the end-stage treatment for knee arthritis. After all conservative treatments and less-complicated surgical procedures have failed, the next step is to perform a total knee replacement.

When do you know if a knee replacement is needed? Helping a patient answer this question is part of the art of medicine. Two criteria must be met in order to proceed with a TKA. First, the X rays must show enough arthritis to warrant surgery. Usually this means there is a bone-on-bone or near bone-on-bone situation between either the tibia and femur or the patella (kneecap) and femur. When viewing a standard anterior-posterior (front and back) bent-knee X ray, most surgeons can tell quickly how much arthritis is in the knee. As the cartilage layers coating the ends of the bones wear away and become thin, the space between the bones on the X ray appears to narrow (Figure 2.3). For those difficult cases where the symptoms are more severe than seems to be indicated by a relatively normal looking X ray, a diagnostic knee scope (arthroscopy) may be necessary.

The second criterion that helps define the need for TKA is the severity of the patient's symptoms. Defining when an individual's pain is serious enough to warrant such a major surgical procedure can be a challenge since each patient perceives pain differently. Also, since every person places different functional demands on his or her knees with daily activity, symptoms that seem minor to one patient may be totally disabling to another. Determining this variable pain threshold for TKA in each patient may require several visits and long discussions with the surgeon to reach a decision. If basic activities of daily living are compromised, then the decision may be easier. For example, if a patient can no longer go up or down stairs, rise from a chair without help, put on shoes, get in and out of a vehicle, walk in the grocery store, sleep through the night, or walk without a cane, these are usually signs that a TKA is needed. Many patients have told us of a "defining moment" when their arthritic knees caused such severe disability that they were no longer willing to live with the dysfunction.

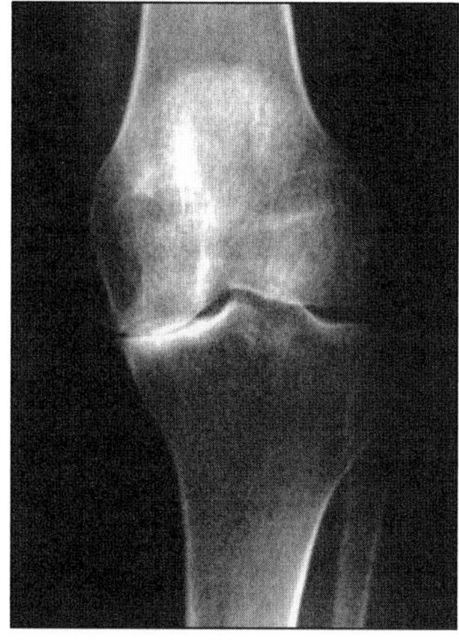

Figure 2.3. The arthritic knee and "bone-on-bone" deformity

There is no specific age to define when it is "too soon" or "too late" to perform a knee replacement. The general principle of timing for a TKA is to wait as long as possible before doing surgery. This is because the average life span of a knee-joint replacement is ten to fifteen years, and then revision surgery is required. Waiting as long as possible shortens the patient's remaining life expectancy, thus theoretically minimizing the chance that a revision arthroplasty will be needed. In addition, as the patient becomes older, less demand is placed on the prosthesis (knee replacement), thus enabling it to last longer. Of course, this treatment principle must be balanced by the severity of pain. It is cruel to allow a patient to suffer with severe pain just because they are young. As the overall results for TKA improve, the relative age threshold for surgery continues to drop.

On the other hand, there is concern about waiting "too long" before undergoing total knee arthroplasty. The longer the wait, the more potential there is for the deconditioning that occurs with inactivity. Advancing age is also associated with more medical problems, thus increasing the risk of major surgery. Defining when is "too soon" and when is "too late" to undergo TKA surgery is another part of the art of medicine. The timing of surgery needs to be a mutual decision between the patient and the surgeon.

Selecting a Surgeon

When a decision has been made to proceed with a knee replacement, the next step is to select a surgeon. The choice may be heavily influenced by an insurance plan. Some managed-care insurance plans have received negative public relations for interfering with this important selection process. It is the responsibility of the patient to know their insurance-plan limitations.

Ask lots of questions! Find out about the surgeon's training. Where did he or she attend medical school and serve their internship and residency programs? Did he or she receive any special training in joint replacement surgery? How many TKAs does the surgeon perform each year? Is the surgeon board eligible, board certified, or board recertified in orthopedic surgery? Do not be afraid to ask your surgeon these questions; usually they are welcomed.

A great way to research a surgeon is to talk with some of the health-care professionals who have seen him or her work. Call the local hospital and talk with the head nurse on the orthopedic floor where all the postoperative patients stay. Call the operating room and speak with the orthopedic nurse coordinator who knows about the surgeon's abilities. Contacting some local physical therapists may also shed some light on how a surgeon's patients do in rehabilitation. Usually, health-care professionals are willing to talk with a prospective patient to help them choose a surgeon. Finally, ask the surgeon for names of former patients who are willing to talk about their experience with this surgery. Former patients are often quite candid about their experiences.

An anesthesiologist should be chosen using a similar method. It is of paramount importance to be in good hands from an anesthetic viewpoint. Your surgeon usually has a core group of anesthesiologists she or he works with. Do not be afraid to ask your surgeon which anesthesiologists are preferred.

During the search for a surgeon, getting a second opinion may be quite helpful. Even if there is no doubt about the diagnosis or choice of surgeon, a second opinion can often bring different perspectives into view. It is critical to gather as much information as possible before surgery. Doing so creates a better-informed patient and will enhance the recovery process.

TKA Surgical Technique

Total knee arthroplasty is not an entirely accurate term. The knee is not totally replaced; rather, the joint is resurfaced. The cartilage surfaces are removed and replaced with metal and plastic components (Figure 2.4). The overall shape and structure of the bones are maintained. In a normal knee joint, the end of the femur (thigh bone), which consists of knuckle-shaped femoral condyles, slides against the upper part of the tibia (shin bone), or tibial plateau. During a TKA surgery, the femoral condyles are replaced with metal, and the tibial plateau is replaced with a component that is a com-

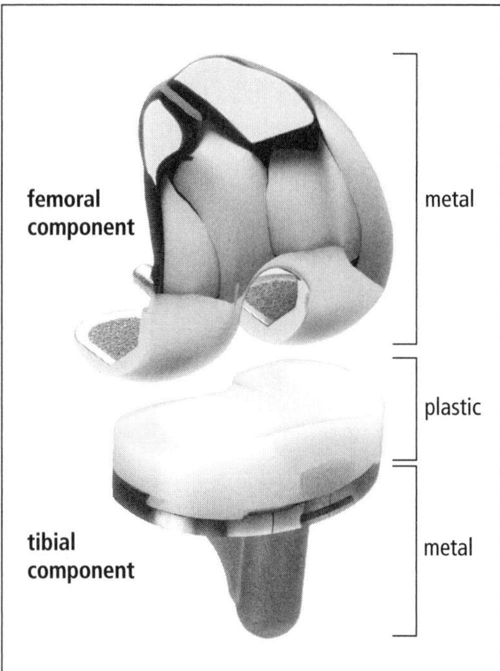

Figure 2.4. Components of the TKA. (Medical Pivot TKA, manufactured by Wright Medical Technology, Inc.)

bination of plastic and metal. In addition, the patella (kneecap), which slides over the front part of the femur, is resurfaced with a round plastic "button." Critical to knee mechanics are the surrounding tendons, ligaments, and muscles; these are all preserved during the procedure. See Figure 2.5 for an X ray comparing a TKA knee (left) to a "normal" one (right).

Several types of prostheses are available for the surgeon to use. A surgeon chooses a prosthesis based on his or her preference and experience. The most common type used for a primary (first-time) TKA is an *unconstrained artificial joint* (see Figure 2.6 on the next page). In essence, the end portion of the femur is resected (surgically removed) and "capped" with a metal surface. The upper portion of the tibia is removed and replaced with a metal tray upon which a plastic insert is placed. The metal is composed of a cobalt-chromium alloy, and the plastic is a high-density, high-molecular-weight polyethylene. The preserved tendons and ligaments are responsible for maintaining proper alignment of the joint surfaces.

A relatively new, second type of prosthesis is the *mobile bearing knee arthroplasty*. This type of prosthesis can be described as a moving, polyethylene (plastic) post and insert, which separates the femoral condyles from the tibial tray. The plastic insert moves along the metal tibial tray in conjunction with normal knee motion. The mobile bearing knee arthroplasty is gaining popularity for use with younger patients because it theoretically causes less wear on the plastic cushion and less stress at the juncture of the

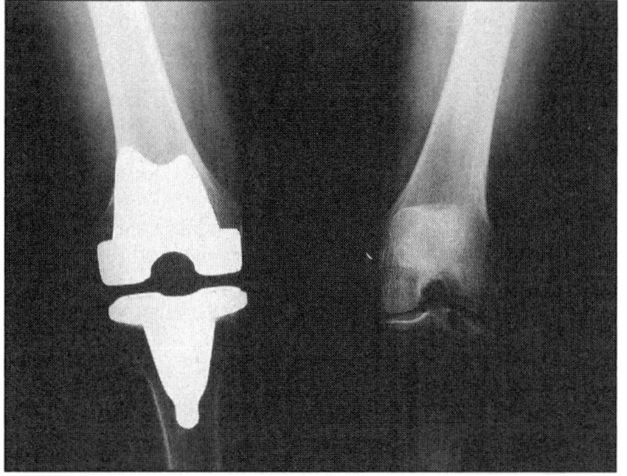

Figure 2.5. X ray showing a TKA (left) and a "normal" knee (right)

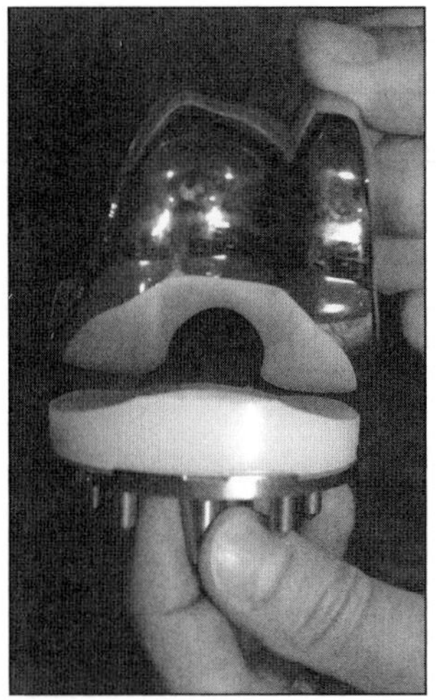

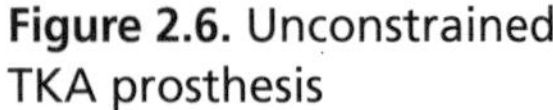
Figure 2.6. Unconstrained TKA prosthesis

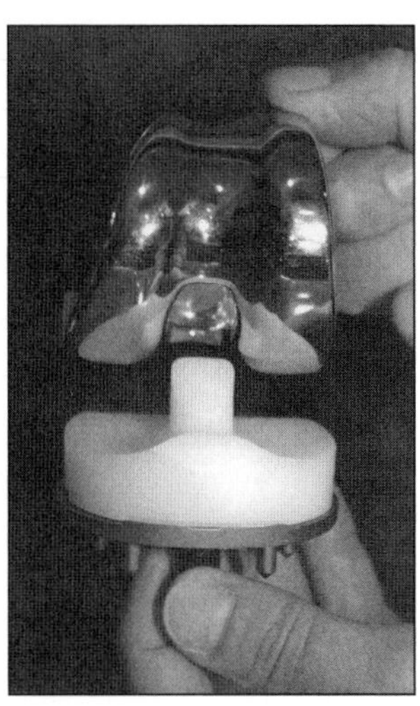

Figure 2.7. Posterior stabilized TKA prosthesis

prosthesis/bone connection. It is hoped that this design will be longer lasting than the unconstrained TKA prosthesis.

Another prosthetic design is the *posterior stabilized total knee arthroplasty* (Figure 2.7). In this design, a plastic post extends from the plastic tibial tray and inserts into a housing on the femoral component between the femoral condyles. The posterior stabilized TKA provides more stability for the knee and is used primarily with knees that have poor ligamentous or muscular support. It is most commonly used on elderly patients.

It is not important for you to be concerned with the "brand name" or exact design of the prosthesis. What is important is that the surgeon is comfortable with the model, that it yields the best results in his or her hands, and that it is a design appropriate for you. There is a significant learning curve involved in getting to know the finer points of any specific brand or make of TKA prosthesis. Surgical mastery of a prosthetic system is the key to excellent results.

Another variable in the technique for TKA is the fixation of the prosthetic components—that is, how to attach the prosthesis to the bone. Fixation of the prosthetic components to the bone is done either with or without cement. The cemented technique involves using methyl methacrylate cement to "glue" the metal to the bone. Cementless fixation is a method that requires precise bone cuts to achieve maximum contact of metal to bone. The metal components used with this technique have a porous surface to allow bone to grow into the prosthesis, thus achieving solid fixation.

The advantage of cement fixation is that the prosthetic components are instantly fixed to the bone, allowing the patient to bear full weight on the leg immediately after surgery. On the other hand, cement is a disadvantage if the prosthesis ever needs to be replaced. It is difficult to chip out all the cement during removal of the old prosthesis. Therefore, cement is typically used in patients over sixty-five. Their bone tends to be more osteoporotic (softer), with less potential to grow into the metal. In addition, there is less likelihood of a revision being needed due to the lower demands on the joint and the overall relatively shorter remaining life expectancy when compared to younger patients. The early days of cement fixation had some problems, but recent results have improved dramatically due to newer pressurizing cement techniques.

Prosthetic cementless fixation is used for younger bone. The younger the patient, the better the bone quality and the better the ingrowth potential. The downside is that it typically takes six weeks for bone to grow into the porous metal backing of the prosthesis. This means that any weight-bearing activity is usually restricted for six weeks postoperatively. The advantage with the cementless technique is that fixation is achieved more naturally, and the metal is fixed directly to the bone without a cement intermediary. With a younger patient, there is a greater chance that future revision surgery will be needed. A cementless prosthesis is easier to revise than its cemented counterpart, as the surgeon does not have to deal with cement removal.

A patient cannot feel the difference between the two types of fixation. The fixation technique is chosen by the surgeon based on the bone quality, age, and demands of the patient.

Bilateral TKA

Another surgical option that must be discussed is the case of the patient with end-stage arthritis in both knees. This situation requires *bilateral TKAs* (surgery on both knees). The surgeon and patient need to decide whether it is best to do one procedure at a time on two different days or to perform surgery on both knees on the same day and during the same anesthetic.

Several things need to be considered when making this decision about bilateral TKA. When one knee is significantly more painful than the other, it is usually the most painful one that is operated on first. In the scenario where a single knee is done, blood loss is minimized and the patient is under anesthesia for a shorter period of time. In the unlikely event that an infection occurs, it will be confined to only one knee. It allows the patient to have a "good" leg to stand on to facilitate rehabilitation of the recently replaced knee. The time interval between total knee surgeries is typically about three months. By this time the first knee to have undergone surgery is usually solid and reliable and can bear the weight in anticipation of the other knee requiring surgery. The downside to separating the knee surgeries is that the patient receives two anesthetics. In addition, the recovery and rehabilitation is prolonged.

In the case where both knees have nearly equally severe symptoms, the patient and surgeon should consider bilateral TKA. The simultaneous bilateral TKA gets everything done at once under a single anesthetic. Doing everything at once may be an emotional and financial necessity for some patients. Rehabilitation can be performed simultaneously on both knees, thus reducing the overall length of the program. The disadvantages to this method are the prolonged anesthetic time and a potential for increased blood loss. If an infection should occur, there is a greater chance of it affecting both knees. In addition, the longer time lying on the operating table increases the risk of blood clots. The same surgeon may perform the surgery on each knee in sequence, or the procedure may be done simultaneously by two different surgeons. If the patient and surgeon both agree to it, simultaneous surgery by two different surgeons may eliminate some of the downside associated with a longer procedure.

Together the patient and the surgeon make the decision to undergo a single or bilateral TKA. The choice must take into account the overall health of the patient as well as patient and surgeon preference. Minimizing the time taken off work must also be considered. There is no "right" or "wrong" decision; the right one is the one that works best for you.

■ ■ ■

The decision to undergo a total knee replacement is a difficult one. Fortunately, the results are consistent and reproducible. Most patients report 90 to 95 percent improvement in terms of pain and function.[21] It is typically a positive, life-changing experience. Only after all the other treatment options have been considered or attempted can the patient and surgeon decide on total knee arthroplasty. Once the decision has been made to undergo the surgery, though, it is important for you, the patient, to gather as much information as possible about the procedure, recovery, and rehabilitation. There is a positive correlation between a well-informed patient and an excellent surgical result.

The patient, family, and home need to be prepared prior to surgery to make the road to recovery as smooth as possible. The next chapter will guide you in your preparation for surgery.

? Common Questions and Some Answers

What kind of anti-inflammatory medication should I take?

It is best to consult your physician to determine which type of anti-inflammatory medication is suitable for you. Your overall state of health as well as potential interactions with other drugs you might be taking are both to be considered when your doctor recommends an anti-inflammatory medication. In general, it is safest to start with over-the-counter anti-inflammatory medications. If these fail to relieve pain, most likely your physician will prescribe Motrin or Naprosyn. They provide a stronger dose of the same over-the-counter medication. If these drugs also prove unsuccessful, the next step is for your physician to prescribe one of the newer-generation anti-inflammatories. The entire process of finding the medication that works for you may take some time—and many trials.

Should I continue taking glucosamine and chondroitin sulfate after surgery?

Although glucosamine and chondroitin sulfate are no longer needed for the replaced knee, they provide certain benefits for other joints. If you have joints other than your knees that are helped by taking glucosamine and chondrotin sulfate, we recommend continuing the supplements. They have no known negative effects on the healing process.

How many steroid injections into my knee are "too many"?

This is a good question, and there is no confirmed limit. We have found that three or four injections in a single joint in a patient's lifetime is a good guideline for a maximum number of injections. Repetitive doses of steroids weaken the connective tissue around the knee joint (i.e., the tendons, ligaments, and cartilage). If a patient requires more than four injections for pain control, a different type of treatment is probably a good idea. There are exceptions to these general guidelines; they can be discussed with your doctor or surgeon.

Can viscosupplementation injections be done more than once?

Viscosupplementation has been shown to be safely repeated in patients who experience good relief after the first set of injections. If no pain relief is obtained after the first set of injections, a repeat set is not recommended. However, if a patient experiences more than six months of pain relief, a second set of injections should be considered.

How many arthroscopic surgeries are "too many"?

Again, there is no definitive number that constitutes too many arthroscopies. A minimum of two years of relief from symptoms following arthroscopic surgery is needed for the procedure to be considered successful and to warrant a repeat procedure. Since arthroscopy provides symptomatic relief, it "buys time" before total knee arthroplasty is necessary. It is more common for arthroscopic procedures to be repeated in younger patients in an effort to delay total knee arthroplasty. In general, arthroscopic procedures that are performed in order to "clean up" arthritis are less successful with each subsequent surgery. The number and timing of the arthroscopies are an individual decision between patient and surgeon.

How long is the surgery for total knee arthroplasty?

In general, it should take an experienced surgeon approximately two hours for the entire procedure, including time for anesthesia and wound closure. The time may vary based on the patient's age, previous surgeries, amount of bony deformity, and size of the patient's leg. Total time for the surgery will vary, and the surgeon will discuss this topic with the patient and her or his family prior to the operation.

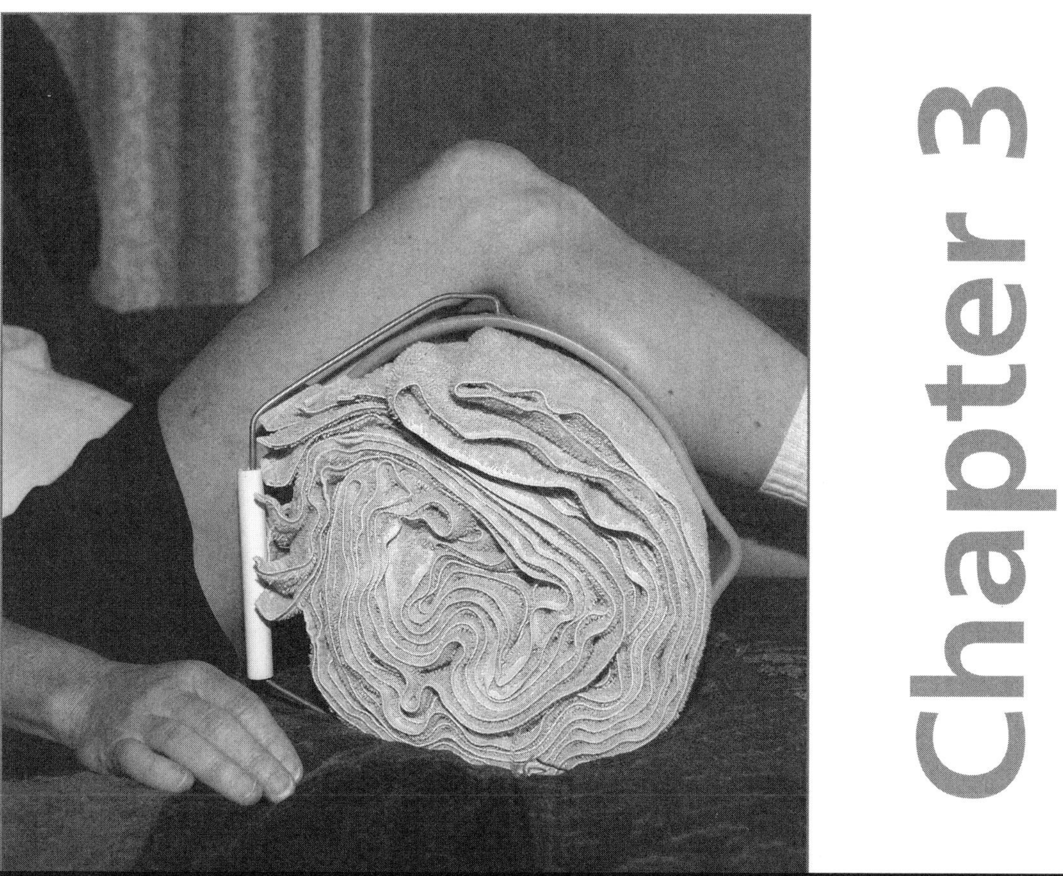

Chapter 3

Getting Ready

Preparing Your Home and Yourself for Surgery

You've made the decision to have your knee replaced. Now it is time to prepare your home for your return from the hospital and to get yourself ready for the surgery. Undergoing a total knee replacement will make your life much better, because the pain you have felt for so long will be gone. Eventually you will be able to do much more than you've been able to do for a while, since your knee will no longer limit your activities. However, after any surgery, and especially after total-knee-replacement surgery, for a time you will require additional assistance to move around in your home. There are several things to do prior to going to the hospital that will make your home more "user friendly" and make the recovery period much easier on you and your family.

Home Preparation

One of the first things to do in preparing for surgery is an assessment of how to get in and out of your home. After TKA surgery, it is difficult to climb stairs, particularly if you have both knees replaced at the same time. At the hospital you will be instructed in stair climbing using either a walker or crutches. This topic is covered in later chapters of this book. If your residence has several steps that do not provide a railing or banister for support, consider constructing a temporary ramp to make getting in and out of your home easier and safer. A ramp is especially convenient after undergoing simultaneous bilateral TKA. It will facilitate entering and exiting the house with minimal difficulty and thus provide more independence. If you, a family member, or a friend is handy with woodworking tools, a ramp can easily be constructed in just a few hours using two-by-four boards and plywood. If not, there are many volunteer groups (church groups, Boy Scouts, etc.) that would assist you in construction of a ramp for a minimal charge. The general rule of thumb to follow when building a ramp is that for every inch of vertical height (from the door to the ground) there should be one foot of ramp length. This creates the proper slope of the ramp to facilitate its use.

The next step in home preparation prior to surgery is evaluating the bedroom. In the initial phase of recovery, a lot of your time will be spent resting in bed. Consider placing a bed of some sort on the first floor or near the main living area of the house. It is important that your bed be on the same level as a bathroom and as close to the main living area as possible. Getting up and down stairs will be difficult in the first few days or weeks after returning from the hospital. Therefore, having a bed or foldout couch to sleep on for a short period of time will make life a lot easier for you and your family. One of the things that becomes obvious after total-knee-replacement surgery is how little effort it takes for you to reach the point of exhaustion. Having a bed on the main living floor will eliminate your having to climb stairs and will make it easier to rest.

A very useful piece of furniture for after surgery is a recliner with a leg rest that can be raised and lowered to different heights.

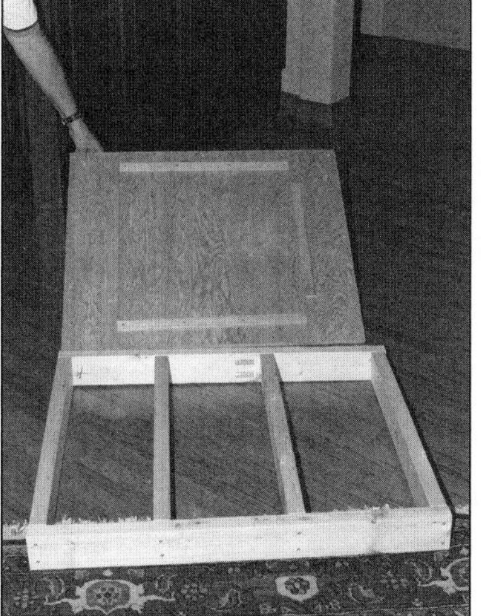

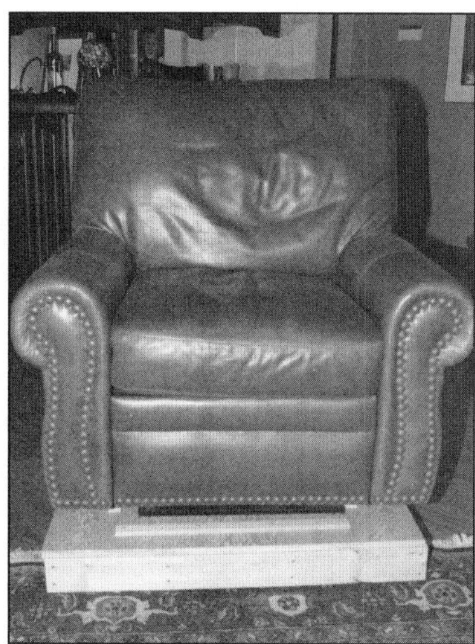

Figure 3.1. Elevation of a recliner on a platform built of two-by-fours and plywood

Many patients find it easier to sleep in a recliner after surgery, or at least to spend part of the night in the recliner. It allows you to elevate your legs, which will help control swelling, and as we will see in Chapter 6, you can even work on increasing your range of motion while in a recliner. If you already have a recliner, consider raising it a few inches off the floor. Do this by placing it securely on a platform of two-by-four boards with a plywood base and top. When it's elevated it is easier to get into and out of (Figure 3.1). If you don't already own a recliner and are considering buying one, several manufactures make "elevated" recliners, some offering electronic controls to tilt the seat, thus enabling you to sit and stand with minimal stress on your new knee.

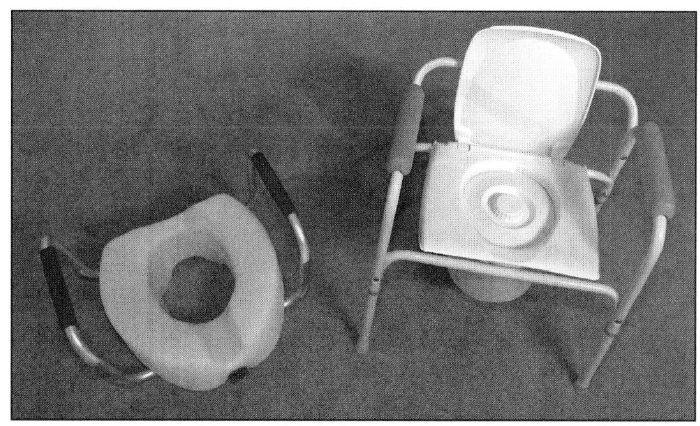

Figure 3.2. Three-in-one bedside commode (right) and elevated toilet seat (left)

Next, we recommend some minor modifications to your bathroom. After surgery, it will take some time to regain a "normal" range of motion in your knee. The lack of motion and increased swelling in the TKA knee make it difficult for some patients to get on and off a toilet. There are two pieces of equipment that facilitate using the toilet after surgery. The first is called a *three-in-one bedside commode chair* (Figure 3.2, item on the right). It is an adjustable bench that fits over a toilet. It has a lid and commode seat, as well as a removable bucket under the seat. It can be used over the toilet in your bathroom by adjusting the height and removing the bucket. Alternatively, it can be used by itself in your bedroom with the bucket in place. The three-in-one commode chair works very well; it conveniently fits over most bathroom toilets with no permanent modification to the bathroom. It can be purchased at a self-help store or hospital-equipment store, or may even be rented or borrowed from a hospital-equipment loan program. Talk to your surgeon about where you can purchase or borrow a three-in-one commode chair.

The second adaptive toilet device is a *toilet seat elevator* (Figure 3.2, item on the left). It is a sturdy plastic extension that attaches to the rim of the toilet bowl and elevates the seat height to allow you to get on and off the commode with less stress on your new knee. The raised toilet seat is less convenient than the three-in-one commode seat but is another option for use after total knee replacement.

The other modification for your bathroom is in the shower. After surgery, it is difficult to stand on your operated leg for prolonged periods of time, particularly in the shower. A simple device for the shower is an adjustable, waterproof shower bench that allows you to sit while taking a shower. This takes the stress off your new knee and minimizes the chance of falling while showering.

Some patients find that a hand-held shower adapter is another useful piece of equipment for the shower. It includes a flexible hose that attaches to the shower pipe on one end and to a large hand-held showerhead on the other. Once the water is turned on, it runs through the hand-held showerhead, allowing you to control where the water is being sprayed while sitting on the shower bench.

Yet another modification for the shower is a grab bar. This is a large stainless-steel bar that attaches to the wall of the shower, enabling you to stabilize yourself while showering and getting into and out of the shower. A grab bar is an excellent safety feature, and many newer homes and apartments already have grab bars installed in the shower. The only caution about a grab bar in the shower is that in order for it to be safe, it has to be installed correctly. Contact your local plumber or contractor about proper procedures for installation of a grab bar in the shower. All of the items for modification of the shower can be purchased at your local building-supply center, hardware store, or self-help shop.

Several other self-help and assistive devices exist that can make you more safe and independent during your daily activities around the home after your total-knee-replacement surgery. The first is a cordless telephone. Since it can be taken with you anywhere in the house, a cordless phone will not only increase your independence but will also give you a sense of security and safety. It is a convenience that is well worth the investment.

You may want to purchase a long-handled grabber or reacher (Figure 3.3). This device lets you pick up objects without bending over. It comes in many styles and

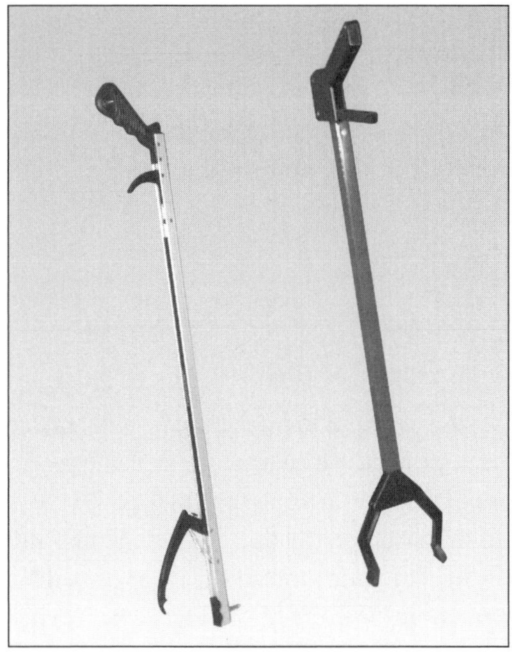

Figure 3.3. Long-handled grabber/reacher

designs and can be purchased at a self-help store or medical-supply company. Your in-hospital physical therapist may even offer you one. The long-handled grabber is a worthwhile investment because it has hundreds of uses around the home even after you are fully recovered from your surgery.

Another item that adds to your independence is a sock helper. This ingenious device allows you to put your socks on without having to bend over or even bend your knee. It is relatively inexpensive, and while it is "standard equipment" for patients who have hip-replacement surgery, it works equally well for knee-replacement patients and is definitely worth considering. Ask your in-hospital physical therapist about purchasing a sock helper.

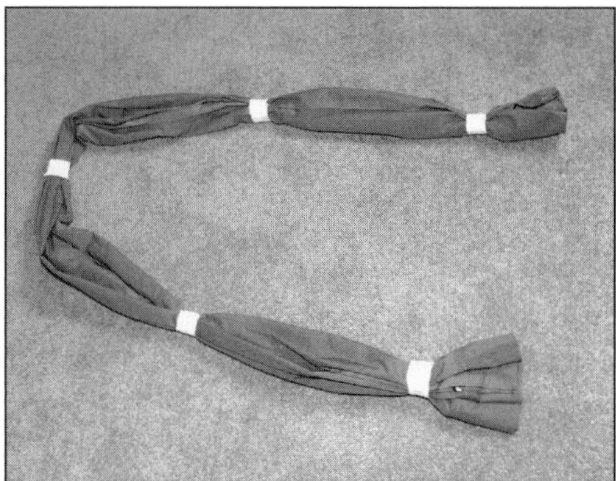

Figure 3.4. Rolled-up sheet to help with moving the TKA leg

Another handy prop to assist you in moving your TKA leg around in bed and in and out of chairs is a rolled-up sheet. Simply take an old sheet, roll it up along its long axis, and then tape the ends and several spots between the ends (Figure 3.4). The rolled-up sheet can then be placed around the bottom of your foot, and by lifting the ends of the sheet with each hand, you can safely move your TKA leg up, down, or sideways without stressing the muscles in your thigh. Once you are able to raise your leg after surgery without bending it, you will not need to use a rolled-up sheet for bed mobility; but until that happens, this simple device works very well. Other items such as a belt, strap, or rope can be used instead of a sheet to assist in moving your leg. However, we find that the sheet works best for cradling the foot and doesn't slip off the heel while you're moving your leg.

Basic Presurgery Home Exercises

Preparing the home for your return after knee surgery is only part of the preparation. You need to prepare yourself as well. The better your strength and endurance prior to surgery, the easier your recovery and rehabilitation will be. However, there is a very cruel paradox between the need to improve fitness and strength and the persistent pain in your knee that prohibits exercise. Most likely, your surgeon has told you that it is important to be as strong and fit as possible prior to surgery. At the same time, the pain and dysfunction in your knee prohibit or at least severely limit your ability to exercise. It is ironic that the main cause for knee replacement also hampers the preparation for a knee replacement. Try to do as much exercise as possible prior to your surgery, favoring low-impact activities such as swimming, stationary cycling, rowing, or weight lifting. This section provides some suggestions for preoperative exercises to make your recovery and rehabilitation optimal.

At least one month prior to surgery, go to your local paint store or building-supply center and purchase an empty one-gallon paint bucket and five-gallon paint bucket. These two simple devices will be used extensively after your return home from the hospital for gaining range of motion and strength in your knee. Remove the handles from the buckets and start doing the following exercises at least one month prior to surgery to make the muscles in your leg as strong as possible. Doing the exercises preoperatively provides your muscles with a "memory" that makes it easier to perform the same exercises after surgery, even in the presence of pain and swelling.

Exercise 1

Short-Arc Quadriceps Exercise with One-Gallon Bucket

Lay the one-gallon bucket on its side. Lying on your back, place the bucket under your bent knee while allowing the heel to continue resting on the floor or bed. Slowly lift the heel of your foot off the floor or bed by straightening your knee (Figure 3.5). This exercise will help strengthen the quadriceps muscle (front of the thigh), which helps control the kneecap during walking. Of all the exercises we will present, this simple exercise is one of the most valuable to our patients in helping them learn to walk again. Complete 3–5 sets of 15–25 repetitions each, at least 3 times per day.

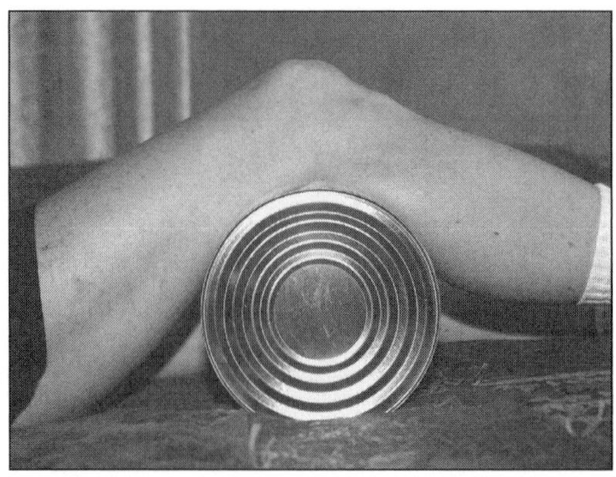

Figure 3.5.

Exercise 2

Short-Arc Quadriceps Exercise with Five-Gallon Bucket

Lay the five-gallon bucket on its side. Lying on your back, place the bucket under your upper thigh. This will result in a greater degree of flexion (bend) in your knee. After surgery, this exercise will help you regain the flexion in your knee by letting gravity pull your foot down toward the floor. For now, repeat the short-arc quadriceps exercise as above, but when your knee is fully extended (straight), hold the position for 10 seconds, and then lower your foot back to the floor or bed (Figure 3.6). Due to its large size in relation to the thigh, people with a short thigh may be unable to use a five-gallon bucket. If this is the case, use a standard-size cleaning bucket with a towel rolled up inside to give the bucket more rigidity (Figure 3.7). Complete 3–5 sets of 15–25 repetitions each, at least 3 times per day.

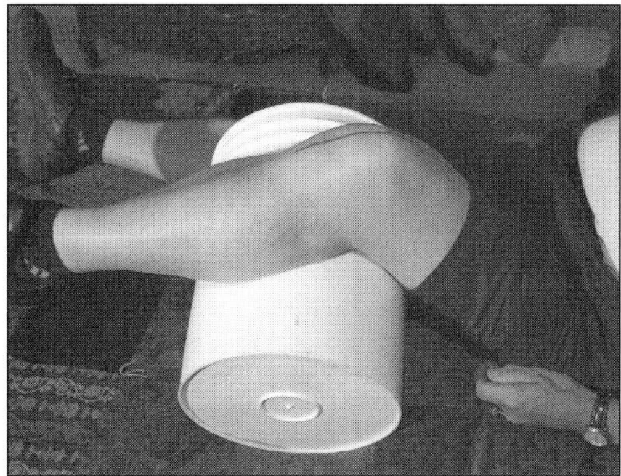

Figure 3.6. Short-arc quadriceps exercise using five-gallon bucket

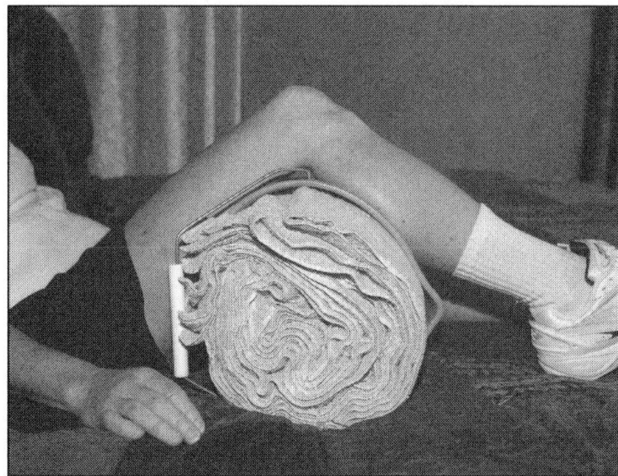

Figure 3.7. Short-arc quadriceps exercise using modified standard bucket

Exercise 3

Hamstring Isometric Exercise with Five-Gallon Bucket

Lay the five-gallon bucket on its side. Lying on your back, place the bucket under your heel. Try to straighten your knee all the way by pushing the back of your knee down toward the floor. After surgery, you will do this exercise to help straighten (gain extension in) your new TKA. After holding your knee straight for a count of 15 seconds, try to roll the bucket up toward your buttock while keeping your heel on the bucket. Don't use your hands to move the bucket; use only your leg (Figure 3.8). This exercise works your hamstring muscle (back of thigh) and is a very important exercise in TKA rehabilitation. Complete 3–5 sets of 15–25 repetitions each, at least 3 times per day.

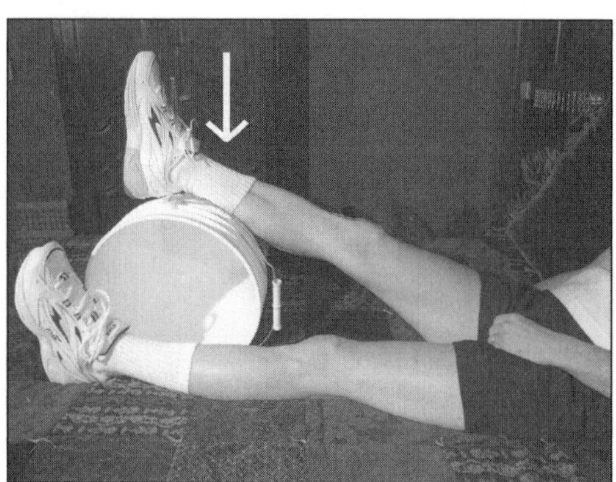

Figure 3.8. Hamstring isometric exercise using five-gallon bucket

Exercise 4

Straight-Leg Raise

If you have ever had arthroscopic knee surgery, this is one of the exercises you did afterward to strengthen your leg. Lying on your back, keep your knee straight, tighten your quadriceps muscle, and lift your foot 8–12 inches off the bed or floor (Figure 3.9a). Hold your leg at this height for a count of 5 seconds, and then slowly lower it back to the bed or floor. This exercise should not be too difficult; however, it is vitally important for you to be able to do it as soon as possible after surgery. The ability to do a straight-leg raise determines when you will be able to get in and out of bed by yourself. Complete 3–5 sets of 15–25 repetitions each, at least 3 times per day.

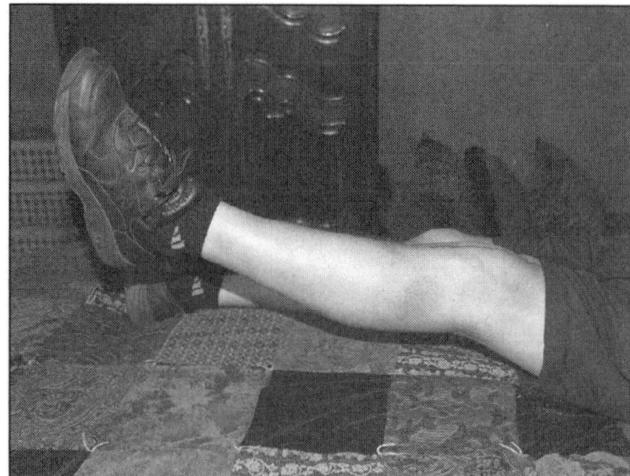

Figure 3.9a. Straight-leg raise exercise without resistance

Exercise 5

Straight-Leg Raise Using Nonoperated Leg for Resistance

One way to make the straight-leg raise more difficult, and thus make your leg significantly stronger, is to follow the instructions for Exercise 4, but this time you should place your good leg on top of the leg you're working (Figure 3.9b). The resistance added by the weight of your good leg will make performing a straight-leg raise after surgery much easier. Again, complete 3–5 sets of 15–25 repetitions each, at least 3 times per day.

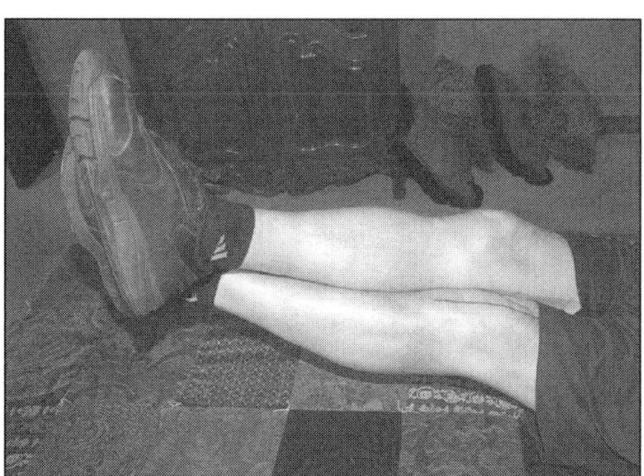

Figure 3.9b. Straight-leg raise exercise using other leg for added resistance

Exercise 6

Armchair Push-Up

This exercise will help you to strengthen your arms before using either a walker or crutches. Sit in a chair with sturdy armrests, place a hand on each of the armrests, and push down with your arms to lift your buttocks off the chair (Figure 3.10). Hold this position with your arms straight for a count of 5 seconds, and then slowly lower your buttocks back to the chair. Complete 3–5 sets of 15–25 reps each, at least 3 times per day. The more you do this exercise before surgery, the easier it will be to use a walker or crutches after surgery.

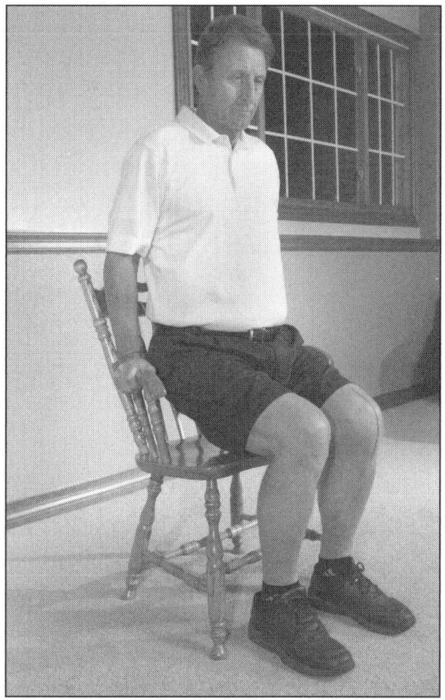

Figure 3.10. Armchair push-ups for strengthening upper arms

Planning Your Postsurgery Exercise Program

The simple exercises outlined above go a long way toward preparing you for surgery and toward making your postsurgery rehabilitation much easier. It is important to realize that the actual knee-replacement procedure accounts for only half of the long-term functional results of your new knee. The components affecting the other half of your overall outcome are the quality of your exercise program and the effort you put forth during your rehabilitation. The pain in your knees has probably prevented, or at least limited, the amount and types of exercise you have been able to enjoy for many years.

Once you have made up your mind to have your knee replaced, you must commit to undertaking an exercise program that will allow you to get the most out of your TKA for years to come. The exercise program you need is a combination of strength training and endurance training. In the book's later chapters we will help you establish such a program. The exercises designed to help you recover from your knee-replacement surgery are considered part of the rehabilitation phase. After rehabilitation has progressed for six months to a year, you will then enter the next phase of your exercise program: the lifelong fitness program. In addition to adding years to your life, maintaining your level of fitness will also enhance your quality of life with your new knee.

The first step in planning your exercise program is finding the best location for you to exercise. The initial location for everyone is the hospital, followed by home. As you progress with your rehabilitation program, however, you may need to use more sophisticated strength and endurance equipment to help you reach your fitness goals. Options to consider include joining a health club or purchasing in-home exercise equipment. There are several advantages and disadvantages to both environments. Many people find they need help from other people to exercise and may therefore benefit from becoming a member of a health club. Health clubs and fitness centers offer a variety of programs for people of all ages. They provide a wide range of exercise equipment for both strength and endurance training. Many offer aquatic therapy, which is very beneficial for total-knee-replacement rehabilitation. Most health clubs also offer fitness trainers to help guide and monitor your exercise program. Many fitness trainers have only limited experience working with TKA patients, so if you are planning to join a health club or fitness center, ask them if anyone on their staff is qualified to assist you with your specific exercise needs. You may also want some advice from your physical therapist on what types of equipment to use, how to set up the equipment, and how to advance your exercise program.

The disadvantage of exercising at a health club is that you have to go to the club to exercise. This requires motivating yourself to get to the club, transportation, and, once you are there, working around other people's workout schedules. Most clubs require a monthly payment schedule. To maximize your investment, try to develop a regular exercise schedule and then plan it out for the next month.

Many people like the convenience of exercising at home. There are no lines for the more popular pieces of equipment, you can exercise any time you like, and you don't have to go anywhere to do your exercise. The biggest disadvantage of setting up a home exercise program is the need for equipment. The membership fees at a health club or fitness facility can be paid monthly throughout the year. However, for approximately the same amount of money that is spent for a year-long health-club membership, several pieces of home exercise equipment can be purchased that you and your family can use anytime. Most companies that sell home exercise equipment will let you amortize your payments for the equipment, and once you have paid it off it is yours forever.

A number of home exercise systems are available on the market today. When used properly, they all do a reasonable job of improving strength and endurance. When shopping for home exercise equipment, some general guidelines may help you in making your decision. Try out the equipment at the store. Make sure the construction is sturdy and that you feel stable while exercising. Check out the noise level: Many people like to exercise while watching TV, and if the exercise apparatus is too noisy, it may not get used. Be sure the equipment can be adjusted to accommodate your height. Later in the book we will show a variety of exercises to gain range of motion using a stationary cycle and rowing machine, two of the best pieces of home exercise equipment you can own for rehabilitation after TKA surgery. To be most effective, these devices need to have adjustments for seat height and leg length. It is also important to be able to exercise against a variable resistance. Test this feature in the store as well to see how smooth the transition is from low to higher resistance. These are the most important features for you to consider when buying home exercise equipment. Many types of equipment are available that offer these and other features, such as electronic monitors, that are "neat" but not necessary, so shop around to find the model that fits you and your budget. It will be easier to go through this process prior to surgery in order to have your exercise equipment ready to go.

We have had considerable personal and professional experience with an assortment of home exercise machines, and we have found that the Total Gym works exceptionally well for total-knee-arthroplasty rehabilitation (see Figure 3.11 on the next page). The Total Gym is an extremely versatile exercise system, enabling the user to perform a variety of exercises with minimal set-up changes. It is commonly used in

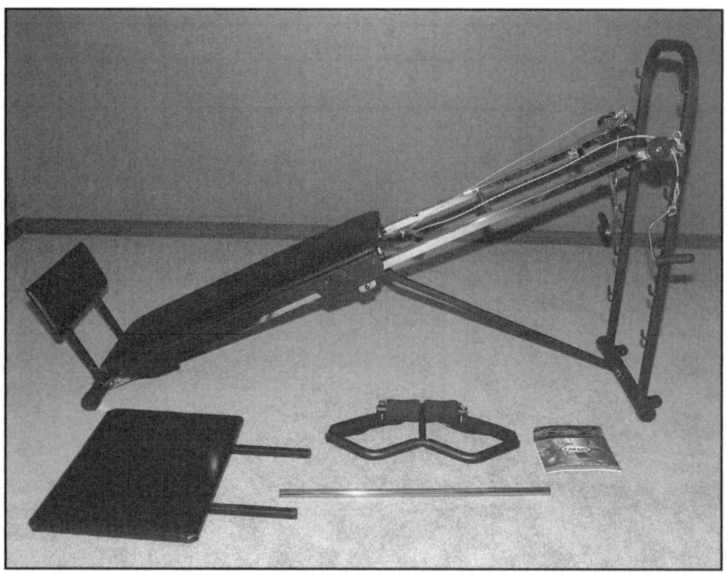

Figure 3.11. Total Gym exercise apparatus

many outpatient physical-therapy clinics, and a unit of the same quality can be purchased for home use. Throughout the book we will provide a number of exercises using the Total Gym for presurgery exercise training, postsurgery rehabilitation, and lifelong fitness training.

One of the features of the Total Gym is that it allows the arms and shoulders to assist with leg exercises. This permits someone with weak lower extremities to accomplish leg exercises with minimal pain. The Total Gym easily changes between configurations for exercises involving the upper body and the lower body. It allows for exercise and rehabilitation by letting patients work against gravity to lift and move a portion of their body weight. It exercises muscles similarly to the way the body naturally moves. It is a low-impact, noncompressive system that allows patients to experience success quickly and safely while stretching and strengthening their muscles. Raising or lowering the slide platform easily varies the resistance. The Total Gym can provide the TKA patient with an optimal exercise experience during preoperative preparation, during recovery, and for lifelong fitness. There are a variety of Total Gym models to choose from, and customers receive a special discount for ordering from the company's website: www.totalgym.com.

Presurgery Exercises Using the Total Gym

Here are a few Total Gym exercises that should be started at least one month prior to surgery:

Exercise 7

Total Gym: Squat with Both Legs

Position the rails at a challenging resistance level. Roll the glideboard toward the ladder and sit at the bottom of the glideboard. Place your feet flat on the squat stand, shoulder width apart. Lie back and bend the knees to approximately 90 degrees (Figure 3.12). Then push against the squat stand until the legs are straight. Complete 3–5 sets of 5–15 repetitions each.

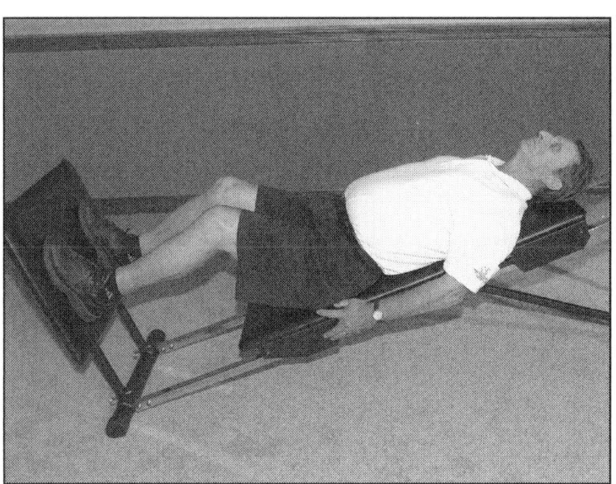

Figure 3.12. Double-leg squat

Exercise 8

Total Gym: Squat with Single Leg

Perform Exercise 7 as described above, except use only one leg at a time on the squat stand (Figure 3.13). Complete 3–5 sets of 5–15 repetitions each.

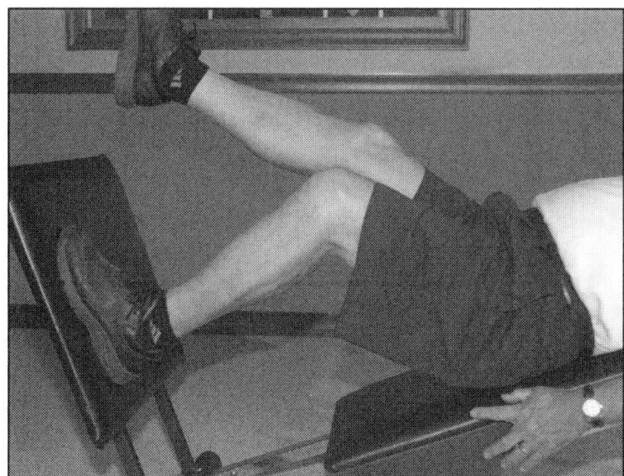

Figure 3.13. Single-leg squat

Exercise 9

Total Gym: Heel Raise

Lie on the glideboard, facing away from the ladder. Place your toes on the bottom edge of the squat stand. Push your heels off the squat stand by rising up on your toes, lifting the heels as high as you can. Return to the starting position. Next, try an advanced variation in which you raise the heel of one leg at a time (Figure 3.14). Complete 3–5 sets of 5–15 repetitions each.

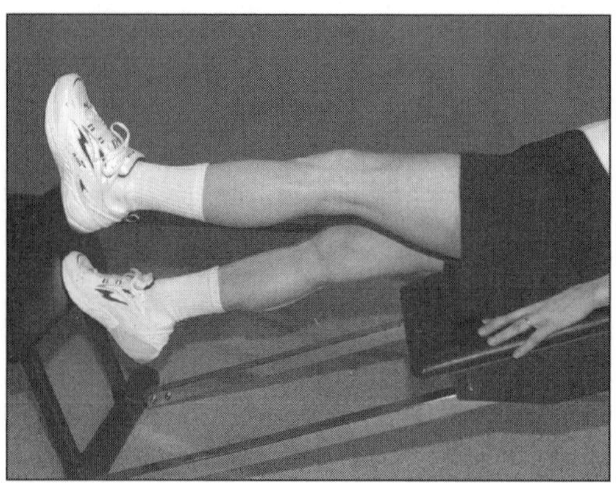

Figure 3.14. Single-leg heel raise

Exercise 10

Total Gym: Hamstring Pull

Secure your feet in the wing. Lie on your back with your legs straight and your buttocks near the top of the glideboard. Point your toes toward the ceiling. Pull the glideboard toward your feet until it nearly reaches your heels. Lower the glideboard slowly (Figure 3.15). Complete 3–5 sets of 5–15 repetitions each.

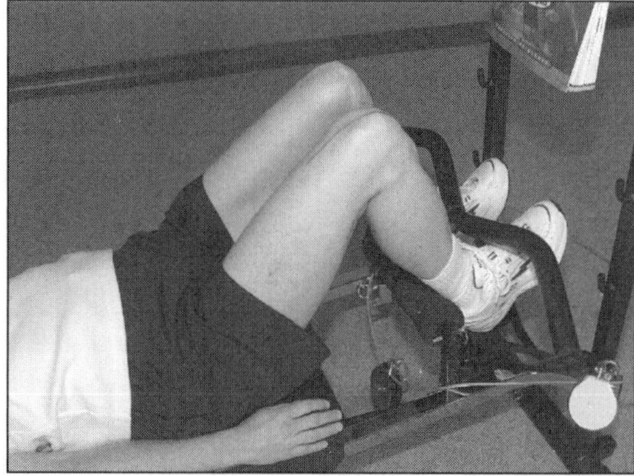

Figure 3.15. Hamstring pull

Exercise 11

Total Gym: Overhead Pull

Grasp the handles and lie on your back with your head at the top of the glideboard. Stretch your arms overhead. Bend your knees and put your feet on the bottom of the squat stand, if needed (Figure 3.16a). Pull your arms in an arc motion forward over your head and torso until your hands touch your thighs (Figure 3.16b). Complete 3–5 sets of 5–15 repetitions each.

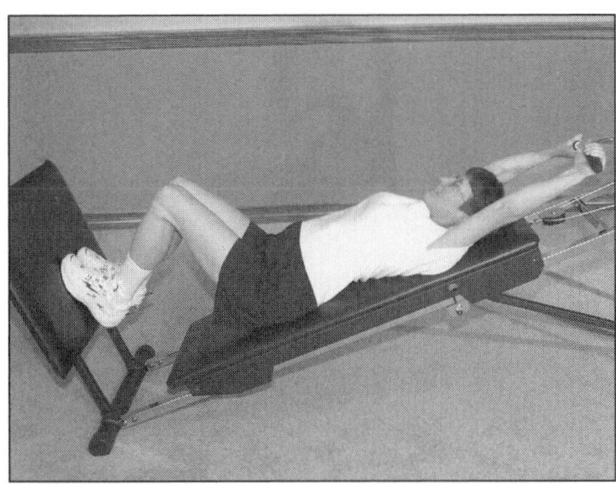

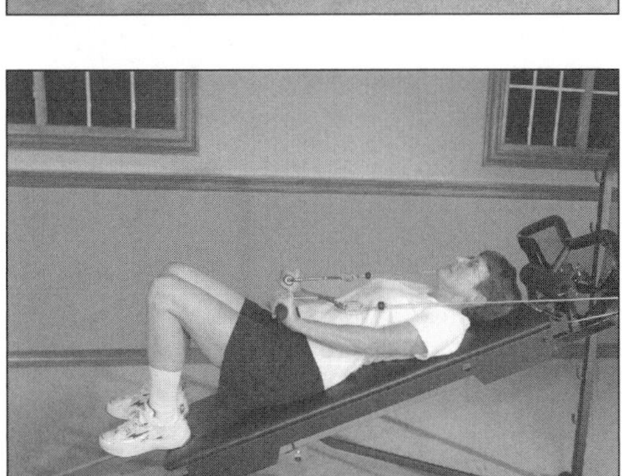

Figure 3.16 a/b. Overhead pull

Exercise 12

Total Gym: Triceps Pull

Grasp the handles. Lie on the glideboard with your head toward the ladder and your feet resting on the squat stand. Place your hands above your shoulders with the palms up (Figure 3.17a). Keep your elbows stationary at your sides, and bring your hands to your lower thighs in an arc motion (Figure 3.17b). Return to the starting position. Complete 3–5 sets of 5–15 repetitions each.

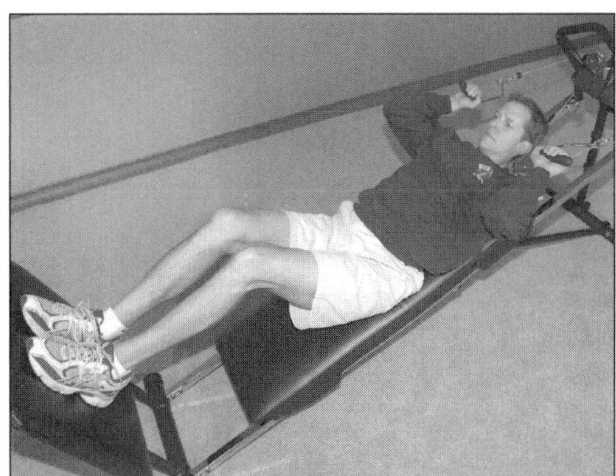

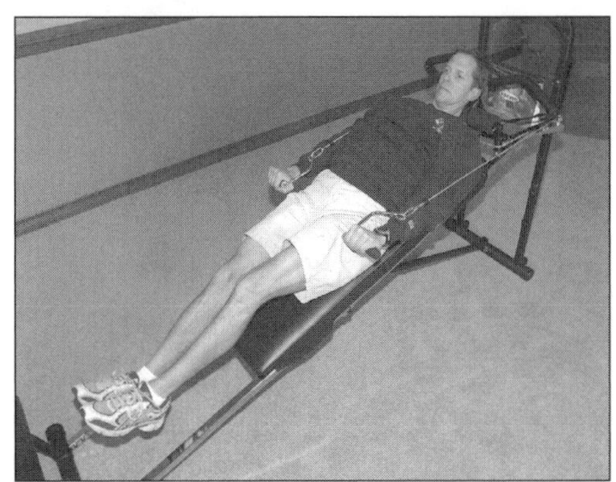

Figure 3.17 a/b. Triceps pull

Exercise 13

Total Gym: Seated Chest Press

Grasp the handles and sit at the top of glide-board, facing away from the ladder. Bend your elbows, and hold the handles with the palms down on either side of your chest (Figure 3.18a). Push forward and slightly upright by extending your arms (Figure 3.18b). Return to the starting position. Complete 3–5 sets of 5–15 repetitions each.

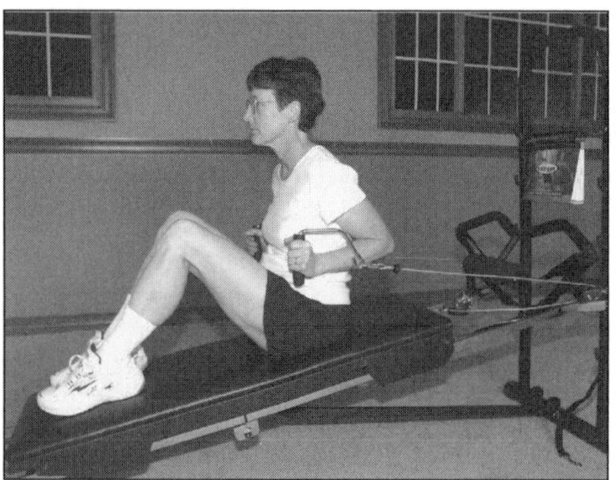

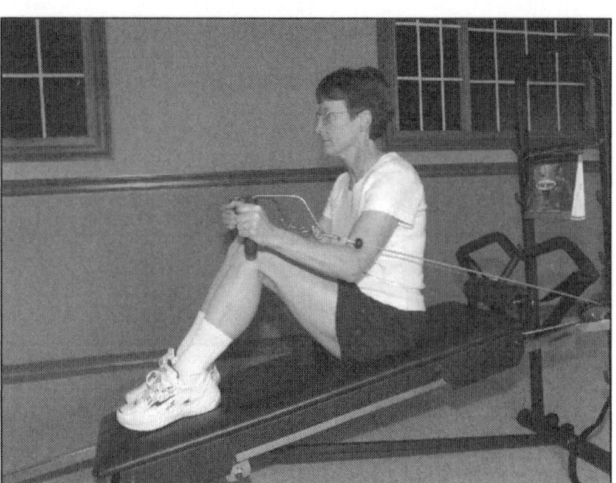

Figure 3.18 a/b. Seated chest press

Exercise 14

Total Gym: Cardio Pull

Position the machine at the highest resistance level. Grasp the handles and sit at the bottom of the glideboard. Lie on your back and place your feet on the squat stand. Stretch your arms overhead (Figure 3.19a). Move your arms in an arc overhead while simultaneously bending your knees and pushing off the squat stand (Figure 3.19b). Complete 3–5 sets of 5–15 repetitions each.

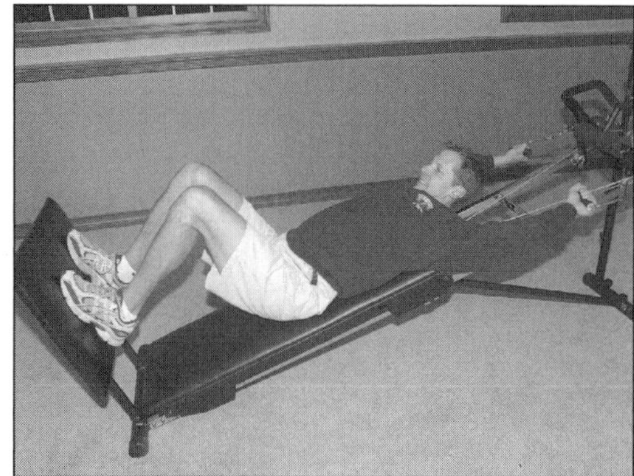

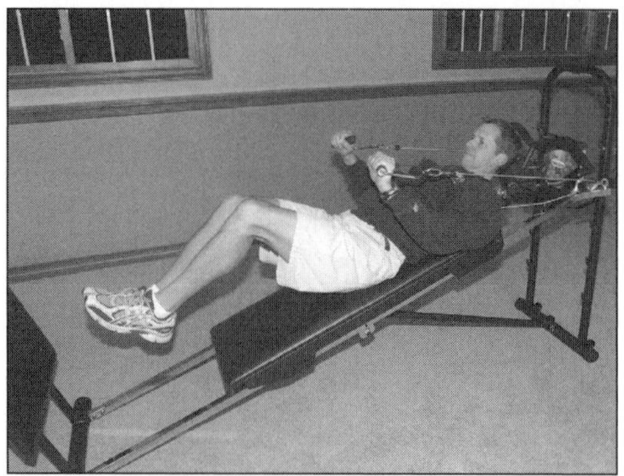

Figure 3.19 a/b. Cardio pull

■ ■ ■

Whether you choose to exercise at home or at a health club, the most important part of any workout program is to make the commitment to exercise—not only for your rehabilitation, but also to enhance your quality of life with your new TKA.

Cardiovascular and Endurance Exercise

Almost universally, our patients can't believe how easily they fatigue after surgery and how the least amount of exercise leaves them totally exhausted. This phenomenon results from several factors. First, the TKA surgery is considered major surgery, as the overall stress to the body and the effects of the anesthetic require a great deal of time for recovery. Second, for many patients, the pain they've experienced in their knee for many years prior to surgery has prohibited them from being very active, and as a result they've become deconditioned. Then, after the surgery, when they do not exercise much for the first few weeks, they become even more deconditioned.

One way to prevent some of the debilitating consequences of deconditioning is to try to perform cardiovascular exercise as much as possible right up to the time of surgery. Many patients feel they are in too much pain to do any exercise prior to surgery. However, they may be able to participate in low-impact cardiovascular exercises such as stationary cycling, stationary rowing, or aquatic/swimming exercises with minimal pain. These types of aerobic exercises provide a good cardiovascular stimulus while avoiding loading the knees as much as weight-bearing exercises such as walking or running do. In addition, stationary cycling and rowing are excellent methods of gaining knee motion, strength, and endurance after the TKA surgery. We will further discuss these activities in later chapters. If you plan to exercise at home, it would be wise to invest in either a stationary cycle or a rowing machine prior to surgery to improve your cardiovascular fitness.

Attempt to perform some form of cardiovascular exercise at least every other day for a minimum of fifteen to twenty minutes. Exercise at an intensity level where you can easily carry on a conversation. Some people can't exercise continually for fifteen minutes; if that's the case for you, try exercising for five to ten minutes, twice a day.

Another option that works very well for many patients is aquatic exercise. Exercising in water places minimal stress on the knees, and cardiovascular fitness can be achieved either by swimming or by aquatic exercises as simple as walking in the water. If there is a pool near your home or office, it may offer aquatic exercise classes specifically for people with arthritis. These classes are fun and will dramatically help to increase your endurance prior to surgery. Again, try to perform some type of aquatic exercise or swimming for at least fifteen to twenty minutes, three to four times per week.

If you have not been exercising regularly, it is important to check with your family physician before starting any cardiovascular exercise. In general, people over the age of forty-five should be evaluated by their physician prior to starting a conditioning program.

Weight Control

The more you weigh, the more stress you place on your knees and lower-extremity joints with every step. One way to increase the life span of your TKA is to keep your weight at the optimal level. For many patients, it is very hard to lose weight prior to surgery because the pain makes it so difficult to exercise. In fact, some surgeons will put off TKA surgery until their patients lose as much weight as they can. However, because of the pain, doing so may be extremely difficult or even impossible.

One of the first steps in weight control is examining your diet. Talk with your surgeon or primary-care physician about setting up a nutritional counseling session with a dietician. A dietician can help analyze your eating habits and can work with you to plan a diet that provides optimal nutrition while assisting you in controlling your weight. After your TKA surgery, weight control may be easier because exercise in general will be less painful, allowing you to participate in a lifelong exercise program.

Walker, Crutches, or Cane?

After surgery, you will need help walking. The amount of assistance needed with walking is based on several factors. The environment in your home—including factors such as types of flooring, number and design of stairs, your new TKA's weight-bearing tolerance (the ability to take all or part of your weight), and how "good" your other knee is—will determine which assistive device to use. Your surgeon may also have an opinion about what type of device he or she wants you to use after TKA surgery.

There are three main types of assistive devices for ambulation (walking): walkers, crutches, and canes. Each has its advantages and disadvantages. Therefore, one of the questions for you to ask your surgeon prior to surgery is what type of assistive device for walking is preferable after surgery. The other influencing factor in selecting the appropriate type of support is your confidence level in using the device. Most patients tell us that their biggest problem after surgery is a fear of falling, or lack of confidence in their new knee while walking. It is very important to gain confidence in whatever assistive device you use.

While you're in the hospital after surgery, the physical therapist will teach you how to use one or all of these devices. However, the physical therapist probably will not be present when you first arrive home. Therefore, it is important to practice walking around your home and entering and exiting your home with these assistive devices before surgery. Many patients who eventually receive a total knee replacement have had to use some form of support during walking after one of their previous knee operations. Typically, these patients find that walking after a total knee replacement is more challenging than it was after undergoing a lesser surgery such as a knee scope. For at least a week prior to surgery, practice entering, exiting, and moving around in your home with an assistive device.

A walker is the most stable assistive device to use after TKA surgery. It provides four points of contact with the ground, thereby providing a safe base of support while walking. If your surgeon does not allow full weight-bearing on your total-knee leg right after surgery, then a walker is initially the best choice. If you have both of your knees replaced at the same time, again, a walker will probably be the best device to use when you first arrive home. However, if you need to use the stairs in your home to get to bed or to the bathroom, etc., a walker can be tricky to use. Make a point to tell the physical therapist in the hospital that you have to use stairs at home, so that he or she can teach you how to use the walker safely (Figure 3.20). It is ideal to be able to practice negotiating stairs while still at the hospital to prepare for your homecoming.

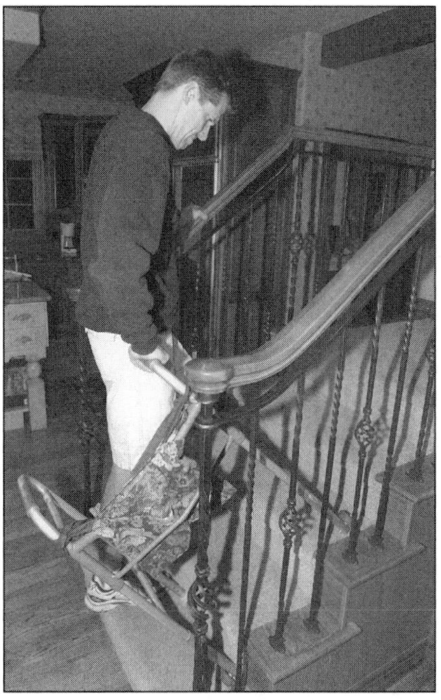

Figure 3.20. Using a walker to ascend stairs after TKA surgery

Crutches are much easier to use on stairs, and they are designed for walking longer distances. One of the disadvantages of crutches is that it is difficult to carry anything in your hands while using crutches correctly. Crutches also require a fair amount of upper-extremity strength, coordination, and balance. If you have successfully walked with crutches before, if your home is designed in such a way that using a walker is not appropriate, and/or if you have sufficient strength, balance, and coordination, consider using crutches to assist with ambulation. It is prudent to practice walking around your home and up and down the stairs with the crutches for at least one week prior to surgery. While practicing with crutches at home, try to simulate putting only partial weight on the leg that will

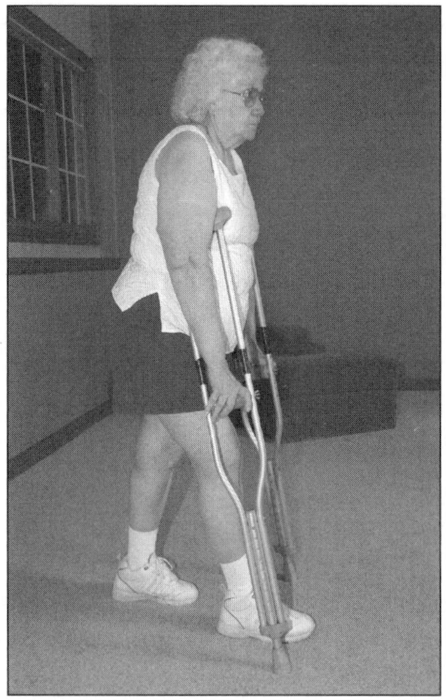

Figure 3.21. Crutch walking

receive the TKA. This will accomplish two things: First, it will provide the confidence you will need to use crutches, and second, it will help you develop the endurance required to be able to walk around the house. You will be amazed how incredibly weak and tired you become after knee-replacement surgery. To minimize this weakness and fatigue, "training" your muscles will help with mobility after surgery. Practicing crutch walking is a great way to develop confidence and endurance (Figure 3.21).

? Common Questions and Some Answers

- **Do I need to have a ramp to get into my house?**

In general, it is necessary for patients to be able to get into and out of their house on their own in case of an emergency. Some patients have difficulty getting up or down stairs for the first few weeks after surgery. If your house lacks handrails or the stairs are steep, installing a ramp is a safe and convenient way to provide easy access to the house.

- **Which assistive device—walker, crutches, or cane—will be best for me?**

There are many factors that go into determining which assistive device is right for each patient. These include balance, coordination, upper-extremity strength, weight-bearing status, pain, home obstacles, and confidence level. The decision is usually made by your surgeon and therapist. It is ideal to try out each form of assistive device before surgery to see which one works best for you.

What happens if it hurts too much for me to exercise before surgery?

It is very important to try to do as many exercises as possible prior to surgery. While it may be painful to walk or lift weights, exercise in the water should be tolerable. This includes water walking, swimming, or aquatic-exercise classes. The more exercise you can tolerate prior to surgery, the easier your recovery and rehabilitation will be. Enduring the short-term pain of exercising preoperatively will pay off in the long run.

How do I know how much exercise to do?

It is important for each patient to set functional goals for themselves. Success of the TKA surgery is measured by how functional patients are after surgery with their normal activities of daily living. Exercise is a critical part of the formula for success. There is a delicate balance between getting enough exercise and preventing it from dominating your everyday routine. In the beginning of the TKA rehabilitation, exercise will be the main focus of all your activities. As time progresses, exercise will become a smaller percentage of your daily lifestyle. Achieving this balance occurs with time and is different for every individual.

Which piece of home exercise equipment is best for me?

The best piece of equipment is the one that you will actually use. Try different devices; find the one that fits your home and your budget. But the most important consideration is determining the exercise system that you like best. If the piece of equipment you have chosen sits in the corner collecting dust, it's not the right one for you.

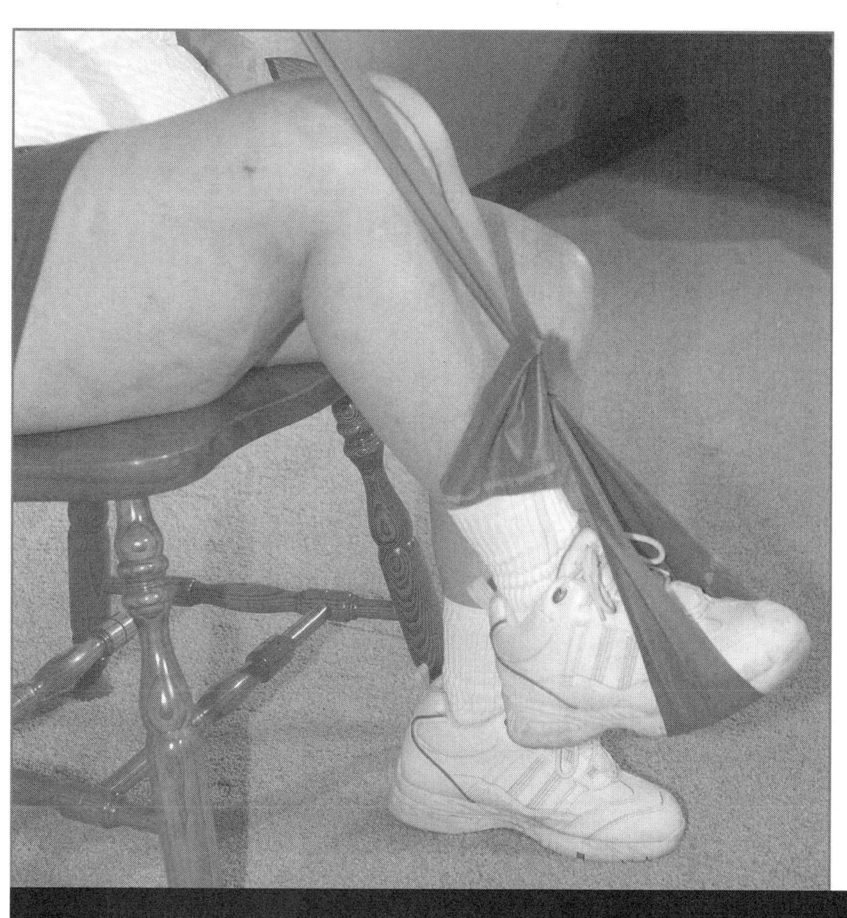

Chapter 4

The Total Knee Operation

What to Expect Before, During, and Immediately After Surgery

Preoperative Preparation

Besides setting up your home and doing your presurgery exercises, certain other preparations need to be made prior to the total knee operation to achieve the best possible result. Participating in a patient-education class can be quite helpful in preparing for the entire experience of knee replacement from start to finish. These classes are usually taught by a nurse and are sponsored by the hospital where your surgery is to take place. The goal is to explain the step-by-step journey from admission to discharge, so you know what to expect. Most patients become less fearful of the whole "ordeal" when they know what will happen to them. Ask your surgeon whether any preoperative total-joint classes are available in your area.

Often, your surgeon will have a videotape that you can borrow that explains the steps of a TKA. The videotape may provide a detailed explanation and may graphically depict the actual surgical procedure. If you feel unable to view a real surgery or if you can't handle "blood and guts," then it is best to pass on the videotape. Some patients find the surgery fascinating, while others don't want to go there.

Your surgeon will want you to undergo a preoperative examination, or "history and physical" examination (H and P). This is an evaluation done by your primary-care doctor, internist, or cardiologist to make sure you are healthy enough to withstand the stress of surgery. No one likes surprises in the operating room. Your anesthesiologist may require, or strongly recommend, a preoperative H and P by an internist or cardiologist if significant medical problems exist. An evaluation of your overall state of health will help in choosing the best anesthetic for you. It will also help the anesthesiologist anticipate any necessary adjustments during surgery. Not all patients will require a preoperative evaluation by a primary-care physician, internist, or cardiologist. For younger and healthier patients, the surgeon or assistant will often perform his or her own history and physical.

Preoperative laboratory testing is typically performed approximately one week prior to surgery. This includes blood tests, electrocardiogram (EKG), urinalysis (U/A), and chest X ray (CXR). The blood tests check the patient's electrolyte balance, blood-sugar level, and liver and kidney function. The EKG checks the heart, primarily looking for ischemia, that is, areas where the heart muscle is not getting the proper blood supply. It also looks for arrhythmias, heartbeat patterns that are abnormal or unhealthy. The U/A checks for any urinary-tract infection. An infection elsewhere in the body can potentially infect the knee prosthesis and may be a reason to delay the surgery until the infection is resolved. A preoperative CXR is done depending on the health of the patient. Any older patient, as well as any patient with a history of smoking, cancer, or lung disease, usually requires a CXR preoperatively.

Blood Donation

Blood transfusions may or may not be needed during or after surgery. This is determined by blood loss during surgery as well as the patient's state of health and preoperative blood count. Intraoperative blood loss (blood loss occurring during surgery) is influenced by the size of the leg, the thinness of the patient's blood, and the length and complexity of the procedure.

A pneumatic tourniquet is routinely positioned on the patient's upper thigh prior to making the incision. This device is similar to a large blood-pressure cuff. When filled with air, it constricts blood flow to the leg. During surgery, the pneumatic tourniquet prevents any blood from going into or out of the leg, therefore minimizing blood loss at the operative site. The tissues of the leg can typically go without blood for approximately two hours without any problem. Normally this is enough time to perform a primary TKA. Pneumatic tourniquets operate much more effectively on a thin, muscular leg. By contrast, more blood loss occurs with a larger leg even when a tourniquet is used due to the necessity of a longer incision and the larger area of dissection needed to expose the knee joint.

The relative thinness of a patient's blood influences the total amount of blood lost during surgery. People with "thin" blood, or blood that does not clot readily, will tend to lose more blood. Having thinner blood can be normal for some people, or it can be caused by long-term use of anticoagulants (e.g., Coumadin) or of nonsteroidal anti-inflammatory drugs (NSAIDs). "Thin" blood increases the chances of a patient needing a transfusion during or after surgery. Drugs that affect the thinness of blood are discussed in the later section titled "Medication Adjustments."

Blood transfusions are unnecessary for some patients. Theoretically, such a patient is healthy enough to tolerate blood loss, has a high preoperative blood count to provide a safety net, has a thin leg, and requires a straightforward, uncomplicated TKA. In this case, when a tourniquet is used, there is not enough blood loss to warrant a transfusion. However, in some patients with a low preoperative blood count or a poor state of health, even a small amount of blood loss is poorly tolerated. In addition, a more complex procedure requires more time to complete, thus causing greater blood loss. If patients have relatively thin blood, have a larger leg, and/or require a more lengthy, complicated procedure, a blood transfusion is more likely.

When a significant blood loss is anticipated, your surgeon may want one or two units of packed red blood cells available at the time of surgery. There are three common ways to obtain blood for surgery. The first is to use packed red blood cells from the blood bank. A sample of your blood is typed and screened so that compatible blood from the bank can be matched to yours and then made available for the operation. Another method is to use donor-directed blood. In this case, a friend or family member can donate blood to be used for a specific patient, provided that the two types of blood are compatible. Autologous blood donation is the third method.

Autologous blood donation involves donating your blood to be used later for your own blood transfusion. Essentially you are donating blood to yourself. When two or more units are donated, ideally they are drawn at least one week apart. The final unit will be donated one or two weeks before your surgery. Usually the blood can be safely stored for two months before expiring. This is a popular method of blood donation, as it minimizes the risk of contracting any blood-borne diseases. And if a patient is receiving her or his own blood, the risk of incompatibility is avoided. All units of blood, regardless of the method of donation and transfusion, are routinely tested for hepatitis B and the AIDS virus. The chances of getting AIDS from a blood transfusion are about one in a million.

There are some circumstances when the surgeon does not feel that preoperative blood donation is necessary, but for some reason the patient experiences more blood loss than is anticipated. If this scenario arises, compatible blood from the hospital blood bank is usually available for transfusion. Even in this circumstance, the stored blood is routinely tested to ensure its safety.

Smoking

Once the decision to undergo surgery has been made, if you are a smoker, now would be a good time to quit. Quitting as soon as possible prior to surgery is helpful, while quitting for good is ideal. Studies have shown that smoking constricts the small blood vessels, thus impeding circulation to the body's tissues. This increases the risk of wound breakdown and infection as well as the time it takes for the wound to heal. And because of the significant stress that smoking places on the cardiopulmonary system, smokers definitely have an increased risk of anesthetic complications during and after surgery. If quitting is impossible, even cutting back is beneficial.

Medication Adjustments

Making adjustments in the medications you take may be necessary prior to your surgery. A high percentage of patients requiring TKA are on some form of NSAIDs (nonsteroidal anti-inflammatory medications) to help with pain, swelling, and inflammation. The majority of these medications to some degree inhibit platelet function, and therefore may cause excessive bleeding during surgery, even with the use of a tourniquet. (Platelets are a component of the blood that assists with clotting.) For this reason, it is ideal to stop taking all NSAIDs five to seven days prior to surgery. Although stopping your NSAIDs may lead to an increase in pain, it is worth the discomfort to minimize any complications from surgical bleeding. Aspirin also inhibits platelet function and thus can cause excessive bleeding. For patients using aspirin for pain control, this too should be stopped five to seven days preoperatively. However, if you are taking one "baby" aspirin (81 mg) a day to improve circulation and reduce the risk of heart attack or stroke, this is not a problem. Such a small amount of aspirin is not enough to significantly increase bleeding during surgery.

Patients on long-term Coumadin (warfarin) therapy to reduce the risk of blood clots or strokes may also need to modify their dosages before surgery. This medication is designed to thin the blood in order to prevent blood clots, and it may potentially cause excessive bleeding during surgery. It is ideal to stop taking Coumadin five to seven days preoperatively to allow the blood to become "thicker," or to clot more efficiently. However, sometimes the primary-care physician, internist, or cardiologist may feel it is too risky to interrupt the Coumadin therapy, especially in patients taking it for stroke prevention. If this is the case, it is still possible to proceed with surgery without discontinuing the Coumadin. Special precautions can be used during the operation to minimize blood loss. Be sure to tell your surgeon and anesthesiologist if you are still taking your usual Coumadin dosage right up to the surgery date.

Insulin is another medication that commonly needs adjustment for diabetic patients planning to undergo surgery. Insulin doses are calculated for a specific patient's caloric intake. Therefore, when a patient does not eat or drink anything for eight hours before surgery (as is almost always required), the usual insulin dose becomes inappropriate. The anesthesiologist or internist will ask the patient to reduce the insulin dose the morning of surgery, according to the patient's needs. Most times the insulin dose is cut in half.

Although dosages of several medications are reduced or eliminated preoperatively, blood-pressure medications do not need to be interrupted. Blood-pressure medications are needed to keep blood pressure at an even and acceptable level. This is particularly important during the stressful time of anesthesia and surgery. Your anesthesiologist or internist may ask you to take your blood-pressure medication in the morning as usual. Even though you are not supposed to eat or drink anything for eight hours before surgery, you will be allowed to take your blood-pressure medications with a small sip of water prior to the operation.

Anesthesia

There are different anesthetic options to choose from, based on patient preference and recommendation by the surgeon and anesthesiologist. The most common type of anesthesia is a general anesthetic. The patient is given an anesthetic drug through the vein (intravenously, or IV), followed by an inhalation agent through a mask or endotracheal tube (tube down the throat). This is all painless. Under a general anesthetic the patient has no awareness of the surgery. The most common side effects are nausea/vomiting and a groggy, "hangover" sensation after surgery. A commonly asked question is "Can I die from general anesthesia?" The answer is yes; it is possible, but extremely rare. There is a greater chance of dying in a motor vehicle accident than from general anesthesia.

The second most utilized form of anesthesia for TKA is a regional anesthetic such as a spinal or an epidural. A spinal principally involves an injection of a combination of local anesthetic medications inside the dural membrane of the spinal cord. The anesthetic is injected with the patient awake. A spinal involves a one-time injection, and then the needle is removed. It anesthetizes all the nerves coming out of the spinal cord at that specific level, rendering the patient entirely numb from approximately the waist down. An epidural is a similar technique, although the needle tip is placed in a different spot, only millimeters away from where the needle is inserted during a spinal. A long, thin, flexible tube called a *catheter* replaces the needle, and the catheter is used to deliver medications. The catheter tip, and thus the medication, is placed in the epidural space, an area composed mostly of fatty tissue surrounding the spinal cord just outside the dural membrane. The drugs bathe the layer of fat all around the cord, also causing numbness from approximately the waist down. Medications can be administered intermittently through the long, thin catheter when needed. Intravenous sedation is used in conjunction with a spinal or an epidural to facilitate relaxation.

A regional anesthetic is preferred for patients who do not want a general anesthetic or the side effects associated with it. Typically the "hangover" following general anesthesia is minimized with a spinal or an epidural. Nausea and vomiting are also diminished with these regional techniques. Some people would rather have more control over their senses by having a spinal or an epidural. These anesthetic methods routinely cause less stress on the cardiopulmonary system. Therefore they may be the anesthetic of choice for patients with heart or lung problems.

The spinal and epidural techniques also help with postoperative pain control. When a spinal is administered, a long-acting local anesthetic can be given so that the numbing effect will last for hours after surgery. In the case of an epidural anesthetic, after the catheter is placed, it can stay in position for twenty-four to forty-eight hours after surgery. Anesthetic pain medications can be put through the catheter as needed to help with pain control after the operation. This may reduce or eliminate the need for other pain medications.

A disadvantage of the regional methods is that they may fail to achieve complete anesthesia in every patient. It is difficult to hit the right spot with a needle in some patients with severe arthritis of the lower lumbar spine, with lumbar scoliosis, or in those who have had a previous spine surgery in the same area. Also, obese patients can prove to be a "difficult stick" for the anesthesiologist trying to achieve correct needle placement. Even when these procedures go smoothly they can be somewhat unpredictable. Occasionally, areas of "patchy" anesthesia are achieved, wherein not all areas of the leg are sufficiently numb. This may occur even when the technique is done properly. If this should occur, a general anesthetic is usually necessary.

An infrequently used anesthetic for TKA is a regional nerve block. This is performed by the anesthesiologist injecting local anesthetic drugs around the major nerves of the leg. It involves a number of needle sticks. The success of the technique is dependent on the skill of the anesthesiologist. This method is usually reserved for patients with a compromised cardiopulmonary system (making general anesthesia too risky) or a spine with abnormal anatomy (making a spinal or epidural injection difficult). For patients with a history of pain-control problems, a regional nerve block can be used as another tool for postoperative pain management.

NPO

Your surgeon and anesthesiologist will ask you not to eat or drink anything at least eight hours prior to surgery. This is termed *NPO*, or nothing by mouth, and it includes no coffee, juice, tea, or even water for at least eight hours prior to surgery. Your anesthesiologist and surgeon must approve any exceptions to the NPO restriction. Sometimes you will be allowed to take medication before surgery with a small sip of water. This is discussed further later in the chapter. Failure to observe this general rule will result in your surgery being cancelled and then rescheduled at a later date. The purpose is to have the stomach as empty as possible to reduce the risk of vomiting. Vomiting while under general anesthesia is a significant concern since the contents of the stomach can be aspirated into the lungs, causing pneumonia. Under general anesthesia the gag reflex is eliminated, and with the patient in the supine position (lying on the back) it is easier for vomiting to lead to aspiration pneumonia.

The TKA Surgical Procedure

A detailed description of the entire surgical technique is beyond the scope of this book; however, a general understanding of what is involved can be helpful. Actual operative time for a primary TKA will vary from approximately one hour and thirty minutes to two hours and thirty minutes, depending on the complexity of the procedure, bony deformity in the knee, size of the leg, and experience level of the surgeon.

Typically, a straight or slightly curved incision is made over the front of the knee,

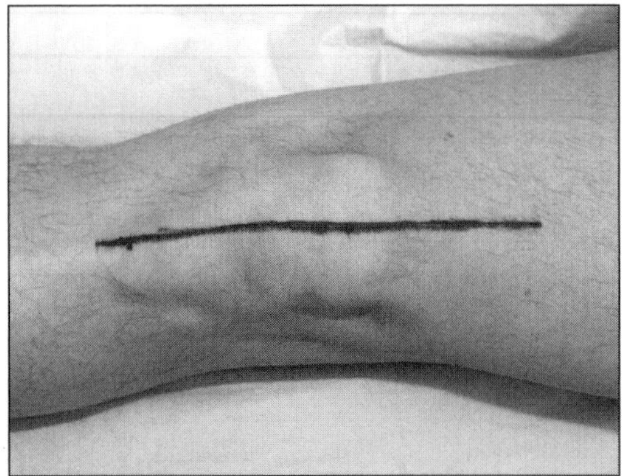

Figure 4.1. Skin incision to start TKA surgery

centered over the patella, or kneecap (Figure 4.1). The incision may need to be modified to incorporate old surgical scars around the knee. Next, the quadriceps muscle, tendon, and fascia are incised longitudinally around the patella. The patella is everted (flipped over) to expose the cartilage undersurface, or joint surface, of the kneecap.

Bone cuts are made on the end of the femur (thigh bone), upper end of the tibia (lower leg bone), and the undersurface of the patella (kneecap). These bone cuts are made precisely to accept the prosthetic components (Figures 4.2 a and b). When the bone cuts are made, most of the ligaments around the knee are preserved. It is during this step that any alignment problems of the leg are corrected. Upon performing the bone cuts, the orthopedic surgeon functions as a "carpenter" under sterile conditions. The prosthetic components are then sized and put into position. The size and type of components are chosen based on bone size, knee motion, and joint stability. Then the components are "press fitted" (cementless technique) or "glued" (cement technique) into position.

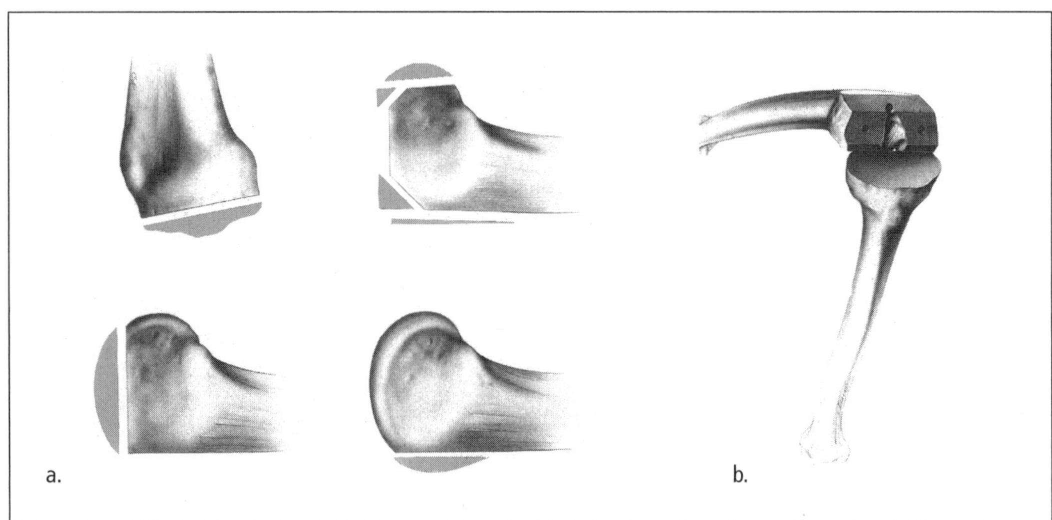

Figure 4.2 a/b. Cuts during TKA surgery. (Illustrations courtesy of Zimmer, Inc.)

Once the components are in position, the surgeon will check the range of motion and stability of the TKA. At that time, any ligament balancing will be performed if necessary. This may require releasing or tightening the collateral ligaments on the sides of the knee. Ligament balancing is needed primarily with patients who have significant bony deformities that affect the alignment of the leg. In severe cases of bony deformity of the knee joint, it may be necessary to reconstruct or tighten one of the collateral ligaments.

As the surgeon moves the knee in flexion and extension (bending and straightening), the tracking of the patella (kneecap) is assessed. Patellar tracking refers to kneecap movement over the end of the femur during joint motion. Quite commonly, a procedure called a *lateral release* is done to improve the tracking of the patella. This involves dividing the tight fibrous layer of tissue on the outer side (lateral side) of the patella, allowing the patella to glide directly over the center of the femur. The lateral release is similar to making an incision in the soft tissue alongside the patella, but it is invisible underneath the skin. Although invisible from the surface, the lateral release can cause additional swelling, bruising, and pain on the lateral (outside) portion of the knee. Finally, the layers of the knee are closed with sutures, drains are inserted, and dressings are applied.

The Recovery Room

Following surgery, you are immediately taken to the recovery room. This is a critical time as you emerge from anesthesia. A nurse monitors the transition process to make sure you breathe properly and have adequate pain control. Your blood count, electrolyte, and blood-sugar levels are checked.

Once you are awake and stable, you will be transferred to a hospital room designated for surgical patients. The recovery-room stay is usually one or two hours, but will vary depending on your state of health, reaction to anesthesia, and length of the surgical procedure. Nurses who staff the recovery room are critical-care nurses and are trained to handle any emergency situation.

The ICU

When a prolonged stay in the recovery room is anticipated, you may go directly to the intensive care unit (ICU) from surgery. Or, if complications arise either during surgery or in the recovery room, you may go to the ICU instead of to a regular hospital room. Patients who end up in the ICU are typically elderly or have unstable medical problems. In the ICU, you receive one-on-one nursing care to carefully monitor your cardiopulmonary system, blood count, and pain control. This setup allows the nurse to provide immediate treatment in response to changes in your medical condition. The length of stay in the ICU is usually a day or two, but it may be several days depending on the circumstances. Once you improve and the ICU is no longer needed, you are transferred to a regular hospital room.

The Hospital Room

It is in the surgical hospital room that the nursing staff attends to your everyday needs while you recover from surgery and begin your rehabilitation. At first it is important to rest, as your body has endured a significant stress. Total knee replacement is major surgery, and while it might be less life-threatening than open-heart surgery or brain surgery, it is still a major procedure that affects your entire body, not just your knee. Pain management is one of the first, and most important, duties of the nursing staff. Techniques of pain management will be discussed later in the chapter.

It is important to begin eating again. You may eat whenever you feel hungry. Restoring caloric intake is critical to helping the body heal. Now is not the time to restrict your diet to lose weight. Several studies have shown that the body requires more calories and nutrients than normal to aid in the healing process. Usually patients start with clear liquids (juice, Jell-O, clear broth, etc.) followed by full liquids (soup, milk shakes, etc.). If this is tolerated, the diet is advanced to a soft diet and eventually to a general diet (regular food). There are those who may argue that hospital food is never regular. However, the dietary staff of the hospital designs the menu to provide optimum nutrition for your recovery, and it is very important to eat the "right foods" while you're healing.

The knee dressing is usually not changed until two or three days postoperatively. It is important to keep the dressing clean and dry, and it will be reinforced as needed by the nursing staff. After three days, a dressing may no longer be necessary as long as the incision stays clean and dry. If some leakage persists or if the incision is overly sensitive, the incision will be redressed.

Prior to sewing up the incision at the end of the operation, the surgeon may have placed a drain (sterile tube) deep in the knee joint or in the subcutaneous tissue layer. This allows the blood to drain out of the knee, which will help reduce swelling and improve motion. Usually the drain is removed on the second or third day after surgery, depending on the amount of drainage. The drain is simply pulled out while you are lying in bed. The removal of the drain may hurt, but it only takes a few seconds to remove, and the discomfort subsides quickly. Some surgeons choose not to use a drain, particularly if only minimal bleeding occurred during surgery.

Blood transfusions, when necessary, are usually given on the day of the operation or one or two days afterward. The blood transfusion may be administered in the operating room, the recovery room, or the hospital room. The output of blood in the drain from your knee is carefully monitored by your nurse. Your blood count is also checked at regular intervals. If your blood count drops too low, your surgeon will order you to receive one or more units of autologous blood (your own blood), donor-directed blood, or banked blood. As discussed before, postoperative transfusions are often unnecessary.

Another activity that is vital to your recovery is using an incentive spirometer. This is a small plastic device with a hose attached to a mouthpiece. You will be instructed to inhale as deeply as possible so the spirometer can measure the amount of air you are moving into your lungs. This breathing exercise should be done a minimum of once an hour while you're awake. After surgery, your breathing capacity may be less than normal due to the anesthesia, pain medication, and general inactivity. This condition is called *atelectasis*, and it occurs when small portions of the lungs collapse because they are underinflated. Using the incentive spirometer opens up these collapsed portions of the lungs. Failure to use the incentive spirometer on a regular basis to treat the atelectasis may result in fever, pneumonia, and delayed recovery.

You'll be given sponge baths for the first few days after surgery. Once you're ready to shower, at first you'll need to cover the surgical site in plastic to keep the incision completely dry. If there is any drainage coming out of the incision, theoretically water can seep under the skin, potentially causing an infection. As early as postoperative day number three, the incision may be sealed enough to allow you to get it wet in the shower. Soaking in a bathtub is not recommended until three or four weeks after the operation to make sure the incision is completely sealed and experiencing no drainage.

A Foley catheter may be used after TKA. This is a plastic tube inserted through the urethra into the bladder to empty urine from the bladder, making it unnecessary to use a bedpan. It may be placed during surgery for longer procedures, for patients with urinary incontinence, or for use with a spinal or epidural anesthetic since the numbness from the waist down can make normal urination difficult. If a patient experiences urinary retention following surgery, the Foley catheter may be inserted to relieve bladder pressure. The Foley gives the patient a reprieve from having to hop on and off the bedpan. For most TKA patients the Foley catheter is not used.

Dealing with Pain and Other Potential Complications

The Marcaine pain pump is sometimes used to help with postoperative pain management. Marcaine is a long-acting, local-anesthetic medication. As a local anesthetic, it is administered directly to the surgical incision. The medication is placed in a reservoir designed to deliver a slow and constant amount of the drug through a small, thin plastic catheter. The catheter is put in the knee joint or in the subcutaneous tissue layer at the time of surgical closure. It is then attached to the pain-pump reservoir.

The pump can be effective for twenty-four to forty-eight hours, depending on the rate of delivery of the medication. Although this setup does not completely eliminate pain, it may allow the patient to use oral narcotics sooner or to use less pain medication overall.

Management of postoperative medications is very important to your recovery. The first medications you will become familiar with are pain medications. Typically, pain medications are narcotics administered intravenously (IV) or intramuscularly (IM). They work quickly when given by these routes, but tend not to last very long. A PCA (patient-controlled analgesia) machine is a device that administers IV pain medications. It allows the patient to push a button to deliver a programmed dose of IV pain relief. To prevent overdosing, restrictions are built into the machine to limit the amount and frequency of narcotic the patient can "self-deliver." Some common pain medications used with the PCA machine include morphine, Dilaudid, and Demerol. The obvious advantage of the PCA is that it delivers pain medication quickly to the patient when needed, without the patient having to wait for the nurse to administer the medication.

After one or two days patients are encouraged to take PO (oral) pain pills. Oral pain medications take longer to work, but they also provide longer pain relief. Typical pain pills include Dilaudid, Percocet, Percodan, Vicodin, Tylenol #3, and Darvocet N-100. To stay on top of the pain in the early days of recovery it is important to take the pain pills on a regular basis, approximately every three to six hours. If you get behind in pain control it may be difficult to "catch up" with the pain. It is also important to keep up with your pain medications so that you can be more effective in the rehabilitation of your new knee joint. Because of the painful nature of the TKA procedure, postoperative pain management is critical to the overall success of the recovery. If your knee hurts "too much," you will be unable to give your best effort during the rehabilitation exercises. Movement of your new knee starts the first day after surgery, so it is important to take your pain medication on a regular schedule for best results.

Nausea, vomiting, constipation, itching, and lethargy are some of the more common side effects experienced with these analgesics. If these symptoms occur, your surgeon can order a different type of medication. Sometimes, trial and error are the only way to find the right medication for you.

Antibiotics are routinely used preventively during and after TKA. An infection of the knee joint can be a devastating complication requiring multiple surgical procedures and followed by months of IV and oral antibiotics. Therefore, orthopedic surgeons do everything possible to prevent an infection. Even with meticulous sterile technique during surgery, IV antibiotics are given during and after the TKA procedure. A broad-spectrum antibiotic such as Ancef is usually used intravenously for twenty-four to forty-eight hours following surgery.

It may be used longer than that, depending on the duration of the operation and on whether drains or catheters are needed for longer than usual. It is always important to watch for allergic reactions when using antibiotics. Other common side effects with antibiotic medications include nausea and vomiting, which make it necessary to change or discontinue the antibiotics.

Nausea and vomiting are common side effects not only of the antibiotics and narcotics used after surgery, but also of the anesthetic agents used during the procedure. If this happens, your doctor will most likely prescribe an antiemetic (a drug to relieve nausea). Usually the anesthesiologist will give you an antiemetic during surgery or in the recovery room to minimize the chance of nausea or vomiting in the immediate postoperative period. Then, once you're in a regular hospital room, the nurse will give you similar antiemetics IV, IM, or orally, if needed. For the antiemetic to work most effectively, it is best to take it at the early onset of nausea, rather than waiting for violent vomiting.

Constipation is another common problem following surgery. This seemingly trivial problem has the potential to make you miserable. Constipation is a side effect of the analgesic medications used for pain control. In addition, a reduced level of activity coupled with a change in eating habits can reduce bowel motility. These factors can lead to significant postoperative constipation. To prevent constipation you will be encouraged to drink a great deal of water and to eat lots of fruits and vegetables. If you do experience difficulty moving your bowels, you should notify the nursing staff sooner rather than later. Treatment alternatives include various combinations of fiber, stool softeners, and laxatives. Moving around and exercising soon after surgery, as well as keeping bed rest to a minimum can also aid in preventing constipation. With a careful approach to prevention, an enema is rarely needed.

Preventing Blood Clots

Some form of anticoagulation therapy is typically used for all patients after TKA in order to prevent deep-vein thrombosis (DVT, or blood clot in the leg) and pulmonary embolism (PE, or blood clot in the lung). Blood clots can form in the legs or pelvic region during or after surgery because of the tourniquet used during the procedure and the relative inactivity of the patient during the recovery period. A blood clot in the leg may be a minor nuisance that causes pain and swelling. However, it can turn into a potentially fatal situation if the clot breaks free and travels to the lungs (PE). Because a PE can cause death, a great deal of effort is directed to the prevention of blood clots. The two methods of anticoagulation most widely used are pills and shots.

If your surgeon chooses to use pills, you will be given warfarin (Coumadin) daily, beginning shortly after surgery. Your blood will be drawn daily to check your protime/INR level (a measure of the blood's thinness), and the dosage of warfarin will be adjusted as needed. Because the proper warfarin dosage varies in each individual, finding just the right dosage is part of the art of medicine. Warfarin may be prescribed for as long as six weeks postoperatively even following a routine surgery, depending on the judgment of your surgeon.

The other type of anticoagulation involves injections of Lovenox or Fragmin, low-molecular-weight heparins. These subcutaneous injections are usually given one or two times per day in the abdomen and are continued for approximately two to four weeks after surgery. Even though patients may dislike receiving the injections, this method does not require regular blood draws to check the blood's thinness. No matter what method of anticoagulation is used, there can be a fine line between achieving optimal thinness of the blood to prevent clots and causing bleeding complications if the blood gets too thin.

Because a PE can be a devastating complication, other devices besides anticoagulant medications are used to prevent blood clots. Surgical stockings, or T.E.D. hose, are used on both legs postoperatively. These are tight compression stockings that usually extend to mid-thigh. They minimize swelling in the legs so the circulating blood isn't impeded by the swollen tissues surrounding the surgical site. The stockings also help with muscle compression, which assists in pumping the blood out of the legs to the heart. They are worn for several weeks until the swelling is at a minimum and the patient is mobile enough to restore normal blood flow in the lower extremities.

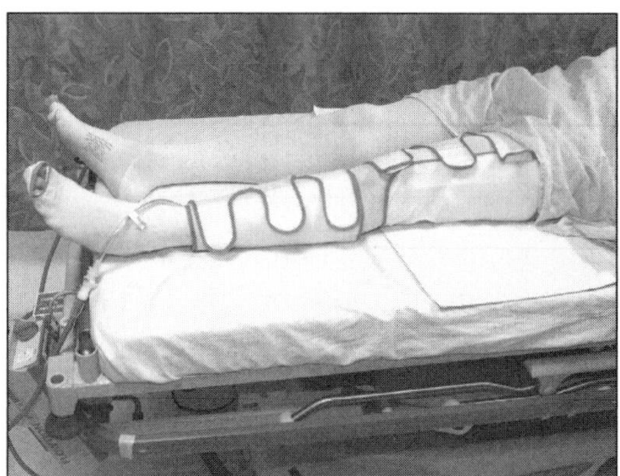

Figure 4.3. Sequential air stockings to assist with circulation after TKA surgery

Many surgeons use a mechanical pump to help blood circulate through the lower extremities. The most popular pumps are sequential air stockings and foot pumps. Sequential stockings are plastic wraps with air bladders that encircle the legs in rings (Figure 4.3). The bladders inflate and deflate sequentially, from the ankle upward to over the knee, thus helping to push the blood out of the leg toward the heart. The foot pump is a slipper-like device that wraps around the foot with an air bladder along the sole of the foot (Figure 4.4). The bladder inflates and deflates, thus emptying the blood from the foot and pushing it up the leg toward the heart. Both devices have been shown to decrease the incidence of blood clots, especially when used in combination with warfarin or low-molecular-weight heparin.

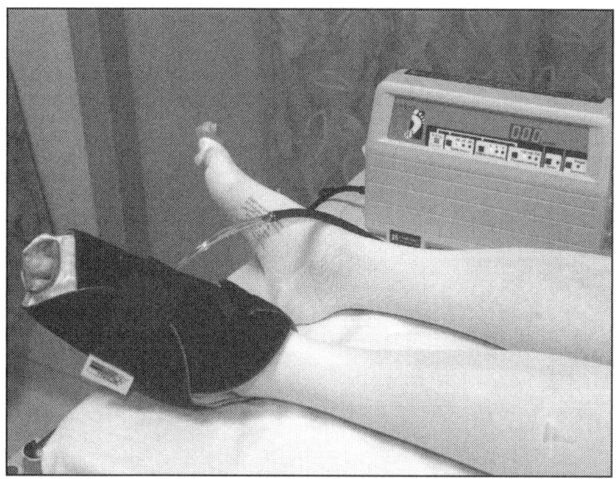

Figure 4.4. Foot pump to assist circulation after TKA surgery

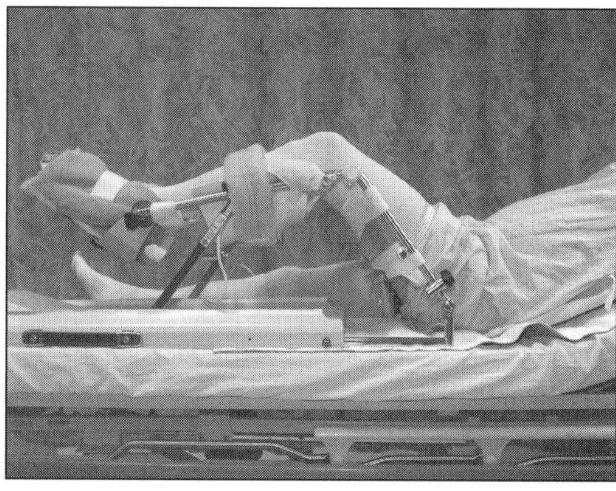

Figure 4.5. Continuous passive motion (CPM) machine, used to improve range of motion after TKA surgery

The CPM Machine

Gaining range of motion in the knee as soon as possible after surgery is critical to obtaining an excellent functional result following TKA. A great deal of discussion in the later chapters is devoted to outlining an exercise program designed to achieve maximum range of motion in your new knee. In an effort to get a head start on encouraging knee motion, many surgeons use a continuous passive motion (CPM) machine (Figure 4.5). This device has a carriage, or sling, that holds the leg as the carriage slowly moves to flex and extend the knee in a passive manner. The CPM machine moves the knee so slowly that you can sleep while your leg is being moved for you. The CPM machine is typically used as much as the patient can tolerate, with the degree of flexion increasing as much as possible. It demonstrates to the patient that it is possible to move the knee just hours after surgery. Fear of knee motion after a surgery of this magnitude is a difficult psychological barrier to overcome. In addition to improving range of motion, the CPM machine offers the benefit of reducing knee swelling. Reducing the swelling helps to prevent blood clots. Sometimes the machine may be used at home for several weeks postoperatively, based on your surgeon's instructions. Although the CPM machine may not be appropriate for every patient, when it is fitted properly most patients provide positive feedback about it. Ask your surgeon if a CPM machine is appropriate for your situation.

Common Questions and Some Answers

Do I have to go to the preoperative joint-replacement class?

No, it is not mandatory that you attend the preoperative joint-replacement class. However, it is our experience that the more educated a patient is prior to surgery, the better he or she understands what is being done and why. This usually translates to a better overall result after TKA surgery.

Is the surgery video very graphic or bloody?

Some videos are actually filmed in the operating room, so they show in vivid detail the steps of the surgery. If you are uncomfortable with the sight of blood, you may choose not to view these teaching tapes.

Why do I have to donate blood if I am not going to lose very much?

It is not uncommon for a patient to lose more blood than the surgeon expected. If this occurs, blood may be needed immediately. In general, it is best to receive your own blood in transfusion, and it is optimal to have it readily available if it is needed during the operation. It is wise to be prepared for the potential of a greater than expected amount of blood loss.

Are you sure I can't have my morning coffee on the day of surgery?

You should not have *ANYTHING* to eat or drink, including coffee, for at least eight hours prior to surgery. If there is anything in your stomach when you get to the operating room, your surgery may be cancelled. The exception is taking medications with a small sip of water as instructed by your anesthesiologist.

Will I get to meet the anesthesiologist prior to my surgery?

Most anesthesiologists will either call you the night before surgery to discuss your anesthesia or will meet with you in the preoperative area before the surgery starts. This is the best time to have all of your questions about anesthesia answered.

What is my new knee made of?

The femoral and tibial components are made of a cobalt-chromium metal alloy, and the plastic is a high-density, high-molecular-weight polyethylene.

How much does my new knee weigh?

While each prosthesis is different, the average weight is between three and five pounds. Although the prosthesis may add to the weight of your leg, your surgeon had to remove bone and cartilage from the knee joint for the prosthesis to fit correctly. Therefore, when the removal of bone and cartilage is measured against adding metal and plastic, there usually is no appreciable change in the weight of the leg.

Will I be either taller or shorter after surgery?

The vast majority of patients experience no change in height after TKA surgery. In order to maintain the proper mechanics of the joint, the size of the prosthetic components are designed to keep the ligament tension as it was before the arthritic collapse of the knee cartilage. Bone and cartilage are removed and replaced with an equal amount of metal and plastic to maintain proper ligament length. Some patients may gain a few millimeters in height by the restoration of the degraded cartilage cushion with the plastic component. The other group of patients who may gain minimal height are those with a severe varus (bowlegged) or valgus (knock-kneed) deformity prior to TKA surgery. For these patients, the lower extremity is aligned properly during the surgery, allowing the patient to stand taller.

Will I be able to feel my new knee after surgery?

Once the swelling goes down, many patients tell us they have the sensation of having an artificial knee. They lack the arthritic pain that was present prior to surgery, but they notice that their new knee "feels different" from the other knee. You will be unable to feel any of the artificial knee's components from the outside, because there is too much soft tissue around the joint. It may take a year or two before you no longer think of your knee as being an artificial knee.

Can I have a private room in the hospital?

Most of the time, the availability of a private room varies depending on how full the hospital is. The best time to request a private room is upon admission to the hospital. Another issue is your insurance company's willingness to pay for a private room. It is important for you to check on this prior to surgery, as some insurance companies will make the patient pay the difference between a private and a semiprivate room.

Will the same nurse take care of me the whole time I'm in the hospital?

The nursing staff typically changes shifts two to three times per day. While every effort is made to keep the patient/nurse relationship consistent, this is not always possible.

Do I need a special diet after surgery and/or during the recovery period?

Even though you may feel hungry after surgery, your nurse will advance your diet slowly. You will begin with clear liquids, progress to full liquids, and eventually return to a general diet. This is not the time to begin a diet to lose weight, as your body needs quality calories to aid in the healing process. The good, "old-fashioned" balanced diet is the optimal diet at this point. If you require a special diet for other reasons, a consultation with a dietician while you're in the hospital is advised.

Will I get addicted to my pain medications?

It is important to keep your postoperative knee pain under control. Your surgeon will prescribe a medication that will help you control the pain as a part of the postsurgical treatment. The goal is to take the minimum amount of pain medication needed for pain control, allowing you to perform the rehabilitation activities effectively. This delicate balance is different for each person. You must rely on the advice of your doctor and the nursing staff to help you achieve this balance. Adhering to these general guidelines, along with the advice from your doctor and nursing staff, will almost never result in an addiction to narcotics. If you are a recovering alcoholic or drug addict, discuss this issue with your surgeon prior to being admitted to the hospital. He or she may modify the pain medications prescribed to you based on this information.

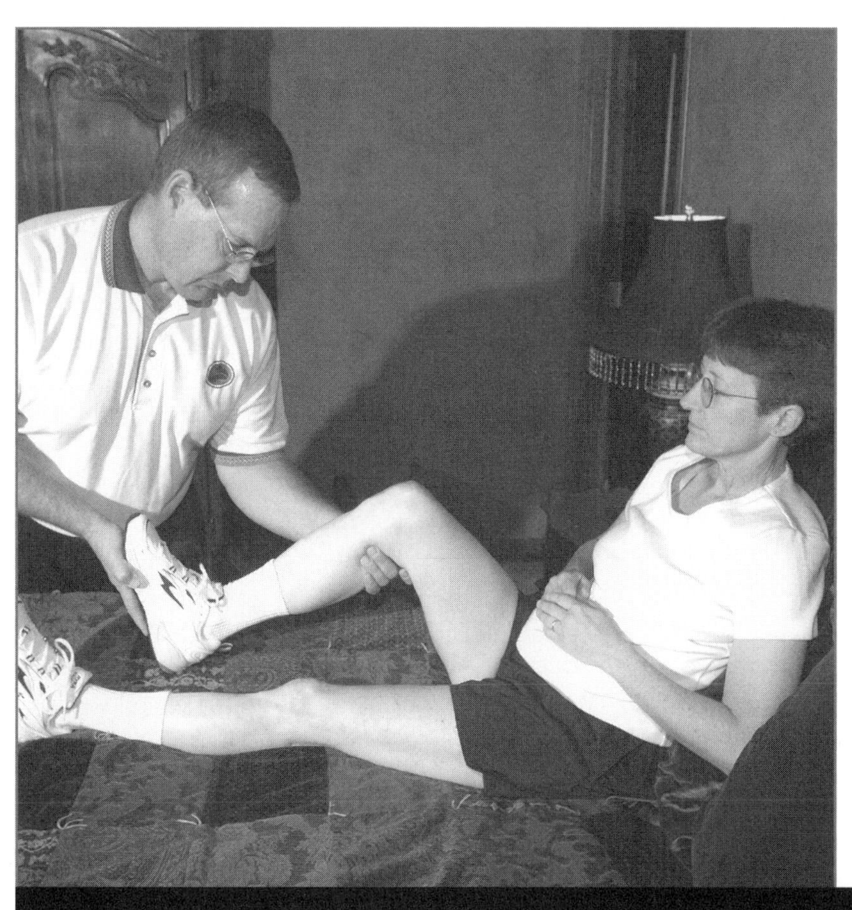

Chapter 5

Postoperative Days One Through Five

Am I Ready for Rehab?

Day One: Beginning Physical Therapy

On the first day after major surgery you may think that you will be resting and recovering in bed. Not so after total knee arthroplasty surgery! Most surgeons want their patients to be up and moving as soon as possible after surgery to get the TKA working right away. Many surgeons actually start the movement of the new TKA in the recovery room, using a continuous passive movement (CPM) machine. Other surgeons want to see if their patients can get the knee moving on their own without a CPM machine. As we mentioned in Chapter 4, discuss this aspect of rehabilitation with your surgeon prior to surgery.

As you lie in bed, try to move your leg. It may be difficult or even seem impossible! Don't panic. As a result of the TKA surgery, there will be significant swelling around the new knee because the muscles and ligaments surrounding the knee have been traumatized during the surgery. Therefore, your leg and new knee may fail to respond to your brain's command to move. This is normal and usually subsides in the first day or two after surgery. It is important to keep trying to move your knee several times every hour while lying in bed to help reestablish the "brain–knee connection." As discussed in Chapter 3, one method of self-assistance is to use a rolled-up towel or sheet as a stirrup or sling around the bottom of your heel and foot. This technique allows you to pull on the sling to assist your muscles in moving your leg (Figure 5.1).

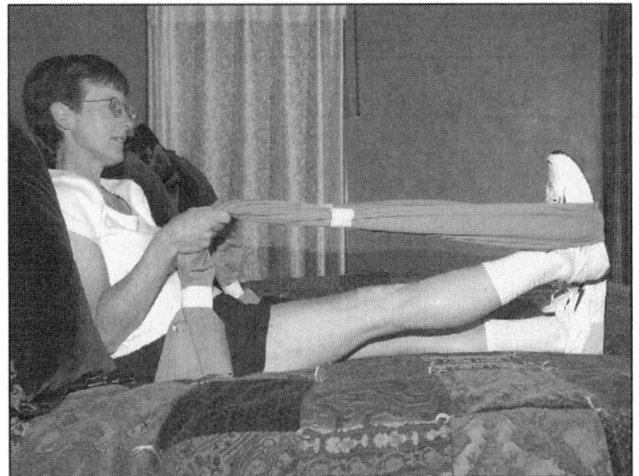

Figure 5.1. Use of a rolled-up towel to assist in movement and control of TKA leg

Sometime during the first day after surgery, expect a visit from a physical therapist (PT). The PT is there to teach you how to move in bed, how to get out of bed, and how to ambulate (walk) with some form of assistive device (usually crutches or a walker). As you can imagine, moving the leg that has been operated on will be painful. Whenever possible, the nursing staff and physical-therapy staff will attempt to coordinate the administration of your pain medication so that you take it approximately thirty to sixty minutes prior to your scheduled therapy. This makes therapy more comfortable and time efficient, allowing you to get the most out of each session.

One of the first exercises the PT routinely reviews with you is the straight-leg raise. If you have been practicing the straight-leg raise at home prior to surgery, this should not be too difficult. However, if you did not work on it, there may be difficulty lifting your foot off the bed while keeping your knee straight. This exercise is critical for mobility in bed, getting in and out of bed, and negotiating the obstacles in your room. If you cannot do a straight-leg raise, the PT can instruct you in additional exercises to assist in developing the strength to perform the straight-leg raise before leaving the hospital.

The straight-leg raise is an example of an isometric exercise. Isometric exercises involve tightening a muscle and holding the contraction in that muscle for several seconds without using the muscle to move the leg. In addition to the straight-leg raise, there are three more isometric exercises that are commonly given to total-knee patients:

Exercise 15

Gluteal Sets

While lying in bed, squeeze the muscles of your buttocks together and hold for 5–10 seconds. Be sure to keep breathing while doing the exercise (Figure 5.2).

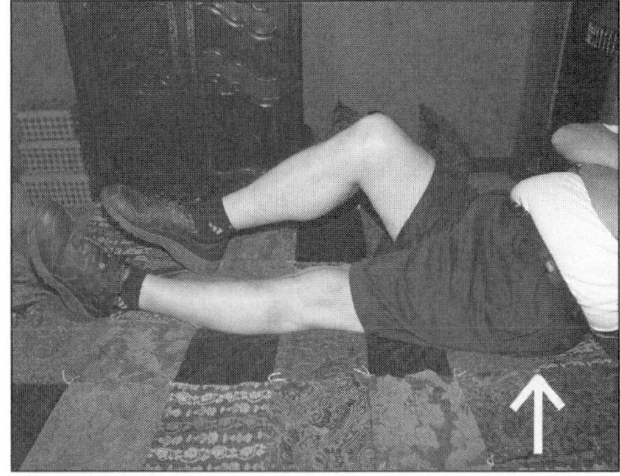

Figure 5.2. Gluteal set exercise for strengthening buttock muscles after TKA surgery

Exercise 16

Quadriceps Sets

While lying in bed, tighten the muscles on the front of your thigh by pushing the back of your knee against the bed, and hold for 5–10 seconds (Figure 5.3). Be sure to keep breathing while doing the exercise.

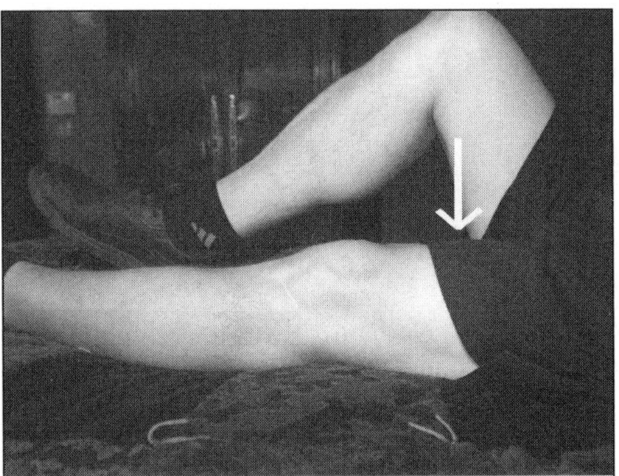

Figure 5.3. Quad set exercise for strengthening thigh muscles after TKA surgery

Exercise 17

Hamstring Sets

While lying in bed, pull your heel into the bed by tightening the muscle under your thigh, and hold for 5–10 seconds (Figure 5.4). Be sure to keep breathing while doing the exercise.

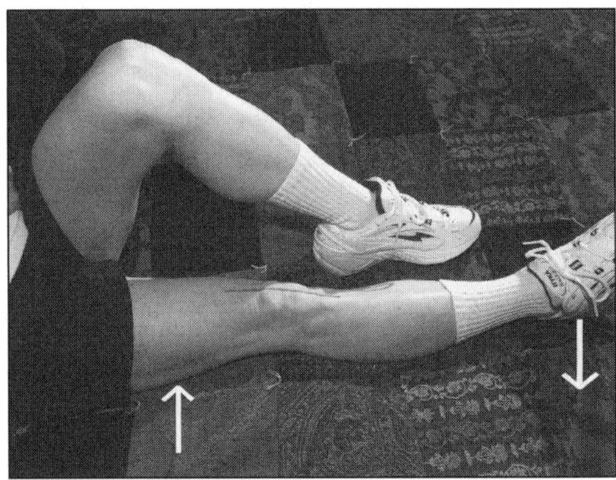

Figure 5.4. Hamstring set exercise for strengthening thigh muscles after TKA surgery

Exercises 15 through 17 should be done at least 10 times during every hour when you are awake. Here's a trick to establishing a regular exercise regime: While watching TV, do these three exercises during the commercials. The more often these simple exercises are performed, the sooner you will be able to move your TKA leg without difficulty.

■ ■ ■

On the first day, the PT also typically demonstrates a few other exercises to help control swelling in the leg:

Exercise 18

Ankle Pumps

While lying in bed, keep your leg straight and repeatedly flex and point your foot by bending and extending your ankle (Figure 5.5). Repeat 25 times for each ankle. This exercise assists with circulation.

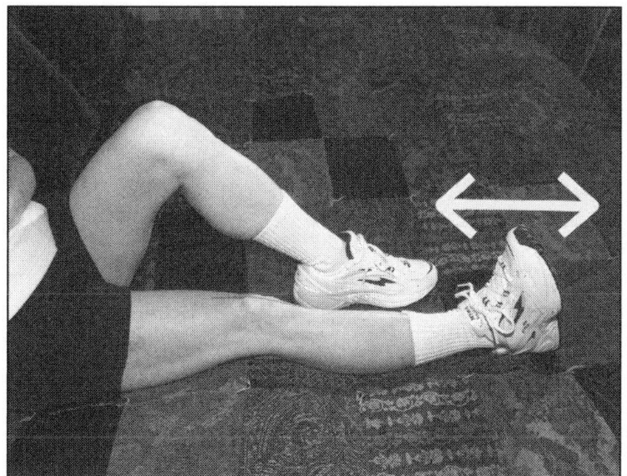

Figure 5.5. Ankle pump exercise to assist circulation after TKA surgery

Exercise 19

Heel Slides

While lying in bed, bend and straighten the knee of your nonoperated leg as far as possible by sliding your heel back and forth along the sheet (Figure 5.6). Repeat 25 times. Now, try to do the same thing with the operated leg. This will be a lot harder and may even be impossible, but try to complete 25 heel slides with your operated leg. Heel slides assist in increasing range of motion in the knee.

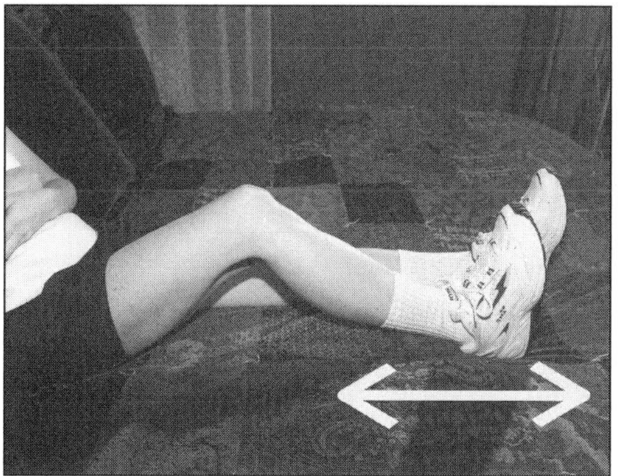

Figure 5.6. Heel slide exercise to assist in gaining range of motion after TKA surgery

Exercise 20

Short-Arc Quadriceps Exercise for Range of Motion

Again, if you have been practicing this exercise with the one-gallon paint can or the five-gallon bucket, it will be much easier to perform on the first day after surgery. While lying in bed, place a rolled-up towel, a one-gallon paint can, or even a five-gallon bucket under your operated knee and lift that foot off the bed by straightening your knee. Keep the back of your thigh in contact with the towel roll, can, or bucket. The larger the roll, can, or bucket, the more range of motion and strength you will develop. Hold the foot up for a count of 3–5 seconds and then lower the foot back to the bed. Complete 1–3 sets of 5–15 repetitions each (Figure 5.7).

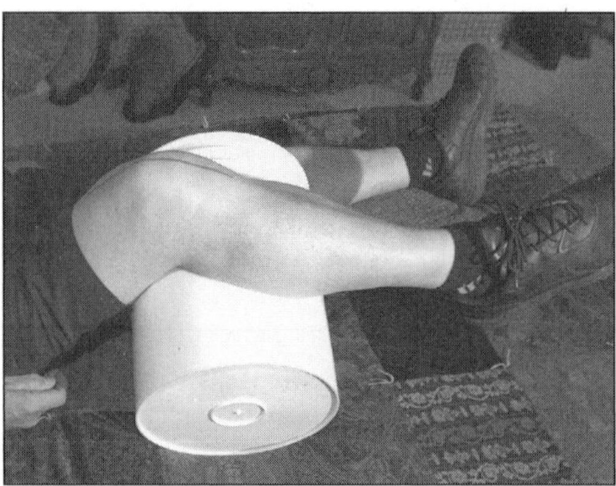

Figure 5.7. Short-arc quadriceps exercise for range of motion

First Attempts to Walk

Now it is time to get out of bed and try to walk. This is initially done only with the supervision of a physical therapist. While you're doing a straight-leg raise, the PT will gently guide your foot over the bed and onto the floor. If you cannot accomplish a straight-leg raise, the PT will have to move your leg for you. Although this is okay for the first time you're getting out of bed, you need to learn to do it by yourself. It is critical to practice the straight-leg-raise exercise as often as possible while you are in the hospital.

Once you're out of bed, the PT will instruct you in the proper amount of weight to bear on your total-knee leg. Some surgeons allow their patients to immediately put as much weight as they can tolerate on the TKA; other surgeons will limit weight bearing. Factors such as how the prosthetic components are attached to the bone, the need for ligament reconstruction, and the presence of bony defects will influence your surgeon's decision regarding weight-bearing status on the new knee. Your surgeon probably discussed this with you prior to surgery, but if not, your PT knows your weight-bearing status.

Next you will be fit with both a walker and crutches. Hopefully you have practiced walking with either a walker or crutches at home prior to surgery, so this inaugural walk on your new knee will be a piece of cake! If you are not allowed to put your full weight on the total knee right after surgery, a walker is probably the safest device to use for the first few days in the hospital. However, if you have practiced with the crutches at home, and if there are many stairs to conquer at home, you may be more comfortable using crutches. Don't despair if you can't get the hang of the crutches immediately. The PT will visit daily while you are in the hospital and will teach you the best way to walk with a walker and/or crutches.

As you read this book before your surgery, these exercises and movements may seem far too simple to spend much time on, or to even consider as exercise. Do not underestimate how difficult these simple exercises can be after major surgery. It is amazing how tired you can become after your first physical-therapy session, and you haven't even started walking! The first time Dr. Falkel tried to walk on the day following his TKA surgery, he was able to walk only about eight feet with a walker, and then he was totally exhausted. In fact, the PT had to bring the bed to him because the eight feet he'd walked was seven feet too far for him to walk back to his bed! Believe it or not, many patients sweat profusely after doing these simple bed exercises and after walking only a few feet. This is totally normal, so don't be alarmed. Most patients are usually so exhausted after their first attempt at exercising and walking that they stay in bed for the remainder of the day.

Range-of-Motion Exercises

The PT may visit twice a day while you are in the hospital. During the second visit of the day, the PT will generally repeat the same exercises as before, assist you in walking slightly farther, and begin range-of-motion exercises. As difficult as the simple strengthening exercises and the walking may be, movement (bending and straightening) of your new TKA will be even more difficult. In fact, it will just plain hurt! The pain is due to the swelling, the surgical removal of the ends of the femur and tibia, and the incisions into the skin, connective tissue, and muscles around the knee. Taking your pain medication is critical. In fact, if you have no pain medication in your system, you most likely will be unable to do the work needed to get your knee moving and to improve your function. For some patients, the pain of the arthritis in the knee was actually worse than or different from the postoperative pain. Still, in order to work your new knee to gain range of motion, it is imperative to take pain medication on a regular basis. The optimal pain-control regime is different for each patient. The type of medication, the method of administration (IV, IM, or orally), and the dose and frequency of the medication can be adjusted to achieve effective pain control. This process may require some experimenting, which involves feedback and coordination between the patient, nurse, and surgeon. If one medication fails to achieve the pain control you need to participate in your PT exercises, notify your nurse and/or therapist so that appropriate modifications can be made.

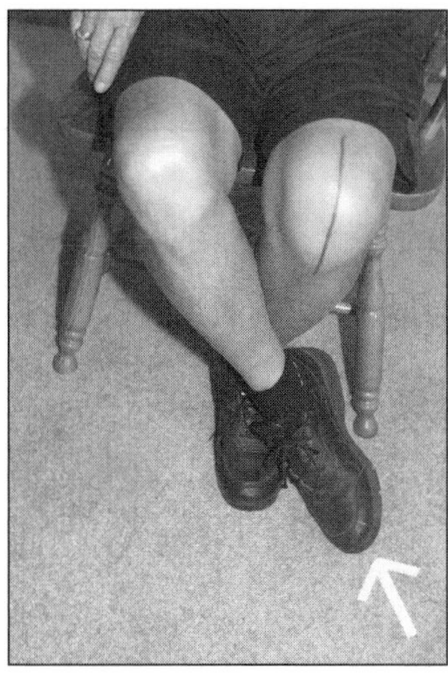
Figure 5.8. Range-of-motion exercise using nonoperated leg for assistance

The PT may utilize several methods for moving your knee. The first technique is to have you sit upright in a chair and then see how much movement, or bend, you can achieve in the new knee by sliding your foot on the floor. Another method of gaining range of motion is to place the nonoperated foot over the foot of your TKA leg while sitting in a chair. Then, push back on the TKA leg by bending the nonoperated knee, moving your feet toward you (Figure 5.8). Once you reach the point where the knee begins to hurt and get stiff, hold that position for as long as possible (up to 60 seconds) and then release the pressure on the TKA leg (Exercise 21; see Chapter 6). Of all the range-of-motion exercises we have used over the years, this simple exercise has proven to be the most effective for the vast majority of our patients. Upon returning home, if you perform this exercise several times a day, you will see rapid results.

The PT may also manually move your leg for you, similarly to how the CPM machine works. This is a tough one. The PT supports your leg by placing one hand under the knee, at the same time placing his or her other hand on your ankle. Then he or she proceeds to bend your knee (Figure 5.9). For this exercise to be successful, you, the patient, need to clearly communicate your limits to the PT. Many PTs learned this technique in school or in continuing-education workshops. This method of manual mobilization, as it is called, can be effective, but it can also cause the patient more pain than he or she expected. Good communication is needed between the PT and the patient. Telling the therapist the amount of discomfort you experience helps guide him or her to avoid going too far with mobilization of your TKA knee. Ultimately it is the patient's responsibility, not the therapist's, to get as much motion out of the TKA as possible. The PT can only spend a limited amount of time

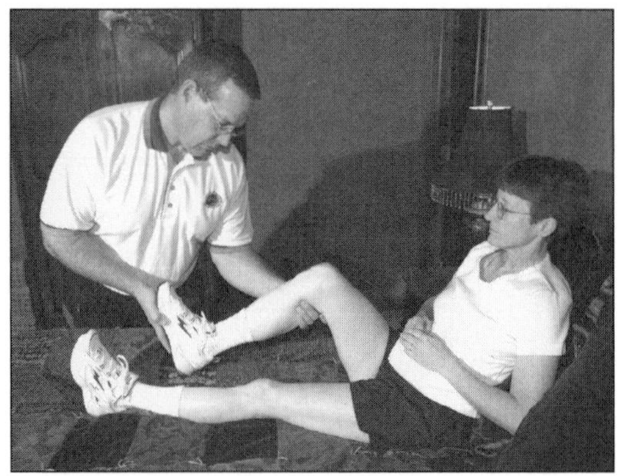
Figure 5.9. Manual mobilization by PT to assist in gaining range of motion

with the patient. Therefore, the more the patient is able to do his or her own range-of-motion exercises, the less discomfort he or she will experience and the more independent functional mobility he or she will achieve.

Breathing Exercises

Breathing exercises are the other key activities that start on day one postoperatively. These are done using an incentive spirometer, which is a small plastic device with several cylinders and a hose attached to a mouthpiece (Figure 5.10). To use the incentive spirometer, place the mouthpiece in your mouth, close your lips around the mouthpiece, and breathe in as deeply as you can. As you breathe in, a plastic piece in the spirometer will move up the cylinders, indicating how much air you have inhaled. After you reach your full breathing capacity, take the mouthpiece out of your mouth and exhale.

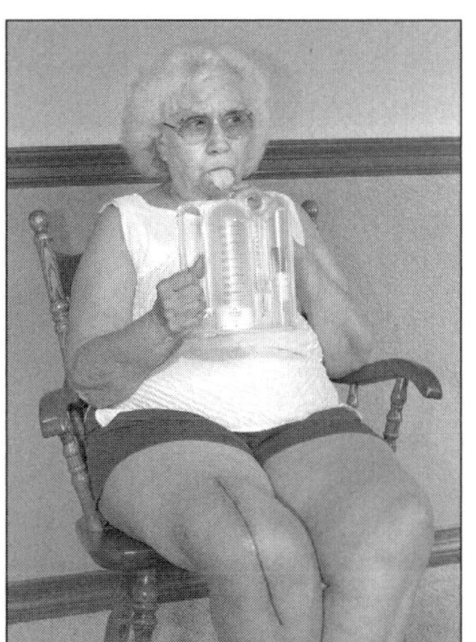

Figure 5.10. Breathing exercises using an incentive spirometer

It is essential that you use the incentive spirometer for five minutes every hour while you are awake to assist in recovery from the anesthesia and in prevention of pneumonia. After surgery, the body is less active than it was prior to the operation. Fluid can build up in the lungs from the inactivity as well as from the diminished lung function that follows anesthesia. With the use of inhalation anesthetics for general anesthesia, atelectasis of the lungs typically sets in. This condition occurs when the small sacs of the lungs collapse during anesthesia. Utilizing the incentive spirometer forces you to use your lungs more vigorously, thereby opening up the collapsed sacs in your lungs. This quickly assists your return to normal lung function, immediately improving your stamina. It is a relatively simple activity, but one that is very necessary for your recovery.

Enough fun for one day! Try to get some rest, because tomorrow is another big day.

Days Two Through Five: Continuing Physical Therapy

On the second day after surgery, your PT will visit again. He or she will continue with the simple exercises in bed and may increase the number of repetitions and the number of sets for each exercise. The PT will routinely take you for a walk, hopefully out of your room and down the hall. You may experience light-headedness once you start walking more. This is a typical response to walking upright and occurs quite commonly. As you lie in bed for a prolonged period of time, gravity tends to cause the blood to pool in your legs. Also exacerbating the situation is the diminished blood volume circulating as a result of surgical blood loss. The prolonged bed rest and reduced blood volume make it difficult for your body to pump the blood up to your head when you're in the upright position, resulting in light-headedness. Once you start to feel light-headed, it is important to sit down quickly. If you don't, you may actually pass out.

Many TKA patients experience excessive sweating with even very minimal exercise, walking, or activity. Again, this is a normal reaction to the physical stress of surgery and nothing to worry about. However, it can occur just prior to the feeling of light-headedness, so be aware of this warning symptom. As you become more mobile and walk longer distances, these sensations diminish and eventually subside completely. Be sure to notify your PT when you feel light-headed, nauseated, or start to sweat excessively so he or she can quickly sit you in a chair until the feeling disappears.

Although you may be eager to take a shower by yourself, be aware of the potential for feeling light-headed and nauseous when doing so shortly after surgery. Be sure to have ready access to an alarm cord or switch when you are in the shower so that you can call the nursing staff for assistance if you start feeling poorly. It is also important to ask for assistance if you feel the incision getting wet.

At day two or three, you and your surgeon should start talking about your leaving the hospital. For most people, this means going home. However, some patients may not reach a minimum level of independence or may not have anyone at home to assist them with their daily activities. These patients leave the hospital for a temporary stay at a rehabilitation center or nursing-home facility in order to improve their strength, endurance, and mobility. Once there, these patients continue with their exercises, range-of-motion training, and walking with crutches or a walker until they have the functional independence needed to return home. As we discussed in Chapter 3, making arrangements ahead of time and preparing your home for your arrival after surgery will facilitate your path to independence, thus significantly reducing the stress to you and your family.

The PT routinely works with patients on using the walker or crutches around the house, especially while ascending and descending stairs. Before your return home, the PT will review with you the pros and cons of using a walker or crutches. The decision to use a walker or crutches is based on your home environment, your ability to put weight on the TKA leg, how "good" your other knee is, and how safe or comfortable you feel with the walker or crutches. Normally within the first three to four weeks after surgery you will progress to using only one crutch or a cane. Eventually you will not need any assistive device while walking. For the first few days or weeks after TKA surgery use whatever device makes you feel most safe and secure.

By day three many patients are able to get up and out of bed by themselves. The more you can get up and walk, and the more you can get out of bed to sit in a chair, the better you will feel. It is much easier to work on range of motion in the TKA knee while sitting in a chair than it is while lying in bed. An increased activity level also helps prevent constipation and reduces the risks of blood clots.

By day three you may no longer need the CPM machine. Many surgeons want their patients to use the CPM machine until the patient achieves 90 degrees of flexion in the TKA. Other surgeons do not use a CPM machine for an uncomplicated TKA. Sometimes CPM machines are used only for a few days, for the psychological advantage of showing the patient that her or his new knee does move. The use of the CPM machine is very dependent on the individual situation of the patient and the philosophy of the surgeon.

Once you're able to safely get out of bed by yourself, try to eat all of your meals sitting in a chair. While sitting up, work on bending your TKA knee as much as you can. The only drawback to sitting in a chair is that doing so may promote more swelling in your TKA. Your TKA becomes swollen as part of the normal healing process. However, with more swelling comes less motion and more pain. Therefore, you need to find a balance between sitting and doing the range-of-motion exercises, and lying down in bed to assist in reduction of swelling. One method of reducing swelling is to keep a bag of ice (in cubes or chips) or a cryotherapy unit (discussed later in this chapter) on your new knee once you get back in bed, while keeping the knee elevated above the level of your heart.

If you are unable to get in and out of bed by yourself on about day three, then you need to work more with the PT on the control of your TKA leg with a modified straight-leg-raise exercise. If you cannot perform a quad set and then a straight-leg raise on your own because of weakness or pain, here is a simple way to develop the strength and endurance of the muscles in your upper leg to allow you to do a straight-leg raise independently.

First, perform a quadriceps set (Exercise 16) and hold the contraction of your quadriceps muscle. Then have the PT, nurse, or a family member support your leg by placing one hand under your knee and the other hand under your heel. While you continue to hold the quad set, have your helper slowly raise your straight leg about 8–12 inches off the bed. Now comes the fun part: You will try to hold your leg straight, 8–12 inches off the bed, while your assistant slowly lowers your leg down toward the bed, *very gradually* removing the support of their hands from under your leg. This might sound incredibly easy, but it can and does hurt a great deal in the quadriceps muscle just above your new knee. It is critical that the person assisting you with this exercise *DOES NOT **DROP** YOUR LEG!* Dr. Falkel speaks from personal experience when he says that words cannot describe how much this hurts! Rather, the person assisting you needs to gradually *lower* your leg.

After several trials of this assisted straight-leg-raising exercise, you will be able to hold your leg straight with less and less effort from the assistant. It may seem to happen all of sudden that on one particular repetition you are able to hold your TKA leg straight, 8–12 inches off the bed, while the assistant removes all support. Once this happens, slowly lower your leg to the bed and immediately repeat a quad set and attempt a straight-leg raise on your own. This seemingly small step is worth a big congratulations! Once it's accomplished, you can do so much more for yourself.

It took Dr. Falkel almost three weeks to be able to do a straight-leg raise with either leg by himself. Until that time, he needed assistance to get in and out of bed, to and from the bathroom, and in and out of a car. It was a *very long* three weeks. This may have been because he had both knees replaced simultaneously—or perhaps it was because he did not work on training his quadriceps to do straight-leg raises *before* surgery. To this day he regrets not doing more preoperative strength training!

Care of Your Surgical Incision

There are many ways that your surgeon can close the skin incision over your total knee arthroplasty. Most surgeons use small staples to close the incision. The main reason for using staples is speed of closure of the incision. Every second that can be saved during the operation is best for the patient. Although the staples are prominent on the skin, their removal is relatively easy. The drawback of the staples is they may catch on dressings, clothes, or bed linens and cause minor discomfort. They may also leave dot-like scars along the main incisional scar.

Another type of incisional closure uses nonabsorbable sutures (stitches) such as nylon or wire on the skin surface. These are similar to staples in terms of ease of removal, but they may also catch on dressings, clothes, or bed linen.

The other popular type of skin closure is a subcuticular suture, meaning a suture that is underneath the skin. With this technique, a dissolvable suture is placed in the dermal layer (the layer just underneath the visible layer of skin). The incision is reinforced with Steri-Strips, which are small sterile pieces of tape applied directly to the skin to add strength to the suture line. This closure technique makes stitch or staple removal unnecessary. The Steri-Strips fall off the skin on their own after one or two weeks. The patient does not have to deal with any staples or stitches catching on objects around the incision, and some surgeons feel it leaves a thinner scar. Unfortunately, this incisional-closure technique takes more time during the operation.

Each surgeon has her or his own preference about closure techniques based on philosophy and experience. The general goal in incisional closure is to do the fastest job possible with the best cosmetic appearance of the scar. In later chapters we will discuss scar management—that is, what is required in order to have the "best-looking" scar.

When you recover from the anesthesia, you will see that your operated leg has a large, bulky dressing over the entire incision. The dressing is held in position with either tape, an elastic wrap (ACE bandage), or a thigh-high surgical stocking (T.E.D. hose). The dressing is kept clean and dry by the nursing staff. It is not uncommon for the incision to leak small to large amounts of blood into the dressing. When this occurs, the dressing is either reinforced or changed. If possible, the dressing will remain undisturbed for the first three days post-op, because the risk of infection is reduced if the incision is left alone immediately after surgery. Dressing changes are done at the discretion of the surgeon or nursing staff. However, if you feel the dressing getting wet, either from bleeding or a leaky ice bag, let the nursing staff know right away.

Ice and Elevation

It is normal for your knee to swell after surgery. However, control of the swelling will improve pain control, range of motion, and circulation in your leg. Enhancing the circulation not only helps with wound healing, but also aids in prevention of infection. With less swelling, there is better circulation and less chance of developing a blood clot in the leg. The best method for controlling swelling is the use of ice and elevation of your operated leg(s).

There are several methods of applying ice to your knee. The simplest is an ice bag. This can be made by placing ice cubes in a reclosable plastic bag wrapped in a terrycloth towel. In some cases the surgeon orders a cryotherapy unit to circulate cold water around your knee. There are several different cryotherapy (cold) units on the market. They circulate cold water by using either an electric pump or a siphoning technique. They offer the advantage of providing a more constant temperature.

When using cold-therapy devices or ice bags on the knee, it is important to protect the skin from direct exposure as excessive cold may cause a minor skin irritation or even a skin burn. The normal sensation around the knee has been altered by the surgery and the swelling. Therefore, if the skin is directly exposed to a cold surface for too long, it may cause a burn. Skin problems can easily be prevented by keeping one or more layers of dressing or fabric (towel, gown, washcloth, etc.) between the cold source and the skin.

Elevation of your leg or legs will also help reduce the swelling in your total knee after surgery. Raising your legs above the level of your heart enables gravity to assist the circulatory system in reducing the fluid in your knee. In the hospital, this can be done with an electric bed and/or pillows. A CPM machine can also be used to assist in elevation of the operated leg.

Swelling in the knee is a normal reaction to total knee arthroplasty. However, an excessive amount of swelling may increase the risk of complications after surgery and delay your recovery process. Ice and elevation should be used as much as possible when you're not exercising. It is important to use ice and elevation for swelling control while in the hospital, and it is equally important that you continue their use at home. We will discuss this topic more in the next chapter.

Personal Care

You will be allowed to take your first shower two to four days after your surgery. This decision is made by your surgeon and nurse, depending on your strength and whether there is any drainage from the incision. The most important consideration for incisional care is the prevention of infection. It is critical that no shower water be allowed to leak into the incision. If fluid is leaking out of the incision, it is possible for bacteria carried by the shower water to get into the incision, causing an infection. Large amounts of drainage may postpone the first shower. With small amounts of drainage, a shower may be permitted with a watertight covering over the incision.

The nursing staff will help you into a wheelchair that fits into a shower. They will cover your incision or dressing with a plastic bag, plastic wrap, or specially designed bag to protect casts from getting wet in the shower (cast guard). Some surgeons may allow you to get the incision wet in the shower as soon as there is no drainage present. Other surgeons do not want their patients to get the incision wet until the staples or stitches are removed, ten to fourteen days postoperatively. If your surgeon permits you get the incision wet in the shower, do not scrub the incision with anything. Simply allow the water to run over the knee and gently wash around the incision. Carefully pat the incision dry with a towel, taking care to not get a staple or stitch caught in the fabric. If Steri-Strips are present over the incision, as they get wet and then dry they will eventually fall off. Once they fall off, you normally do not need to replace them.

As mentioned earlier in the chapter, when taking a shower pay attention to any light-headed or nauseous feelings. Do not hesitate to use the alarm switch or cord if any such feelings come over you. Also pay attention and report it to the nurse if you notice your incision getting wet during a shower (if, that is, your surgeon has requested that you keep the incision dry for now).

Another aspect of personal care that needs to be discussed is having a regular bowel movement. It is extremely common for patients to become constipated after major surgery. As discussed earlier, several factors can contribute to constipation after surgery, including side effects from pain medication, a change in your diet at the hospital, and the effects of prolonged bed rest. This is a very uncomfortable experience and one that may be minimized or avoided. If you do become constipated, notify your nurse and/or surgeon sooner rather than later. Do not be embarrassed. The medications used to assist in keeping your bowels regular are much more effective if used early.

Discharge from the Hospital

What may have only been a few days in the hospital can seem like months. When you are ready to leave the hospital and return home, there are several points to consider:

1. Vehicle size and height are important to think about. Whoever is coming to the hospital to pick you up must have a large enough vehicle to easily accommodate you. Small cars can be very difficult to get into because you may lack enough knee flexion to sit in a seat with limited legroom. Likewise, some larger sport utility vehicles or trucks may be too high to permit you to step up into the seat. Regardless of the type of vehicle, consider sitting across the backseat with your legs on the seat and your back against the door. Support your back and legs with pillows. No matter how smooth the road, you will feel every bump. With your legs across the seat, supported by pillows, much of the shock will be absorbed. It may be necessary to borrow a vehicle from a friend to make the ride home easier. Discuss this with your physical therapist prior to discharge.

2. Getting into the house will be the first obstacle upon your arrival at home. If possible, try to have someone at home to help hold the door open for you and assist with getting you into the house. As discussed in Chapters 3, preparing your house for your arrival prior to surgery makes getting around at home much easier and safer.

3. Stock up on food and personal items so you do not need to leave home for several days. Most patients are shocked at how tired they are when they first get home and at how the simplest of tasks (going to the bathroom, getting a drink of water, etc.) can leave them totally exhausted. Early on, your tolerance for standing up can be measured in seconds. This is normal, and it happens to every TKA patient. Prior to surgery it is helpful to buy frozen dinners or to prepare your own meals and freeze them in individual servings. Then, after surgery, your meals can be prepared simply by heating them in the microwave, with a minimal amount of standing.

Why do patients feel so tired after their TKA surgery? We like to call it the *60-60-24-7-4 syndrome*. Following total knee arthroplasty the patient is involved in rehabilitation of the TKA for sixty seconds a minute, sixty minutes an hour, twenty-four hours a day, seven days a week, for at least four weeks. Everything you do is rehabilitation. There is nothing you can do that does not involve or revolve around your new knee. It is exhausting! Try to imagine spending so much time on any other project. Other causes of fatigue include pain and swelling. The stress of surgery and the lingering effects of the anesthesia also make you tired. Drowsiness and fatigue are a side effect of pain medications. Postoperative anemia due to blood loss during surgery also makes you feel exhausted. All of these factors working against your recovery from TKA surgery present quite a challenge. Our advice to all of our patients is to listen to your body and don't try to fight the fatigue. In the next chapter we will discuss rest as part of the recovery process. For now, when you are tired, rest. Don't feel guilty if you don't get to do all your exercises three times per day; there is always tomorrow. Remember that every second of every minute of every hour you are rehabilitating your new knee, so listen to it when it starts "talking" to you!

? Common Questions and Some Answers

• Why can't I do a straight-leg raise?

After surgery, the quadriceps muscle, in the front of your thigh, will sometimes go into "shutdown mode." Shutdown occurs when there is excessive swelling in or around the knee. In addition, the quadriceps tendon is divided during surgery to gain exposure to the knee. Although the tendon is repaired, a straight-leg raise places the quadriceps tendon under stress and causes pain. As a result, the quadriceps muscle is unable to generate enough tension or force to lift your leg straight off the bed. The best way to minimize this occurrence is to practice straight-leg raises and resisted straight-leg raises, as described in Chapter 3, for a month prior to surgery.

• Why is my leg bruised after surgery?

The bruising you see around your knee is due to bleeding from the bone and soft tissues after surgery. During surgery, a tourniquet is placed on your upper thigh to prevent bleeding into the surgical area. Once the tourniquet is deflated and the incision is closed, there is a slow oozing of blood into the area where the surgery was performed. The blood eventually works its way up to surface of the skin, causing "black and blue" colors. The peak discoloration usually occurs three to five days after surgery. The blood, or bruise, then turns a yellow-green color and will naturally be resorbed by the body within two weeks.

What will my scar look like?

The appearance of the scar is dependent on many factors. These factors include the technique of closure and the type of suture used to close the incision, the amount of swelling, and your ability to heal skin based on your genetic composition. In addition, the fact that the scar is over an area of skin tension due to knee flexion typically causes some or all of the scar to spread. All of these factors can affect the appearance of the scar when it has matured. It may take several years for the scar to fully mature, and as with other parts of your skin, the scar will change in appearance over time. We will discuss scar management in Chapter 8.

Do I have to know before surgery if I will be going to a rehabilitation facility?

No, because the ultimate decision about sending you home or to another rehabilitation facility is determined by your reaction to the surgery and to the hospital physical therapy. Your surgeon will discuss your progress with you, the nursing staff, and the PT to determine what is best for your situation. It is not always possible to predict before surgery if an additional rehabilitation facility will be needed following discharge from the hospital.

Do I need a special diet after surgery and/or during the recovery period?

Since good nutrition is important for your recovery after surgery, the best diet is a well-balanced one. Even if you are not hungry, it is important to maintain your caloric intake. Adequate calories as well as essential vitamins and minerals are required for proper healing. A daily multivitamin is recommended to ensure you are getting the required amount of these essential nutrients. The postoperative period is not the time to begin a diet to lose weight. Restricting calories can slow the healing process. If one of your goals is weight reduction, we suggest waiting until three months after surgery before beginning a weight-loss program. If you have any specific questions about diet or nutrition, consult your primary-care physician.

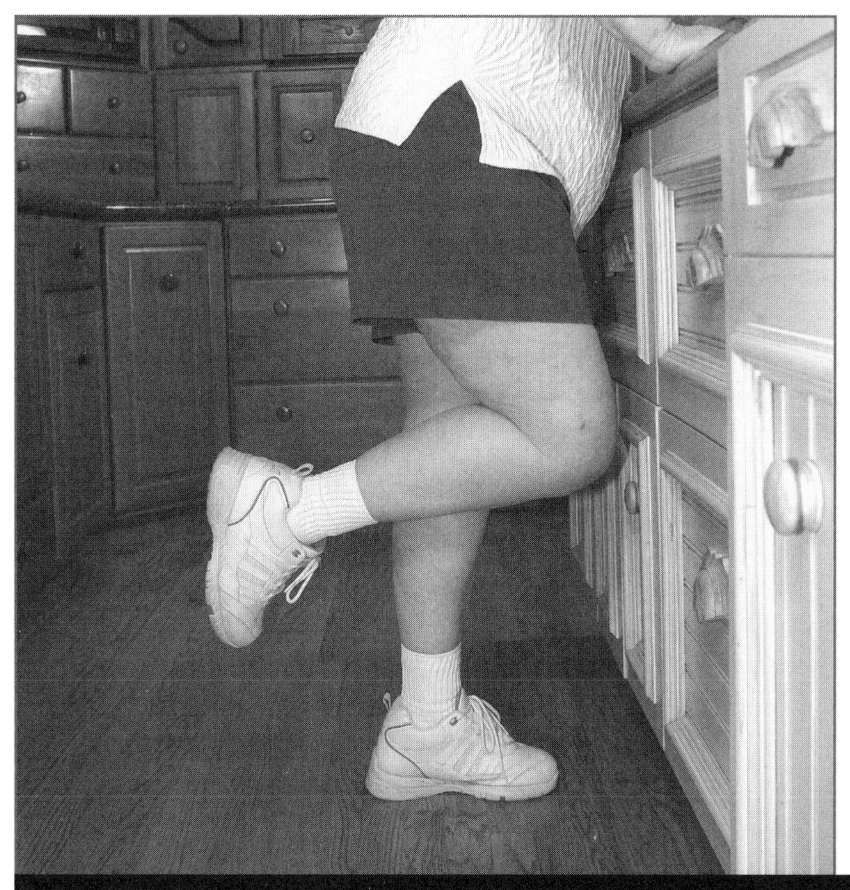

Chapter 6

Week One

You Want Me to Do What?!

Home Physical Therapy

You've made it home. Congratulations! Now the work really begins. More than likely you will have a physical therapist come to your house two to three times a week for the next few weeks. It is important to check on the availability of home physical therapy before the surgery. Consult with your physician about home physical therapy and about the details of your insurance coverage. Most insurance companies will allow for approximately six to ten visits over a period of three to six weeks after you are discharged from the hospital. Dr. Falkel had a total of six visits from his home physical therapist after having had both knees replaced simultaneously.

If your insurance company will pay for home physical therapy, the nurses or PT staff at the hospital should set it up for you prior to discharge. If you lack insurance coverage for home physical therapy, consider paying for it on your own. We feel that home PT is extremely beneficial to the overall recovery process.

Soon after you arrive home, a physical therapist will call to set up an appointment at your home for an evaluation. During the evaluation the therapist will watch how you walk with your walker or crutches, how you get in and out of bed, chairs, and the bathroom, and how you go up and down stairs, if applicable. While many of these tasks are reviewed with you before discharge, the hospital is not exactly like home, so it is important to have some help and guidance upon your arrival home. If you live with someone else, or if a friend or relative will be staying with you for a short period of time, there are several things they can do to make your rehabilitation and mobility a little easier and safer:

1. Have all of your small throw rugs removed from the kitchen, bathroom, and hallway, and from anywhere else in the house. They will move and slip when you place your walker or crutches on them and might cause you to fall.
2. It will be easier for you to stay on one floor. Therefore, as discussed in Chapter 3, consider setting up a temporary bed on the main floor, ideally with access to a bathroom on the same level. Stairs are not impossible, but they are difficult for the first few days. (By the end of week three, you'll find that stairs are no longer the enemy, and you will actually be doing exercises on the stairs to gain strength.)
3. Many people take sponge baths in the kitchen and wash their hair in the sink during the first few days because there are staples in the incision and some surgeons do not want you to get the incision wet in the bath or the shower. Have someone help you get a chair and bathing materials to the kitchen sink if there is not a bathroom on the main floor.

Regaining Range of Motion

In addition to helping with mobility around the house, the physical therapist will also evaluate how much motion, swelling, and strength are present in your knee. Upon your leaving the hospital, the physical therapist routinely measures your knee angle with your leg as straight as possible (measuring knee extension) and again with your knee bent as much as possible (measuring knee flexion). It is helpful to ask your surgeon prior to discharge how much knee flexion is considered optimal. Because every patient, knee, and surgeon is different, there will be different expectations from your surgeon as to the goals for range of motion in your knee.

In earlier chapters we described the continuous passive motion (CPM) machine, used to increase range of motion in the operative knee. Some surgeons do not utilize the CPM machine at all, some order it for use only while the patient is in the hospital, and others have patients use it in the hospital as well as at home. You should be aware of your surgeon's plan with the CPM machine by discussing the matter with him or her before surgery. If your surgeon sends you home with a CPM machine, you will receive instructions about how long it should be used each day. A representative from the CPM company routinely calls once you are home and comes out to your home to set up the machine and instruct you in its use. Since a significant amount of time is spent using the CPM machine, have the representative set it up in a place where you can get comfortable while "working" on the machine by perhaps watching television or listening to music.

Like the PT in the hospital, the therapist who visits your house also works with you to increase your knee flexion and extension as much as possible. Many therapists will ask you to put ice on your knee prior to their arrival at your house. Doing so assists with pain control and swelling, and it is always a good idea as long as you can tolerate the cold on your knee.

Some therapists like to work on gaining range of motion while you lie in bed or on the couch, while others want you to be sitting in a chair. One of the techniques they may use to assist you is a procedure called *mobilization*, which involves the physical therapist's passively moving your knee rather than the CPM doing the movement. Unfortunately, it will be more than a little uncomfortable for someone else to move your knee; it will *hurt*. As discussed in Chapter 5, you need to communicate with your physical therapist about how much discomfort you experience while she or he attempts to move your knee.

The pain you feel when your knee reaches the end of its range of motion—whether it's being moved by you, the CPM, or the physical therapist—is caused by stress on the scar tissue that is forming in your knee as a result of the surgery. Scar tissue is nature's way of healing the muscles, ligaments, and connective tissues that have been forced to accommodate the metal and plastic pieces in your new knee. In order to get normal range of motion in your new knee, you must stretch the scar tissue and actually "break it down." This will hurt. However, there is a fine line between bending and straightening your knee to gain range of motion, and bending and straightening your knee too far. If you bend and straighten it too far, you risk producing too much inflammation in the scar tissue and thus causing even more scar tissue to form. Range of motion that is too aggressive results in excessive pain and causes you to guard against further movement. This cycle of pain is counterproductive, and it is very important to avoid it at all stages of the rehabilitation process. Avoiding excessive pain is part of the art of physical therapy, and it is vital that you communicate excessive pain to your physical therapist. How do you know whether the pain you experience is "excessive" or "acceptable"? We define excessive pain as excruciating, unexpected, or intolerable pain. Acceptable pain can be defined as a pain that is tolerable and that subsides quickly after the cessation of the exercise or activity. One of our patients described acceptable pain as "pain that hurts so good."

The next section of this chapter outlines a number of exercises to do on your own to increase your range of motion. Some of these may have been demonstrated for you in the hospital; some may be given to you by your home physical therapist. The more motion you gain in your knee by your own efforts, the better your knee will feel, thus minimizing the effort required by the physical therapist to move your knee. Remember, ultimately it is *you* who has to move *your* knee. This is how you will eventually be able to do things that were previously impossible because of the arthritis in your knee.

Range-of-Motion Exercises

Before we start a description of the home exercise program, we need to emphasize that it is important to use these exercises as a general guide. Every patient progresses at a different rate for each different exercise. Even patients who have had both knees replaced simultaneously report that each knee heals differently. The progression of exercises in this and the remaining chapters has been developed to fit the needs of the majority of patients, based on our experience. However, some patients will be able to progress through the exercises more rapidly, while others will need more time to get the same results. Don't be alarmed if you are unable to follow each exercise in each chapter. Every patient and every knee is different, and therefore every experience is different. We recommend this particular exercise progression because it has worked for many of our patients; however, if it doesn't work for you, we advise you to progress through the exercises at your own pace.

Here are some simple exercises that you can perform on your own to gain more range of motion in your knee.

Exercise 21

Using Nonoperated Leg for Assistance

Sitting in a chair, bend your total knee as much as possible. Then, place the foot of your opposite leg over the ankle of the operative leg and gently pull the total-knee leg back toward you to achieve even more knee motion. Pull back as far as you can until you feel the stretch, and try to hold it for 20–60 seconds (Figure 6.1a). When you can't hold the stretch any longer, move the top leg forward so you can slightly straighten (extend) the total-knee leg to relieve the stretch pain. Repeat 5–10 times at a single sitting.

Most patients feel this is the *single best* exercise they can do to gain range of motion in their total knee. Repeat the exercise as many times per day as you can. One suggestion for gauging your progress with the exercise is to do it with the back of the chair pushed against a stationary wall or counter (something that is not going to move). Then have someone place a piece of tape on the floor to show how far you are moving your TKA each time you do the exercise (Figure 6.1b). If the floor has some form of design on it (say, tiles on the kitchen floor), you can use it as a "ruler" or indicator to measure your progress in flexing your TKA.

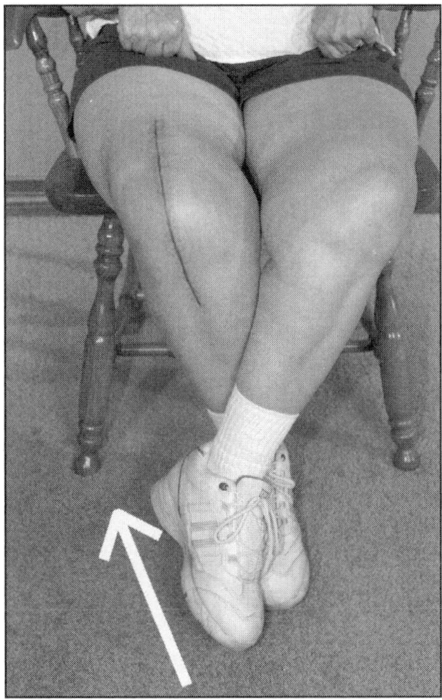

Figure 6.1a. Range-of-motion exercise using nonoperated leg for assistance

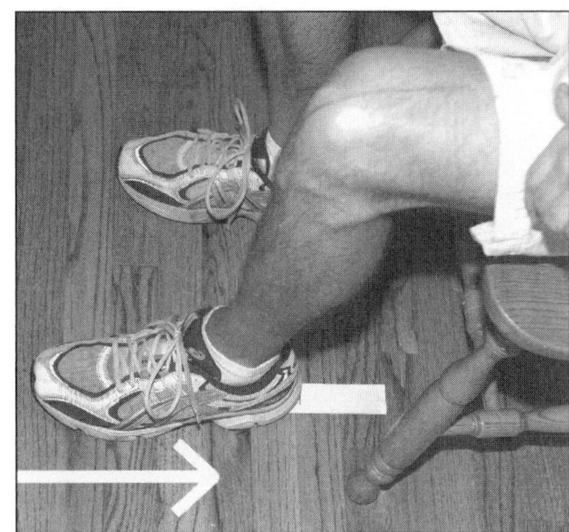

Figure 6.1b. Range-of-motion exercise using floor markings to assess progress in gaining range of motion in the TKA knee

Exercise 22

Using Nonoperated Leg for Resistance

Sitting in a chair as in Exercise 21, bend your total knee as much as possible. Then place the foot of your opposite leg *behind* the ankle of the TKA leg, and, using the hamstring muscles on the operated leg, pull your TKA leg back toward you, pressing against the opposite leg (Figure 6.2). Hold for 20–60 seconds, then relax. This exercise uses the contraction of the hamstring muscles of the TKA leg to get the quadriceps of the TKA leg to relax, thus allowing more flexion of the TKA. Repeat this exercise as many times per day as you can.

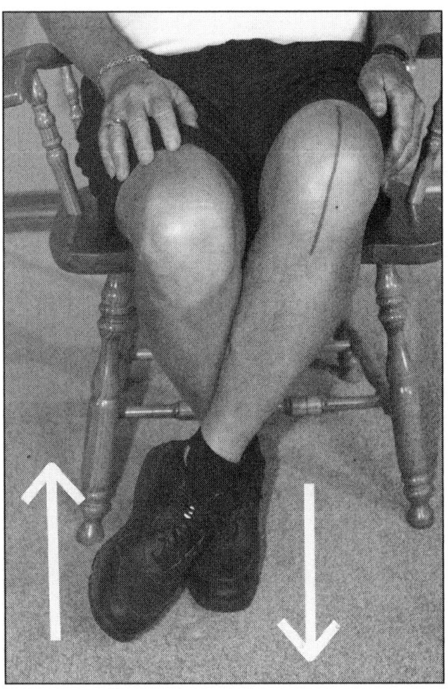

Figure 6.2. Range-of-motion exercise using nonoperated leg for resistance

Exercise 23

Using Block in Front of TKA Foot

Sitting in a chair, bend your new knee as much as possible. Have someone block your foot from sliding forward (or you can block your foot against an immovable object), and then try to slide your bottom forward on the chair, causing your TKA to bend more (Figure 6.3). Hold the position as long as possible, and repeat the exercise as many times per day as you can.

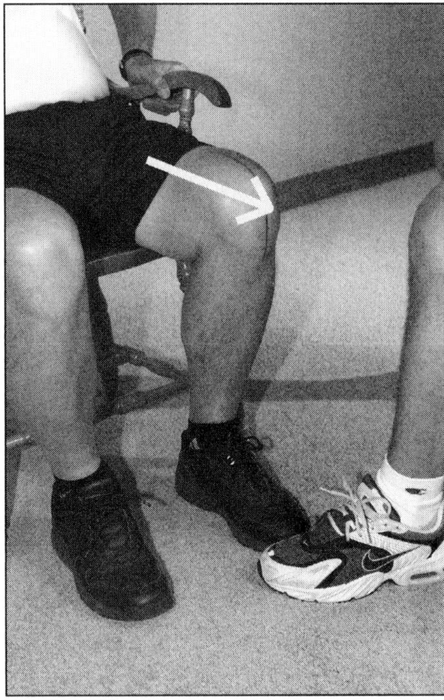

Figure 6.3. Range-of-motion exercise by blocking TKA foot and sliding forward

Exercise 24

Active Knee Flexion

Sitting in a chair, bend the total-knee leg as much as possible. Place your hands under the thigh of this leg, and lift upward with your hands as you slowly straighten and then bend the knee back and forth (Figure 6.4). Complete 3–5 sets of 10–30 reps each, several times per day. This exercise lets gravity help you flex your new knee. In addition, it teaches your new knee that it is "really a knee." Although it may hurt during the first few movements, the exercise encourages the knee to become more limber, thereby decreasing the pain.

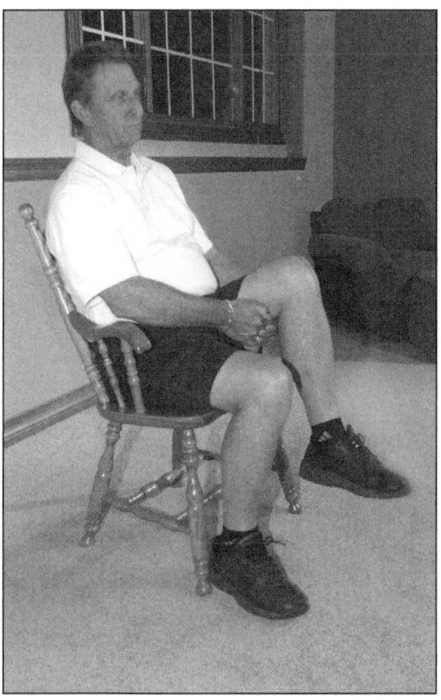

Figure 6.4. Active flexion and extension of the TKA knee

Exercise 25

Passive Knee Extension

Sitting in a chair, prop the heel of your total-knee leg on another chair or table. With nothing behind the total knee to support it, let gravity assist in straightening (extending) the total knee as much as possible. Hold this straight position and occasionally push down on the knee gently with your hands to try to reach full extension (Figure 6.5). Repeat for up to 15 minutes, several times per day.

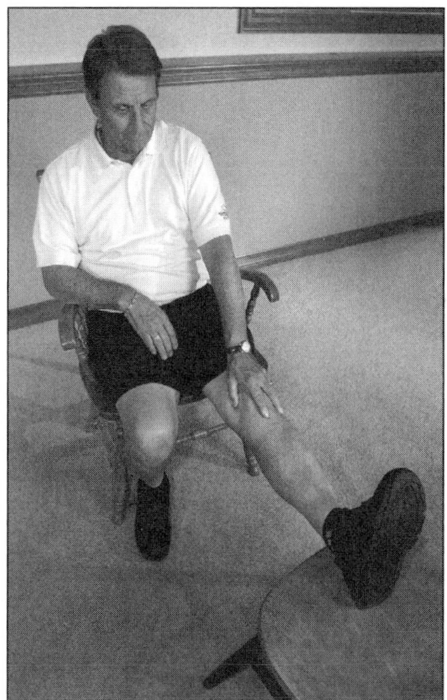

Figure 6.5. Passive extension of the TKA knee

Exercises 26 and 27

Knee Flexion and Extension in a Recliner

If you have a recliner, you can use it for doing two range-of-motion exercises. Raise the leg rest all the way so it is out straight. For the first exercise, slide the heel of your TKA leg toward your bottom, and then try to stop your heel on the edge of the leg rest. Hold this position for 20–60 seconds, and then try to slide your heel even farther back (Figure 6.6a). Repeat as often as possible.

For the second exercise, put a pillow or rolled-up towel on the end of the leg rest, and place the heel of the TKA leg on the pillow or towel roll. As you did in Exercise 25, allow gravity to straighten your knee as much as possible (Figure 6.6b). Occasionally use your hands to gently push down on the knee for even more extension. When you're sitting in the recliner, the pull on your hamstring muscle is different and may allow for more extension than can be obtained in Exercise 25. Hold for as long as possible, and repeat several times per day.

In addition to the two range-of-motion exercises, attempt a straight-leg raise off the pillow or towel roll (Figure 6.6c). Repeat 5–25 times, several times per day.

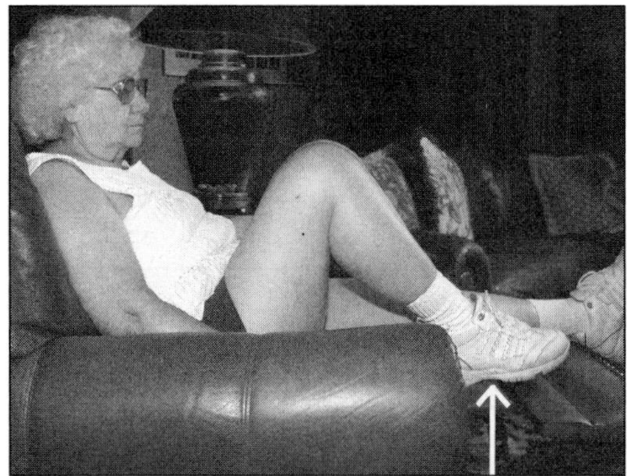

Figure 6.6a. TKA exercise in the recliner: heel slide and stretch

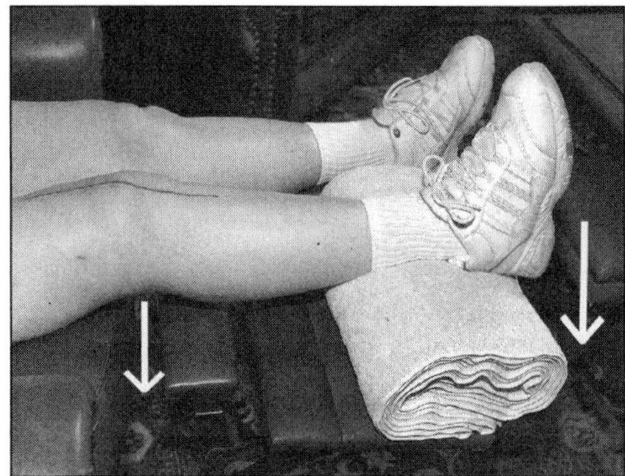

Figure 6.6b. TKA exercise in the recliner: hamstring pull and extension

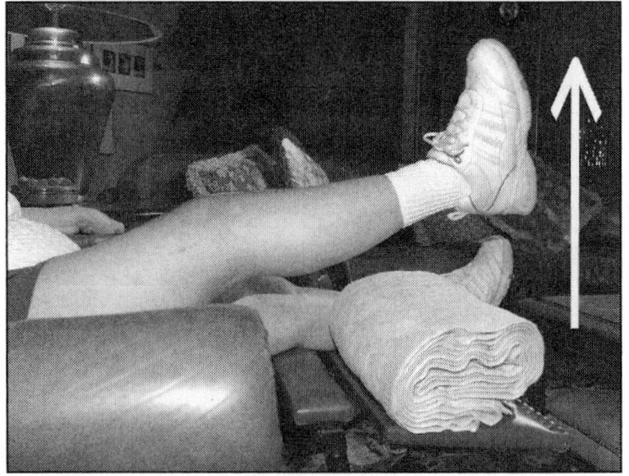

Figure 6.6c. TKA exercise in the recliner: straight-leg raise off pillow

Exercise 28

Active Knee Extension Using Book/Video

Lying on a couch or bed, straighten your total-knee leg as much as possible. Place a VHS videocassette or small book under your total knee. Push down with your entire leg against the video or book, and then have someone try to take the video or book out from under your knee (Figure 6.7). Repeat 10–25 times, several times per day. As you're able to straighten your new knee more, you will be able to hold the video or book in place against significant resistance. Once you've achieved that, try the exercise with a CD case. With a smaller object, more extension is required to secure the object under the knee. The video, book, or other object acts as a target to work toward as such an object helps to quantify how much extension has been gained.

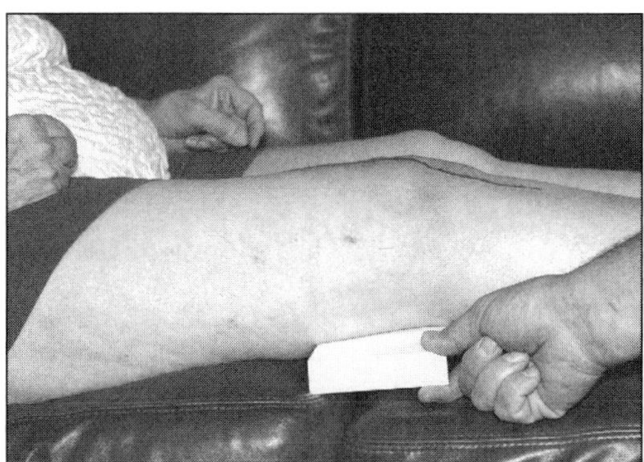

Figure 6.7. TKA extension exercise using "target" to increase extension

■ ■ ■

These simple self-range-of-motion exercises need to be done several times each day. Remember, the physical therapist is only going to see you for a limited number of treatment sessions. You need to move your knee whenever possible when the therapist is not there with you. The more you move your total knee on your own, the better the result will be!

Until you can totally straighten your new knee, you will be unable to walk "normally." Walking normally should be one of the goals of every patient who undergoes total knee replacement. Because of your arthritis pain you may not remember the last time you walked normally. We will spend a great deal of time in another chapter teaching you how to walk normally again.

Pain Control

One of the most important things to do for yourself in order to improve range of motion and function in your knee is to control the pain. Total knee replacement is a painful procedure, but then again, you have endured knee pain for many years. In fact, many patients report that compared to the pain they endured prior to surgery, they experience much less pain after surgery and throughout their rehabilitation. Your surgeon will give you a prescription for pain medications—be sure to take them! If you fail to take your pain medications, it will be very difficult to do the exercises to increase range of motion and return to your desired level of function.

There are numerous types of pain medications available. Most of the ones your surgeon will prescribe are classified as narcotics. See Chapter 4 for a discussion of pain medications commonly prescribed after TKA surgery. If the drug prescribed by your surgeon does not agree with you, or if you feel it is providing inadequate pain relief, call your surgeon to find an alternative medication. Many patients are hesitant to take pain medications because they are afraid of becoming dependent on or addicted to them. However, be aware that taking your pain medications will significantly help you gain motion and get your life back. As the pain subsides, take fewer pain medications. This minimizes the risk of addiction and side effects, which can include drowsiness, lethargy, nausea, and constipation. If severe constipation or nausea results from taking the narcotics, it may be helpful to use a laxative or antiemetic to counteract the symptoms.

The best way to minimize the side effects of narcotics is to use them sparingly. Get off the pain pills as soon as possible and make the transition to acetaminophen (Tylenol). Although any medication can cause problems, acetaminophen has fewer side effects and fewer interactions with other medications. One suggestion for transitioning off the narcotic medication is to use acetaminophen during the day, when pain is typically less severe, and reserve the narcotics for nighttime use, when stronger relief is usually needed. Eventually, the narcotic pain medication can be eliminated altogether.

Anticoagulant Medication

In all likelihood, your surgeon will send you home on some form of anticoagulant medication, as discussed in Chapter 4. The purpose of an anticoagulant is to thin the blood in order to reduce the risk of blood clots, which can be a problem after surgery.

Some of the symptoms of a blood clot include pain and swelling in the calf muscles, swelling in the thigh, and difficulty breathing. If you have any of these complaints, bring them to the attention of your surgeon immediately no matter what time of day or night it is!

The most common anticoagulation medications come in the form of a pill (Coumadin, aspirin) or as home-administered shots (Lovenox, Fragmin). For patients receiving the home-administered shots, the patient and/or family will be instructed in the administration of the shots prior to the patient leaving the hospital. If this is not possible, arrangements can be made for a home health nurse to administer the injections.

With Coumadin it is necessary to monitor the blood's "thinness" with periodic blood tests. At first these blood tests will usually take place daily, and then may reduce to two or three times per week. Their purpose is to ensure that the patient is taking a safe, therapeutic level of Coumadin. The blood test that is performed measures the prothrombin time/INR, and based on the test results, the dosage of Coumadin is adjusted. This is why it is critical that patients who are taking Coumadin do so every day and, preferably, at the same time each day.

The length of time that anticoagulation is needed may vary from two to six weeks. In some rare cases anticoagulant medication may not be used at all, depending on the surgeon's assessment of the patient's situation and medical status.

Restarting Your Regular Medications

If you take regular medications for blood-pressure control, diabetes, heart disease, and the like, they should have been restarted in the hospital and will continue at home. Before discharge, check with your surgeon and/or internist with regard to what medications should be continued, changed, or discontinued. The stress from surgery and the resultant change in activity levels may alter your previous dosage of regular medication. A prime example of this is insulin taken for diabetes. Many diabetic patients report that for several days after getting home, controlling their blood-sugar levels is difficult because of the change in their dietary habits and activity levels as well as the change in their body's metabolic demands as required for healing. Be sure to contact your primary-care physician if you have difficulty adjusting your regular medications.

Another concern about restarting your regular medications is the potential for interaction between regular medications and those prescribed after surgery (anticoagulants and narcotics). For example, patients with systemic arthritis may be on chronic nonsteroidal anti-inflammatory medications (NSAIDs). NSAIDs tend to thin the blood by inhibiting platelet function and should therefore not be taken in conjunction with anticoagulant medications. Narcotic medications can have an adverse effect on blood pressure. This may interfere with the required dose of regular blood-pressure medications needed to maintain adequate blood-pressure control. This is another reason to taper off the narcotics as quickly as possible.

The issue of drug interaction is a complex one. Each patient reacts to medications differently. Patients may be taking certain medications preoperatively, with new ones added following surgery. Complicating matters is that the patient has recently experienced significant stress from surgery, and there is usually a component of anemia due to intraoperative blood loss. The combination of these variables makes drug interactions quite unpredictable. Therefore, it is imperative that you contact your surgeon and internist with any questions about the medications you take.

Control of Swelling

Swelling, or *edema*, is a natural part of the healing process. Therefore, your new knee will be swollen for several weeks due to the surgery. However, too much knee swelling limits motion. It is very important to minimize swelling to gain maximum range of motion in your new knee. The following are several techniques you can use to assist in controlling swelling:

1. Using ice on your knee will significantly reduce the swelling and inflammation. The cold acts to limit active bleeding and the accumulation of fluid in the knee. Cold is probably the most effective way to reduce swelling. There are several ways to apply cold to your knee:
   - Use an ice bag (reclosable plastic bag) filled with ice cubes from the freezer. Wrap the bag in a towel.
   - Use a reusable ice pack, which can be purchased at any drugstore.
   - Use a bag of frozen vegetables, preferably peas or corn. Simply place the bag of vegetables in the freezer, and when it's frozen, place the bag on your knee. Once the vegetables thaw out, all you need to do is place the bag back in the freezer, and in less than an hour you can reuse the frozen vegetables. (A hint: Place the bag in a larger food-storage bag so the original bag does not rip.)

     Three bags are needed to keep a continuous supply of cold packs. As one is thawing out, another is freezing, and the third is ready for use.
2. Another excellent method to reduce swelling is to use the white antiembolic stockings that you probably received in the hospital, called *T.E.D. hose*. These stockings are designed to minimize fluid accumulation and to aid with fluid removal by assisting the muscles in pumping out the fluid. It is important that the stockings come up to mid-thigh, rather than the below-knee variety. The calf-high stocking often provides a tourniquet effect, which may actually produce more swelling. Because you are not walking or moving your legs as much as normal, there is a tendency for fluid to accumulate in your legs. Excessive swelling may predispose you to developing deep vein thrombosis (DVT, or a blood clot) in the lower leg. The stockings work to reduce swelling, and therefore they also lower the risk of blood clots.

   T.E.D. hose are very tight and difficult to put on, but they work well and are highly recommended until the swelling is resolved. It is normally easiest to put them on in the morning, after you have been in bed, when your leg will have the least amount of swelling. You may need help putting them on, and the nurses will show you in the hospital the easiest way to roll them over your toes and up your leg. Be sure to ask your surgeon how long to wear the stockings each day. Most surgeons want you to wear them all the time except while you're sleeping and bathing, and to wear them on both legs for at least the first few weeks.

3. Elevating your leg will assist gravity in controlling the swelling. You can elevate your leg by using pillows or by resting it on the arm of the couch. For this method to truly work, your leg needs to be higher than your heart. Sitting in a reclining chair with the legs extended will not be enough. The best suggestion is to spend at least one hour twice a day lying in bed or flat on the couch with a few pillows supporting your leg. This may seem simple, but it is very effective. In addition, believe it or not, rest is a very important and necessary part of your rehabilitation after total knee replacement. (More on the importance of rest appears below.)

Strengthening Exercises

At this point in your rehabilitation, the main goal is to gain as much range of motion as possible. However, it is also important to begin simple strengthening exercises now, because your legs will be very weak after the surgery. Until your leg muscles regain some of their strength, it will be difficult for you to walk, even with an assistive device such as a walker or crutches. In fact, some surgeons have their patients wear a leg brace for several weeks because the thigh muscles lack the strength to support the knee during walking.

Below are several simple strengthening exercises, a few of which also appear in earlier chapters. Some of them are done in bed, and some while standing up. We recommend standing at the kitchen sink to perform the standing exercises. That way you can hold on to the edge of the sink for stability.

Exercise 16

Quadriceps Sets

(also described in Chapter 5)

Lying in bed, tighten the muscles of your thigh by keeping your leg straight and pushing the back of your knee into the bed (Figure 6.8). Hold for 10–15 seconds, then relax your muscles. This exercise is very important for gaining the necessary strength to control your new knee during walking. It may seem simple, particularly if you practiced it prior to surgery as we recommend, but after your surgeon dissects through part of your thigh muscle to put in the prosthesis, performing it becomes much more difficult and painful. Practice quad sets at least 3 to 5 times per day, and each time do between 10 and 25 repetitions for each leg.

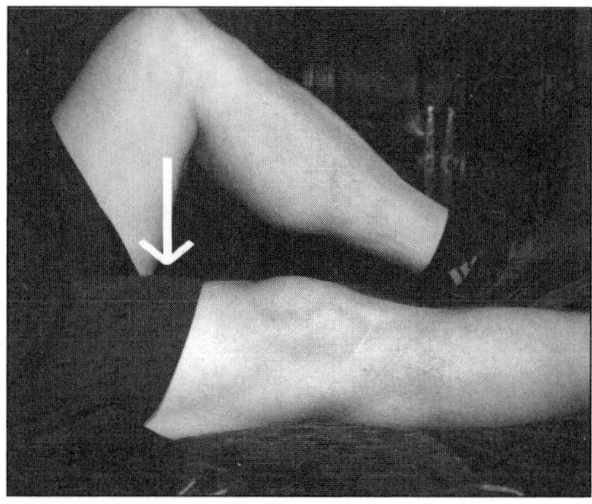

Figure 6.8. Quad set exercise lying in bed

Exercise 15

Gluteal Sets

(also described in Chapter 5)

Lying on your back, tighten the muscles in your buttocks, hold for 10–15 seconds, and then relax the muscles (Figure 6.9). Like the quad sets, glute sets are needed for walking after surgery. Practice them at least 3 to 5 times per day, and each time do between 10 and 25 repetitions.

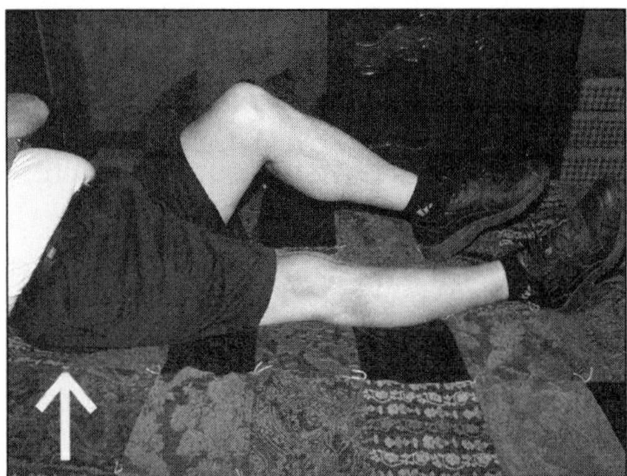

Figure 6.9. Gluteal set exercise lying in bed

Exercise 17

Hamstring Sets

(also described in Chapter 5)

Lying on your back, tighten the muscles behind your thigh (your hamstrings) by pressing your heel into the bed (Figure 6.10). Hold for 10–15 seconds and then relax. Perform this exercise at least 3 to 5 times per day, each time completing between 10 and 25 repetitions for each leg.

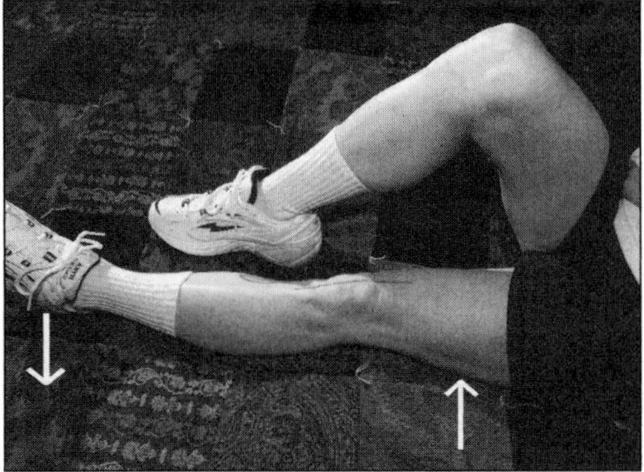

Figure 6.10. Hamstring set exercise lying in bed

Exercise 4

Straight-Leg Raise

(also described in Chapter 5)

Lying on your back and keeping your knee straight, tighten your quadriceps muscle and lift your foot 8 to 12 inches off the bed (Figure 6.11). This exercise is critical for controlling the movement of your leg. Straight-leg raises develop the muscles necessary for using stairs and for getting in and out of a chair, bed, car, etc.

Hopefully you were able to practice straight-leg raises before you left the hospital. If not, you really need to start working on developing the muscle strength and control to do them. Here's a trick that helps if you cannot perform a straight-leg raise: Do a quad set and, while holding the muscles tight, have someone else lift your foot 6 to 8 inches off the bed. Once your leg is lifted to this height, hold your leg there while your helper *slowly* lets go of your foot. *As we said earlier, be sure to tell your helper* not *to let go completely!* You will probably be unable to hold your leg in the air on your own, and if it comes crashing down onto the bed it will *really* hurt! As you get stronger, you will be able to hold your leg in the air with less and less support, and eventually you will be able to hold it there while your helper removes the support completely. Once that happens, slowly lower your leg to the bed, and then try to lift your leg while holding it straight. Most likely you will be able to get it back up to the 8- to 12-inch height.

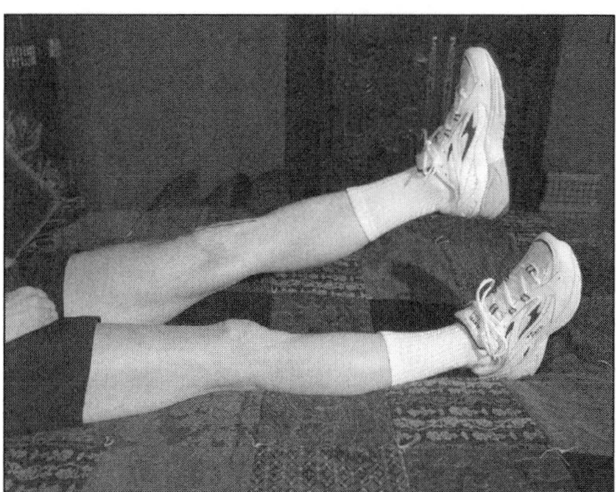

Figure 6.11. Straight-leg raise exercise lying in bed

Again, because the quadriceps muscle was divided during the surgical procedure, this exercise will be very painful; but once you master it, your level of function and movement will dramatically increase. It is common for the quadriceps muscle to shake after a few seconds of holding the straight-leg raise. This is normal and is due to the muscle's weakness. It may occur after only a few seconds or after a few contractions. Once you start shaking, stop and rest. Without rest you will be unable to continue doing this important exercise. Start with only 3–5 repetitions and, as you get stronger, progress to 15–30 repetitions several times a day.

Exercise 1

Short-Arc Quadriceps Exercise with One-Gallon Bucket

(also described in Chapter 5)

Lying on your back, with a one-gallon paint can lying on its side under your knee, tighten your thigh muscles and lift your foot off the bed (Figure 6.12). Hopefully, you were able to accomplish this exercise while in the hospital, but if not it is important to work on it during your first week at home to start gaining strength in your thigh muscles. Perform 3–5 sets of 10–15 repetitions each, several times per day.

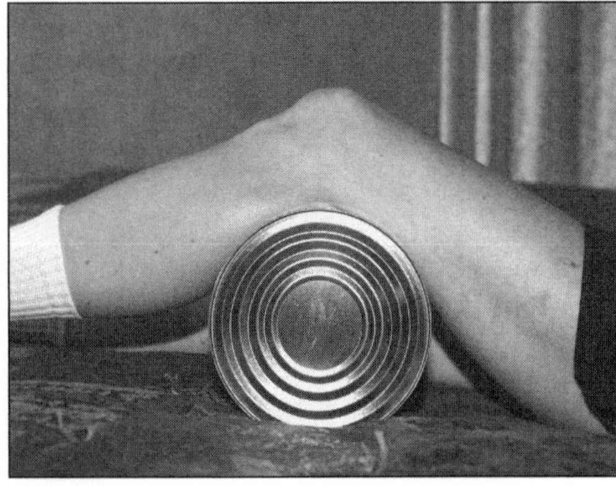

Figure 6.12. Short-arc quad exercise using one-gallon bucket

Exercise 29

Heel Raise Standing at Sink

Standing and facing the sink, hold on to the sink with both hands and rise up and down on your toes, lifting your heels off the ground (Figure 6.13). This exercise is designed to strengthen the calf muscles and to assist with pumping the fluid out of your lower leg. Perform 3–5 sets of 10–25 repetitions each, at least 3 to 5 times per day.

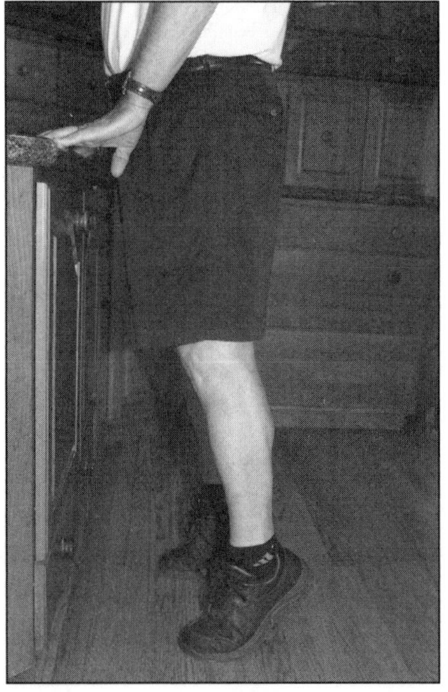

Figure 6.13. Heel-raise exercise at the sink

Exercise 30

Mini-Squat Standing at Sink

Standing and facing the sink, hold on with both hands and perform mini-squats (Figure 6.14). Go as low as you can while still being able to stand up fully straight afterward. You may only be able to lower yourself a few inches at first, and that's fine. This exercise is one of the best there is to increase your leg strength, and eventually you will be doing mini-squats to almost 45 degrees of knee flexion. Perform 3–5 sets of 10–25 repetitions each, at least 3 to 5 times per day.

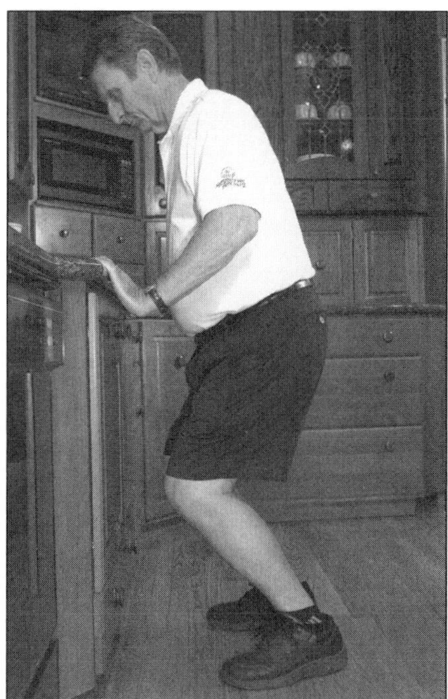

Figure 6.14. Mini-squat exercise at the sink

Exercise 31

Hip Abduction Standing at Sink

Standing and facing the sink, hold on with both hands. While standing on your non-operated leg, lift your operated leg out to the side as far as possible, and then return it to the starting position next to your non-operated leg (Figure 6.15). Keep the knees and toes of the leg you're lifting pointed mostly toward the front, rather than pointed outward away from the body. This exercise serves to get the entire leg moving, primarily the hip. Perform 3–5 sets of 10–25 repetitions each, at least 3 to 5 times per day.

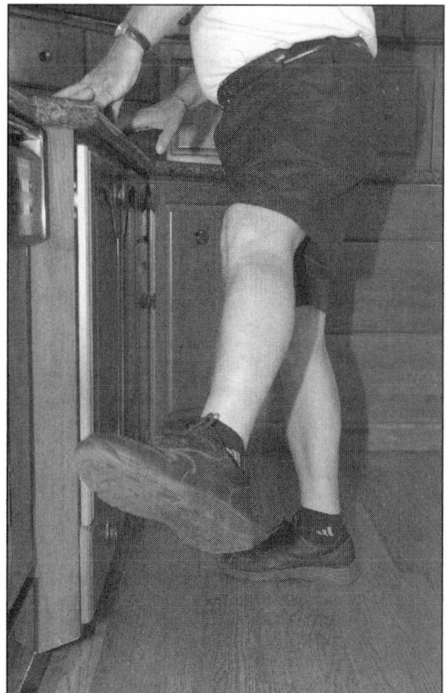

Figure 6.15. Hip-abduction exercise at the sink

Exercise 32

Marching in Place Standing at Sink

Standing and facing the sink, hold on with both hands and march in place. Try to lift your operated knee as high as possible while marching (Figure 6.16). Perform 3–5 sets of 20–50 repetitions each, at least 3 to 5 times per day.

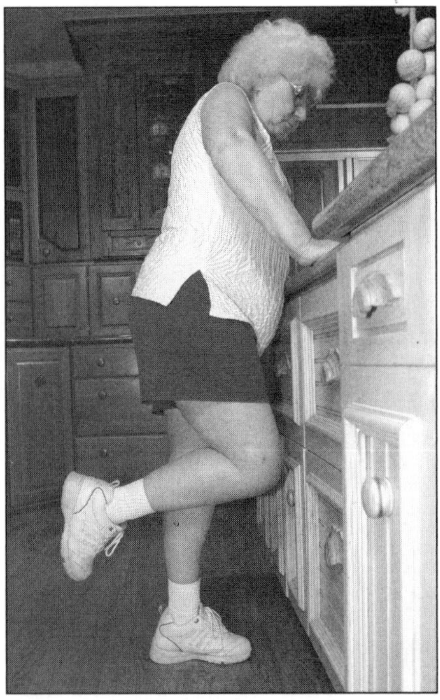

Figure 6.16. Marching in place at the sink

Exercise 33

Hip-Motion Exercise Standing at Sink

Stand next to the sink and hold on with one hand. While standing on the nonoperated leg, slowly swing the operated leg forward and then backward as far as possible (Figure 6.17). Be sure to swing the leg from the hip joint. This exercise develops the strength to do a straight-leg raise if you can't do one when you first get home from the hospital. Perform 3–5 sets of 10–25 repetitions each, at least 3 to 5 times per day.

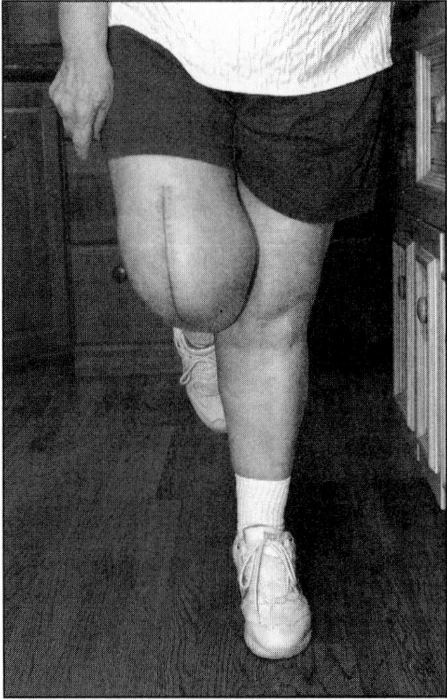

Figure 6.17. Hip flexion and extension exercise at the sink

■ ■ ■

The purpose of these exercises is to get you started on gaining strength in your leg. It is critical to do these exercises several times per day. As you progress in your rehabilitation, you will perform other strengthening exercises that are more rigorous; they are described in the next few chapters.

Getting Around at Home

Earlier in the book we discussed the pluses and minuses of using a walker versus crutches while rehabilitating from TKA surgery. Factors to consider include your home environment (specifically, whether or not you have stairs), your ability to put weight on the operated leg, how "good" your other knee is, and how safe you feel with the walker or crutches. Normally, within the first few weeks after surgery you will progress to using only one crutch, then to using a cane. Eventually you will discontinue the use of any assistive device. But in the beginning, use the device with which you feel most safe and secure.

Once you are confident and comfortable using a walker or crutches, start walking around your home as much as possible. Get up at least once every hour while you're awake, and walk for at least a few minutes. The more you walk now, the better your rehabilitation will be in the future. Be careful going from one type of floor surface to another, such as from carpet to tile or hardwood, as the friction under the walker or crutches will be different between the two. Be aware of objects on the floor such as shoes and newspapers, and try to have them moved out of the way so you have a clear path in which to practice walking. It will be difficult for you to carry food or drink while using your walker or crutches, so plan your meals accordingly.

If your surgeon allows full weight bearing on your total knee, put as much weight as possible on that leg while you are walking with the assistive device. The sooner you are able to put all your weight on the operated leg, the sooner you can reduce the amount of assistance needed while walking. At the same time, don't be in a big hurry to walk without an assistive device. Remember, it has only been a week since surgery, and once you have the confidence in your total knee to support all of your weight, only then are you ready to walk with less assistance.

Get Some Rest: Your New Knee Will Thank You

After total-knee-replacement surgery, rest is something that you will need—and want—more than you could ever imagine. This chapter has talked a great deal about range-of-motion exercises, strengthening exercises, and walking as much as possible. At the same time, however, your total knee will tell you when you need to rest. *Listen to your new knee!* Although exercise is critical to your rehabilitation, rest is just as important. If you don't rest when you need to, you and your rehabilitation program will suffer. Most health-care professionals have not gone through a total knee replacement. It is their job to help you receive the most from your rehabilitation program. But being too fatigued will prevent you from making the appropriate progress. Many patients who have undergone total knee replacements have told us they feel guilty for taking an afternoon off from their exercises. However, if they do so when it's needed, they find that the next day, after having rested and recovered, they actually do better with their rehabilitation.

Do not be afraid to take a day off during your rehabilitation. It has been Dr. Falkel's personal and professional experience that sometimes patients are too exhausted to perform their exercises effectively. The art of physical therapy searches for a balance between the right amount of exercise to increase strength and motion, and the right amount of rest. Achieving this balance will result in the optimal outcome.

■ ■ ■

It's been a long week, but the light at the end of the tunnel is no longer an oncoming train! Keep working at gaining range of motion in both flexion and extension, but also listen to your body and rest when you need to. Next week, we will build upon the exercises and activities you've been practicing so far. And just wait until you feel how good it is to get those staples or stitches out!

? Common Questions and Some Answers

Why is my knee so stiff when I try to bend it?

Your knee is swollen because of the blood and joint fluid that have accumulated from surgery. The soft tissue wall of the knee joint is also swollen because of the surgery. The fluid and swollen soft tissue occupy space in and around the knee and impede normal joint motion. Furthermore, surgical pain is a natural inhibitor to joint motion. The knee joint requires the quadriceps and hamstring muscles to work normally in order to provide joint motion. The quadriceps have been insulted during the surgical exposure of the knee. The large amount of blood in the knee joint and the swelling of the knee joint impair the function of the quadriceps and hamstring muscles, resulting in stiffness and lack of free mobility in the TKA. In addition, both the quadriceps and the hamstring muscle groups are weak due to a lack of normal use for years prior to surgery, and until they regain more of their normal strength, their function will be affected.

Why is there pain above my kneecap (patella)?

As part of the surgical procedure, the quadriceps tendon, located just above the kneecap, is divided longitudinally (lengthwise) in order to gain access to the knee joint. Because it has been cut, it is painful postoperatively. The quadriceps tendon and muscle receive the most stress during walking and knee-flexion exercises. The stress from these activities on the repaired tendon and muscle results in a significant amount of pain. This is normal and will subside over the next few weeks.

Why is there pain along the sides of my knee?

There are two reasons for this pain: First, the bones are cut to accommodate the components of your new, prosthetic knee. Second, the collateral ligaments (located on each side of the knee) are stretched to help the surgeon gain access to the knee joint during surgery. It is the combination of these two factors that typically is responsible for pain on the sides of the knee joint.

Where is my kneecap?

It is still right where it is supposed to be. However, because of the swelling in and around your knee, it may be difficult to see or feel it.

Why won't my knee bend as much as I want it to?

In addition to the stiffness and swelling in and around your knee, discussed in question 1 above, your quadriceps and hamstring muscles are currently much weaker than normal. This combination results in limited motion of the total knee.

When will I be able to straighten my knee completely?

The time that it takes to reach full extension after TKA surgery varies for each patient. It is dependent on pain, swelling, strength, and preoperative deformity of the knee. If the patient was unable to fully extend the knee before surgery, that means the joint capsule behind the knee has been contracted for years. Surgery causes the capsule to temporarily contract even more and will further delay full extension of the total knee.

Why can't I sleep at night?

There are several reasons for postoperative insomnia. The most significant is pain, which is always worse at night. As we fatigue throughout the course of the day, our defenses to combat pain are diminished. In addition, because of the amount of time spent resting during the day in the period shortly after surgery, less energy is expended, resulting in a lower-than-normal sleep requirement at night. Another factor is the lack of noise and distractions at night, which magnifies pain. During the day, life's distractions can draw the patient's focus away from the knee pain. One option would be to use some form of background noise from the radio or TV to act as a distraction while you're sleeping. Taking pain or sleep medications before bedtime can also be helpful.

When should I see my primary-care doctor?

If you have no preexisting medical problems, you should see your primary-care doctor on your regular schedule; there is no need to make a special appointment following knee replacement. However, if you have a preexisting medical condition, such as diabetes, hypertension, or pulmonary or cardiac disease, we advise you to contact your primary-care physician soon after your return home to discuss any alterations in your medication. If you are having any specific medical problems, contact your primary-care physician immediately.

When should I resume taking my normal medications?

Most patients resume their normal medications while in the hospital. If this isn't the case for you, be sure to contact your primary-care physician as soon as you get home to reestablish your medication regime. It is common following TKA surgery for diabetic patents who have not maintained their normal calorie intake to be required to adjust their insulin dosage.

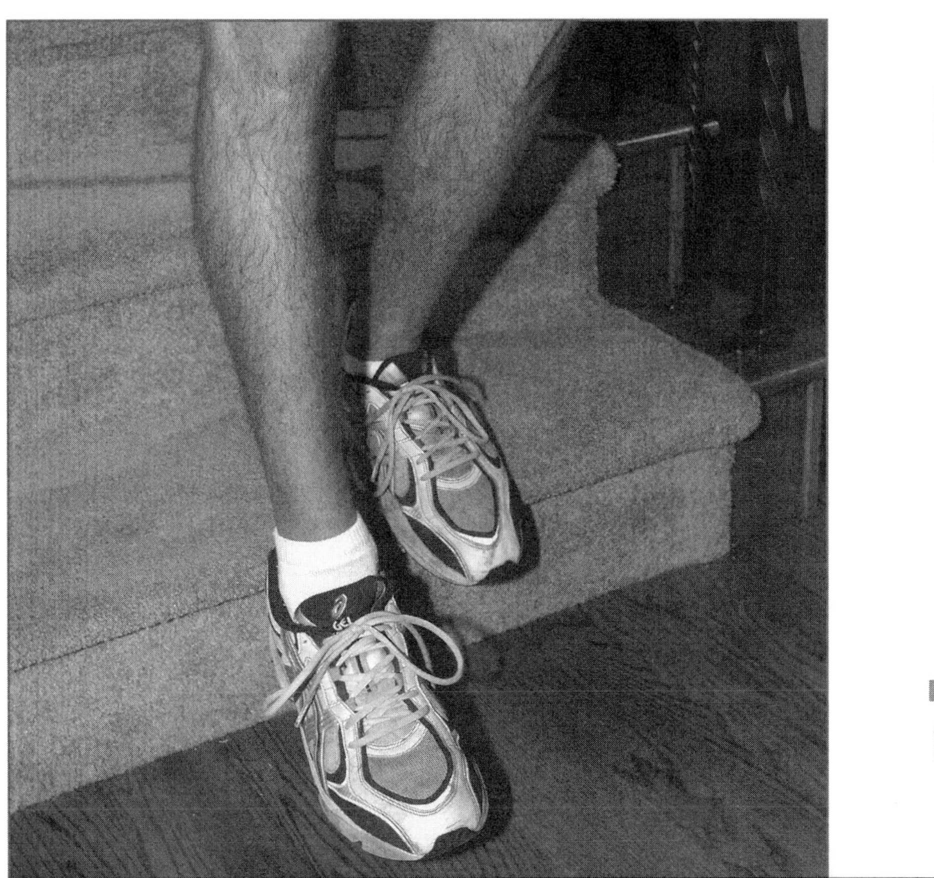

Chapter 7

Week Two

Will I Ever Be Normal Again?

Believe it or not, the first week at home is the toughest. Most of our patients admit that during week two they begin to second-guess their decision to have TKA surgery. Their knees are swollen and don't bend as easily or as much as anticipated, they have a hard time sleeping, and they still have pain, albeit a different type of pain than the arthritis pain. During these early days, the majority of patients tend to have difficulty concentrating on anything but their new knee. These are all normal responses! In this chapter we will cover these topics and also present the next steps in your rehabilitation exercise program.

Follow-Up Visit to Your Surgeon

If you have not done so already, make an appointment with your surgeon for some time this week to have the staples or sutures removed (if necessary) from your incision. If you have a subcuticular stitch that does not require removal, an appointment is still needed for an incision check. This first follow-up visit with your surgeon is scheduled for approximately two weeks postoperatively and can be made prior to your discharge from the hospital. If you do not have a scheduled appointment upon your arrival at home, call the surgeon's office after you've been home about one week and tell them you need to have your staples or sutures removed this week. The removal of the staples is a *relatively* painless procedure (remember, you have just had your knee replaced, so pain becomes "relative"). Dr. Falkel had pain as a "relative" for way too many years. The discomfort of the entire total-knee procedure was just that, a discomfort, compared to the pain he had endured from his degenerative joint disease.

The staples or sutures will probably be removed by a nurse or a surgeon's assistant. To remove the staples they will use a small "staple remover" that may pinch slightly while the staple is being extracted. (Dr. Falkel had sixty-eight staples in his two incisions and only felt the removal of one!) To remove sutures they use a special pair of scissors to cut the suture material and then pull the suture out with a forceps (tweezers). After the staples or sutures are removed, the nurse or assistant will put Steri-Strips over the incision to aid in healing by adding support to the skin. Once the staples or sutures are removed, it is much easier to take a shower because you can get the Steri-Strips wet without worrying about infection or about getting the towel caught on the staples. Steri-Strips are small pieces of sterile tape with a fiber running through them that help keep the skin closed with reduced tension. Steri-Strips are typically used to close the small incisions after a knee arthroscopy. With repeated showering and changing of clothes, the Steri-Strips will start to roll up at the edges and will eventually fall off on their own. As they begin to roll up, trim the edges back until the Steri-Strip comes off all together.

After all the Steri-Strips are gone, you will begin scar management. We will start that discussion in the next section of this chapter. *However, do not take a bath or soak in a hot tub or whirlpool until all the Steri-Strips have come off on their own and there are no scabs anywhere on the incision.* If you soak your new knee in the water for a prolonged length of time, as you would in a bath, there is a chance of infection if some of the water seeps into the incision through a small opening. We tell all our patients to wait at least three or four weeks after surgery before taking a bath or using a hot tub/whirlpool for aquatic exercise to be sure that the incision is sealed completely and there is no risk of infection.

While you're at the surgeon's office, he or she may take an X ray of your knee to see how everything looks. Some surgeons will wait for the six-week postoperative appointment to take the first X ray of your new knee. Another important task during the first visit to the surgeon's office is to get a temporary handicapped-parking permit. These permits normally last for three months and allow parking in designated handicapped spaces. Although walking will be a significant part of your rehab, there may be times when it is best to be able to park close to your destination. When calling for your first postoperative appointment, ask if the surgeon has the appropriate motor vehicle department forms for a temporary handicapped permit. If they do not, have a family member or friend go to the local motor vehicle department and get the required forms to take to the surgeon's office. After the forms are completed by the surgeon or his/her staff, take them back to the motor vehicle department where they will issue you a temporary handicapped-parking card to hang from your rearview mirror when you're parked in a designated handicapped-parking space. It may be easier to perform this job preoperatively, while you are relatively more mobile. Some patients may require a permanent handicapped permit or license plate; however, this decision can be made at any time in the future.

Scar Management

Having the staples or sutures removed is such a relief! Now is the time to start caring for the scar to improve its healing and cosmetic appearance. As discussed above, do not soak your incision in a bath or hot tub/whirlpool for at least three to four weeks after surgery. There is a higher risk of infection when the incision is immersed in water for prolonged periods, especially if the staples or sutures have just recently been removed. By week three or four postoperatively, it will be safe to take baths or to start aquatic therapy to gain range of motion and strength. But for now, be happy to take a shower without the hassle of covering up the staples!

Once the Steri-Strips start falling off, you will be able to get a good look at the incision. If there are any open areas or scabs, keep them dry and avoid using any lotions near them. However, once the scabbing is gone, the open areas become sealed, and the Steri-Strips fall off, you need to start working on scar management. The first component of scar management is performing a massage in small circular motions over the scar. The scar tissue that results after surgery is tough, hard, and adherent to the surrounding tissues. It needs to be loosened and molded into a more normal type of tissue. This can be accomplished by performing small circular massages along the incision line (Figure 7.1). Use your thumb to make small circles about the size of a quarter all along the incision. Change the direction of rotation frequently. Do about 10–15 revolutions in each area, and then move about an inch along the scar and repeat 10–15 revolutions.

Some patients use hand lotion, vitamin E lotion, or cocoa butter on the scar. There are no hard data to support or refute the use of lotion for management of the scar. Some health-care professionals tout the benefits. Regardless of how creams or lotions may affect the appearance of the scar, they certainly reduce the skin irritation caused by friction during massage. Although there may be differing opinions concerning the efficacy of using creams and/or lotions on your scar, there is a minimal downside to their use. The use of lotions or creams is strictly a patient's choice.

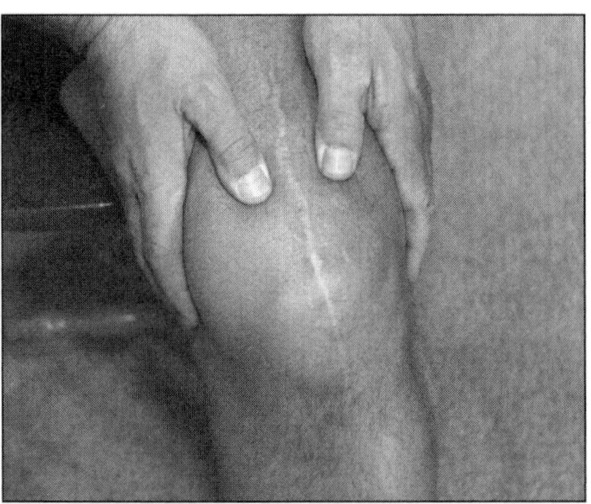

Figure 7.1. Scar-tissue massage along TKA incision

Getting In and Out of the Car

You have already successfully ventured in and out of the car to get home from the hospital, but that trip may have been in a friend's or relative's car. It is time for you to learn to get in and out of your own car. For most patients who have a car with four doors, it is easiest to get in and out of the backseat, particularly if you can extend your leg across the backseat of the car. In this position, your knee is supported by the seat cushion and you are not required to bend the knee to sit comfortably. (Some people still like to place their knee on a pillow to absorb the bumps in the road.)

In a car with only two doors, you will have to get into the front passenger's seat for your trip to the surgeon's office. Here are a few tricks to make getting in and out of a two-door car easier:

1. Have someone (the chauffeur) drive the car to where there are no obstructions

(e.g., no garage walls, bicycles, lawn mowers, etc.) to get in your way.

2. Move the passenger seat back as far as it will go and, if possible, slightly recline the back of the seat to create more room to get into the car.
3. Open the passenger door all the way and have the window rolled down, providing several places to hold onto while getting into the car.
4. Walk up to the space between the door and the car with your crutches or walker, and turn around so your buttocks are facing the car seat.
5. Give your crutches or walker to the driver and, while holding onto the door and the car frame, slowly lower yourself onto the seat of the car.
6. Bend the TKA as much as possible, slide your buttocks as far back into the passenger seat as you can (toward the center of the vehicle), and grab under your knee to help pull the TKA leg into the car. You may need assistance from the driver to get your leg into the car. Try to do it yourself; after all, it is your new knee, and you need to learn how to move it.
7. Once in the car, adjust the seat for comfort, but if you are going to be driving any longer than five or ten minutes, you will probably be most comfortable with the seat as far back as possible so your TKA knee has as much room as possible.
8. At your destination, have the driver park in a handicapped space (temporarily if you do not yet have a handicapped-parking card). Because these spaces are larger, they make it easier to open the car door as wide as possible.
9. Getting out of the car is essentially the reverse of getting in. Slide your buttocks toward the center of the vehicle and grab under the TKA leg to help lift it out of the car. Before you attempt to stand up, be sure the driver has brought your crutches or walker around for support.
10. Once standing, use the crutches or walker to carefully walk away from the car door. Ask the driver to hold the car door open while you stand up and until you have safely walked away from the car in order to prevent the door from accidentally closing on you.

This all seems so simple—until you try it! Even though you have gotten in and out of a car your whole life, doing it with a new TKA is a different experience. You will be amazed how exhausting this simple task can be. When Dr. Falkel went to the surgeon's office for his staples to be removed, he walked approximately two hundred feet with his walker and then went directly home from the office. The whole outing lasted approximately one hour, yet afterward he was completely drained. Once home he slept for twenty-six hours straight without moving! Don't worry—this happens to every TKA patient, and in just a few days even that will get better.

Walking and Endurance Training

During week two, one of the things almost every patient notices is how quickly they fatigue while walking only very short distances. It is shocking how soon after surgery you seemingly lose all endurance and stamina. A loss of endurance and stamina occurs in almost every patient to some degree. Just as it is important to gradually progress with range-of-motion and strengthening exercises, the same is true for walking and regaining endurance. By the end of week two you should be comfortable and confident using crutches or a walker around the house. Now it is time to start walking longer distances outside. If the weather is good and there is no snow on the sidewalks around your home, start by walking for two to three minutes in one direction from your home and then back. As you feel your stamina increase, add a minute or so each way from the starting point of your home. Increasing your walk in small increments reduces the risk of getting "stranded" away from home. Some patients have a lawn chair placed at the end of their driveway to use as a rest station if needed. The key is to gradually increase the distance and time that you walk on a daily basis, rather than all at once.

During the first postoperative visit to the surgeon's office you should ask when you can progress from a walker to crutches or from crutches to a cane. Once the surgeon approves this progression, try to use less assistance while walking around in the house. Get comfortable with the new device inside the house before trying it outside on your endurance walks. We will discuss this progression in the next chapter.

Stairs: No Longer the Enemy!

For most patients with degenerative knee disease, climbing up and down stairs causes as much, if not more, pain than any other type of activity. Prior to surgery Dr. Falkel would only go downstairs once a day (to go to work) and would only go upstairs once a day (to go to bed). If he forgot something, it stayed upstairs until the next day! Beginning in week two, we recommend starting a series of exercises that will dramatically improve your strength and functional mobility for using stairs again like a "normal" person.

In the hospital, the therapist demonstrated how to go up and down stairs. When going up, lift the nonoperated leg up to the step first, and then lift the TKA leg up to the same step. Conversely, when going downstairs, the TKA leg goes down first, followed by the nonoperated leg. A simple saying can help you remember which leg goes first: "The good go up and the bad go down." The reason for this technique is to allow you to control your body weight with the nonoperated leg. When going upstairs, you need to lift your body weight with the nonoperated leg because the TKA leg is too weak. When going downstairs, you need to control your body weight against the force of gravity; thus, the nonoperated leg lowers your body weight onto the TKA leg. Don't worry about memorizing this technique—your body will only be able to go up and down stairs "correctly," because it is physically impossible at this stage to go up or down stairs the wrong way.

"Normal" people, of course, do not go up and down stairs this way; they simply go up and down one foot after the other on each successive step. The following exercises will prepare you to go up and down stairs like "normal" people do:

Exercise 34

Lifting Body Weight Up Stairs

Stand facing the stairs and place your TKA leg up on the first step. Hold on to the banister, and try to lift your body weight by using the muscles of the TKA leg to bring the nonoperated foot up to the first step (Figure 7.2). If you can do this, lower the nonoperated leg back down to the floor, and then complete 3–5 sets of 10–15 repetitions each, several times per day.

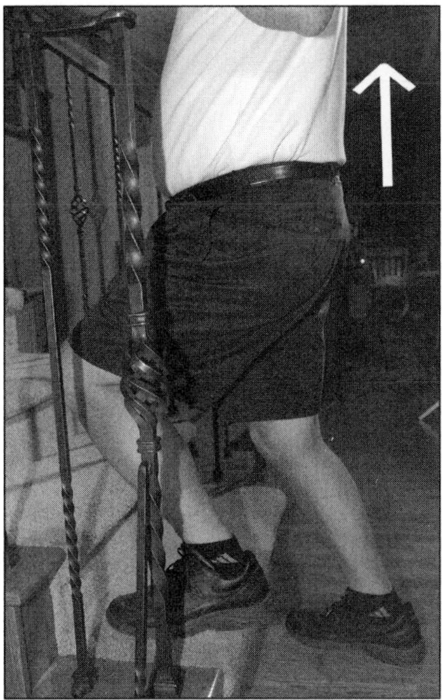

Figure 7.2. Stair strengthening exercise using TKA leg to lift body weight

Exercise 35

Lowering Body Weight Down Stairs

Stand on the first step and slowly and carefully turn around so you are facing downstairs. Hold on to the banister, keeping the foot of your TKA leg on the stair. Slowly try to lower your nonoperated foot off the stair and down toward the floor (Figure 7.3). This may be very difficult and painful, so don't become discouraged. If you can't do the exercise this week, you should be able to do it in week three. Repeat 3–5 sets of 10–15 repetitions each, several times per day.

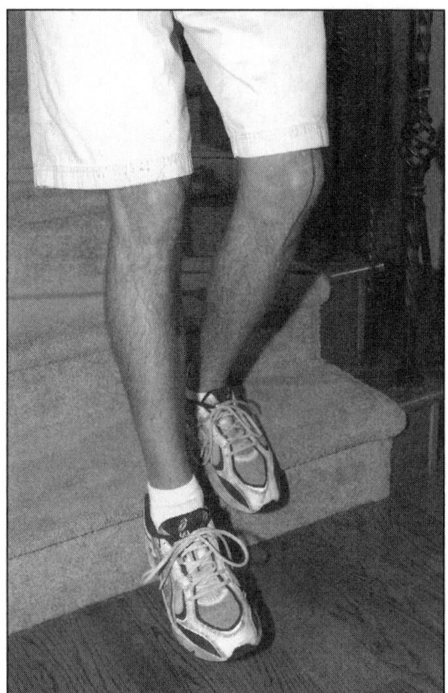

Figure 7.3. Stair strengthening exercise using TKA leg to lower body weight

■ ■ ■

The exercises described in this chapter will take a great deal of your time. However, it is time well spent. By the end of week two, you will notice a phenomenal improvement in your knee's motion, strength, and endurance. Your friends and family will be amazed at your improvement! You should be very proud of yourself for all your effort and hard work.

Home Physical Therapy

If you are receiving home physical therapy during week two, it may be the last week that your insurance coverage pays for a physical therapist to come to your home. Most insurance plans authorize six to ten home physical-therapy visits and then require patients to go to an outpatient rehabilitation facility or continue their total-knee rehabilitation on their own. If a physical therapist is coming to your home, she or he will continue to work on gaining range of motion in your TKA leg. The PT may have you place an ice bag on your knee prior to her or his arrival. The ice is used to control the swelling and is also useful prior to exercise because it has a mild anesthetic effect, numbing the knee before movement and/or exercise. Some patients have a poor tolerance of ice on their TKA and prefer using heat to "loosen" their knee prior to exercise. The use of ice or heat prior to exercise is determined solely by patient preference. After the home PT session is over, it is a good idea to place an ice bag on your knee for twenty to thirty minutes to assist with swelling control. In addition to range-of-motion and mobilization exercises, during week two the home PT will work on strengthening exercises. At the end of this chapter we will describe a variety of strengthening exercises that you may want to share with your home PT.

Home CPM Machine

If you have a CPM machine for home use, your insurance benefits will probably only cover the cost of its rental for two to three weeks following surgery. Ideally you are now able to achieve at least ninety degrees of knee flexion and close to full extension (zero degrees) using the machine. Once you consistently reach this range of passive motion on the machine, you should be able to attain a similar degree of active knee flexion and extension on your own, doing the exercises described in Chapter 6 and later in this chapter. And once you achieve ninety to one hundred degrees of knee flexion and close to zero degrees of knee extension on your own, you no longer need the CPM machine.

Taking Charge of Your Own Rehabilitation

As we have emphasized throughout this book, the person who has the ultimate responsibility for gaining motion, strength, and functional ability in your new TKA is *you*. While it can be helpful to have a home physical therapist or the use of a CPM machine, you need to take charge of your own recovery and rehabilitation. *We strongly encourage you to take charge of your own recovery and rehabilitation, and we strive to empower you to do so!* That is why we present exercises in nearly all of the chapters in this book. Following the regimen we have outlined will allow you to gain as much motion, strength, and function as possible in your new knee.

Range-of-Motion Exercises

Continue with the range-of-motion exercises described in Chapter 6. As you gain more range of motion in your knee, try adding the following exercises to your routine:

Exercise 23

Using Block in Front of TKA Foot

(also described in Chapter 6)

Sitting in a chair, bend your new knee as much as possible. Have someone block your foot from sliding forward (or you can block your foot against an immovable object such as a wall), and then slide your bottom forward on the chair, causing your TKA to bend more (Figure 7.4). Hold the stretch for 60–90 seconds; repeat 10–15 times.

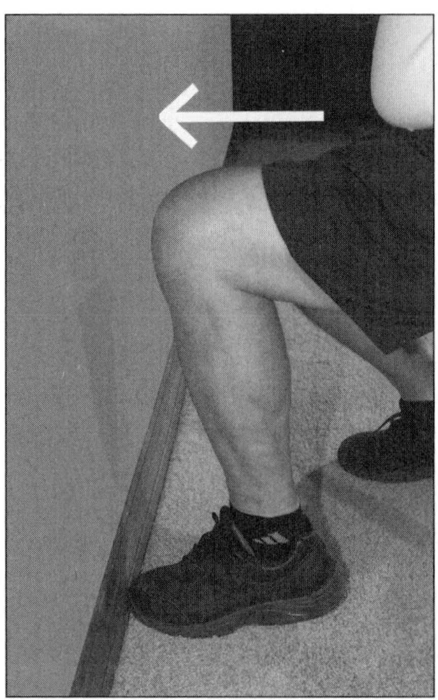

Figure 7.4. Range-of-motion exercise using chair and wall to block TKA foot

Exercise 36

Sitting Using Chair and Wall to Block TKA Foot

Place the back of a chair, preferably one with arms, against a wall, counter, or some other immovable object. Place your heels against the front legs of the chair. Slowly try to sit down, keeping your heels against the legs of the chair. If you cannot lower yourself all the way to the seat, reach back and hold on to the arms of the chair (Figure 7.5), and stay in this position for 60–90 seconds. Repeat 10–15 times.

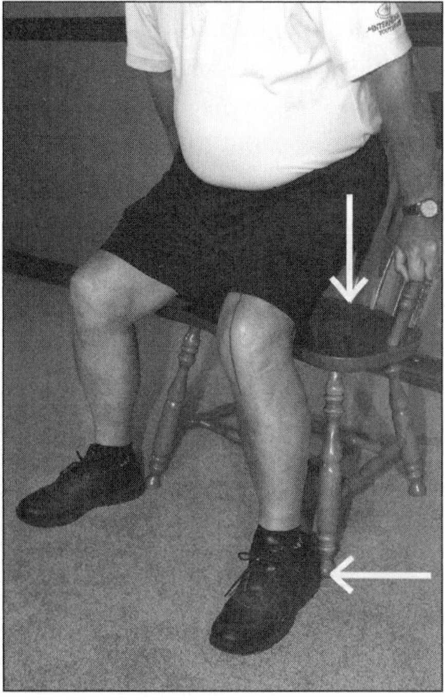

Figure 7.5. Range-of-motion exercise lowering body weight into chair without moving TKA foot away from leg of chair

Exercise 37

Flexing and Extending Using Rocking Chair

Sit in a rocking chair (if you have one), and rock back and forth to flex and extend the TKA knee (Figure 7.6). Try rocking for 25 to 50 repetitions, and progress to rocking back and forth for up to 30 minutes at a time.

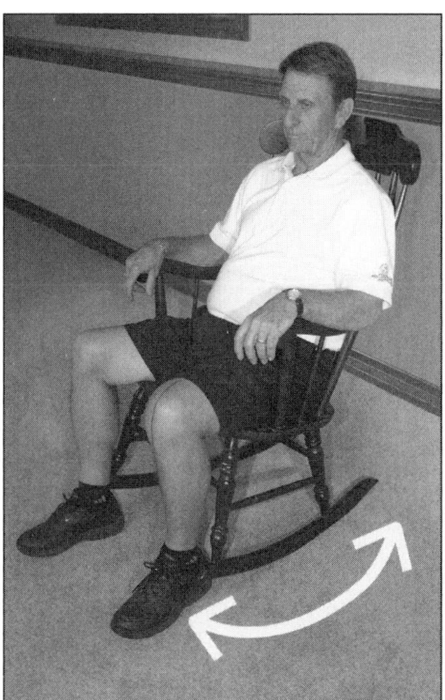

Figure 7.6. Using a rocking chair to gain range of motion in TKA knee

Exercise 38

Using Stair Step for Knee Flexion

For this exercise, use a single step or the bottom step of a staircase, preferably one that has something you can hold on to (such as a banister) so that you do not need to use your crutches or walker for support. Place the foot of your total-knee leg on the step. Keep your other leg straight, and lean forward with your whole body so that your total knee bends more as you move forward (Figure 7.7). Lean forward until you feel a good stretch, hold for 2–5 seconds, and then lean back to relieve the stretch. Repeat 15–25 times.

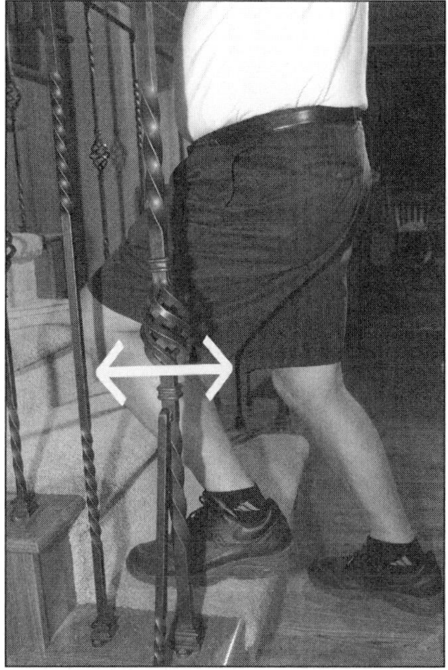

Figure 7.7. Range-of-motion exercise using stair step to rock TKA knee forward and backward

Exercise 39

Using Stair Step and Lowering Hips for Knee Flexion

Place the foot of your total-knee leg on the first step of the stairs (or the second step, if possible). As in Exercise 38, lean forward with your whole body so that your total knee bends more as you move forward. When you reach a point where you feel the stretch but it's tolerable, lower your hips by bending your nonoperated leg (Figure 7.8). This will achieve even more flexion in your total knee. Hold the stretch for 15–30 seconds, and then stand up straight to rest. Repeat 10–15 times.

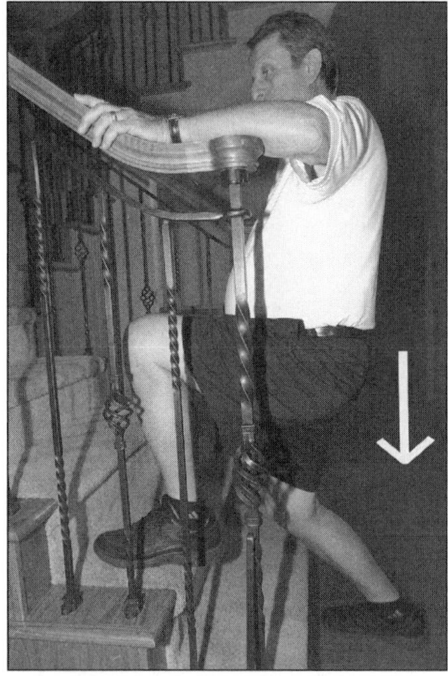

Figure 7.8. Range-of-motion exercise using stair step and lowering hips to get more flexion in TKA knee

Exercise 40

Hamstring Stretch on Stairs

Standing in front of a step or staircase, place the heel of your operated leg on the step or bottom stair. Keep your toes pointing up toward the ceiling. Lean forward slightly at the waist (Figure 7.9a), and then try to straighten your total knee (Figure 7.9b). You will feel a stretch in your hamstring muscle, behind your knee joint and thigh. This muscle gets very tight in most patients with degenerative knee disease, particularly if they had difficulty straightening the knee before surgery. In order to get full extension of your total knee, the hamstring muscle must be stretched and trained to relax while you are attempting to straighten or extend the knee. Hold the stretch for 15–30 seconds, and then stand up straight. Repeat 15–25 times.

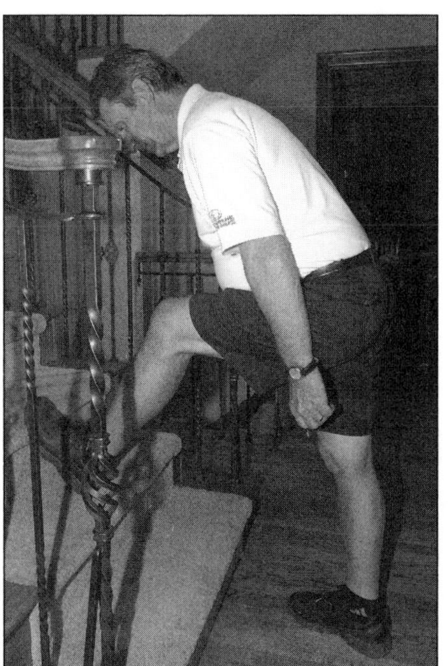

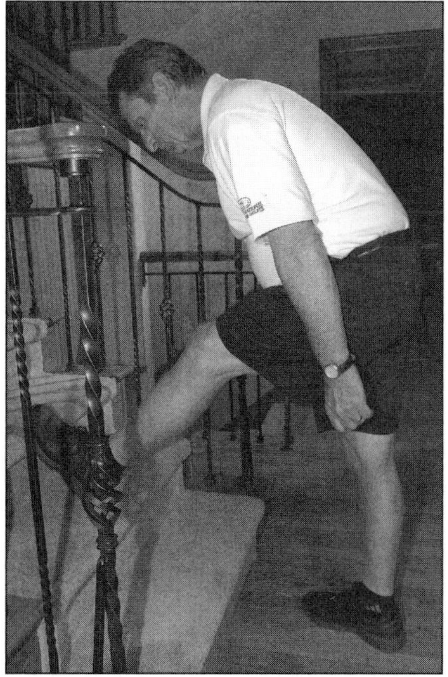

Figure 7.9a/b. Hamstring stretching exercise using stair step

Exercise 41

Hamstring Stretch Variation

After you get proficient at Exercise 40, try this modification. Rather than having your toes pointing up toward the ceiling, roll your leg all the way to the left, and repeat the exercise by bending forward slightly at the waist and then trying to straighten your total knee (Figure 7.10a). Hold for 15–30 seconds, and repeat 15–25 times. Then roll your leg all the way to the right, and repeat (Figure 7.10b). You will feel the stretch in different places in your hamstrings. The hamstring muscle is composed of three separate muscle groups, and these modifications, along with Exercise 40, will stretch all three muscles.

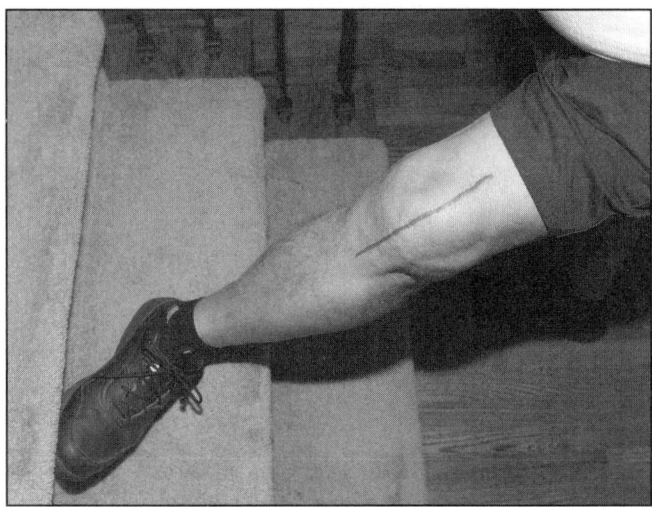

Figure 7.10a/b. Modification of hamstring stretching exercise to stretch all three hamstring muscles

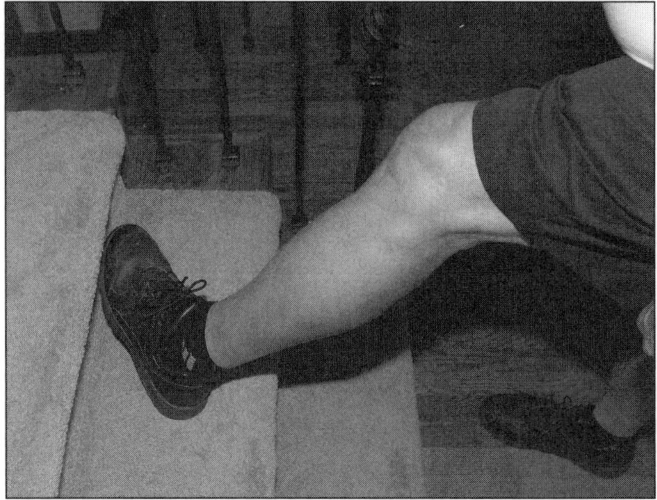

Exercise 42

Using Five-Gallon Bucket for Knee Flexion

Get out the five-gallon bucket you obtained prior to surgery. Lying on your back or sitting up with your back propped against some cushions, lift your total-knee leg as high as you can, and use your hands to roll the bucket as close to your buttocks as possible. Then slowly lower the back of your thigh onto the bucket, at the same time letting your knee bend as much as possible (Figure 7.11). Hold the stretch for as long as you can. When you can't take the stretch any longer, straighten your knee or simply lift your leg up with your hands. Do this exercise for up to 30 minutes, at least three times per day. One suggestion is to do it while watching TV in order to take your mind off the stretch in your knee.

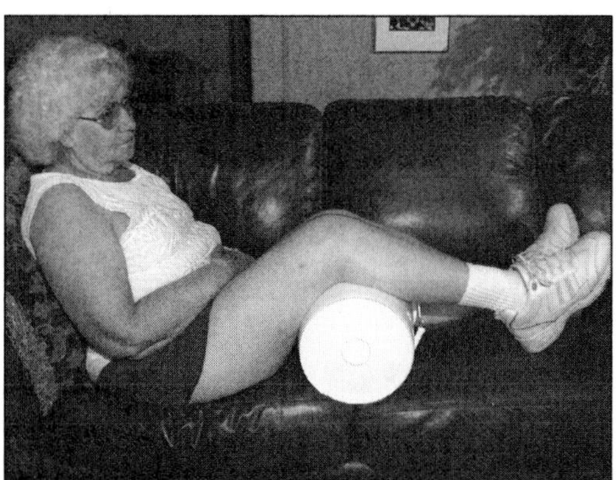

Figure 7.11. Range-of-motion flexion exercise using five-gallon bucket

Exercise 3

Hamstring Isometric Exercise with Five-Gallon Bucket

(Also Described in Chapter 3)

Lying on your back or sitting up with your back propped against some cushions, place the five-gallon bucket under the heel of your total-knee leg. Slowly straighten your total knee, allowing gravity to stretch and improve the extension in your total knee (Figure 7.12). Hold this position for as long as possible, and repeat several times per day.

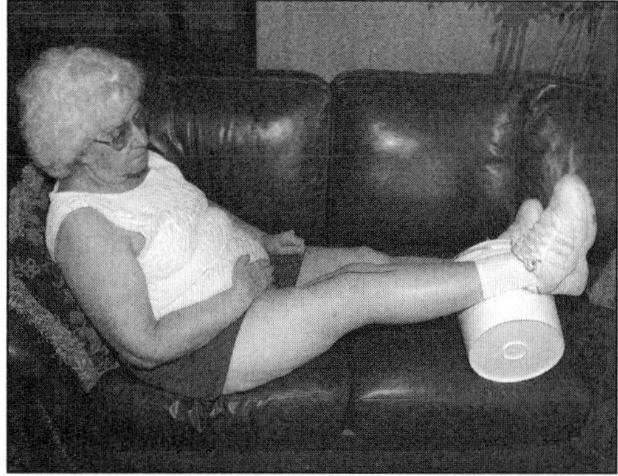

Figure 7.12. Range-of-motion extension exercise using five-gallon bucket

Exercise 43

Using Five-Gallon Bucket for Knee Extension

Here's one final exercise with the five-gallon bucket. With the bucket under your heel as in Exercise 3, try to roll the bucket towards your bottom with your heel, forcing your hamstring muscles to bend your total knee more with each roll of the bucket (Figure 7.13). After getting the bucket all the way to your buttocks, hold the position for 15–30 seconds, then lift your leg and use your hands to replace the bucket at your heel. Repeat the exercise. Take your time rolling the bucket, holding the stretch for as long as you can before trying to roll it farther. If the stretch becomes too intense, simply roll the bucket back toward your heel slightly, rest, and then try again. Repeat this exercise several times a day.

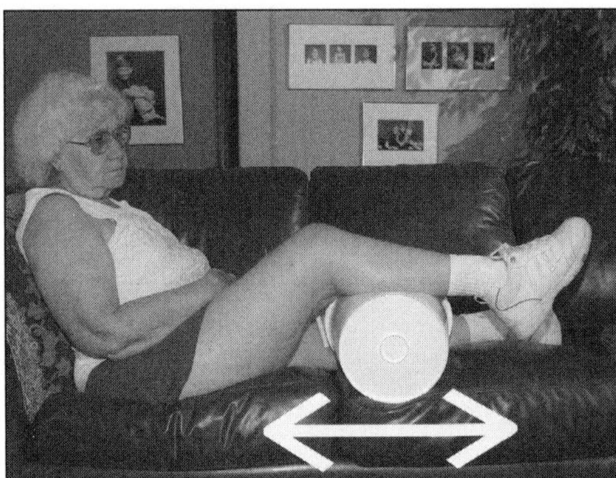

Figure 7.13. Range-of-motion exercise rolling five-gallon bucket for flexion and extension of the TKA knee

Home Strengthening Exercises

In the last chapter we outlined strengthening exercises to perform while lying in bed and standing at the sink. The following are additional strengthening exercises. They will not only help you gain strength in your total-knee leg, but will also facilitate more dynamic motion of your new TKA.

Exercise 44

Single-Leg Balance Exercise at Sink

Stand facing the sink and hold on to it for support. If possible, put full weight on your total-knee leg and try to lift your other foot off the ground, holding it in the air for 10–25 seconds (Figure 7.14). This exercise will enable you to begin walking again in a few weeks without any assistive device. Repeat 15–25 times.

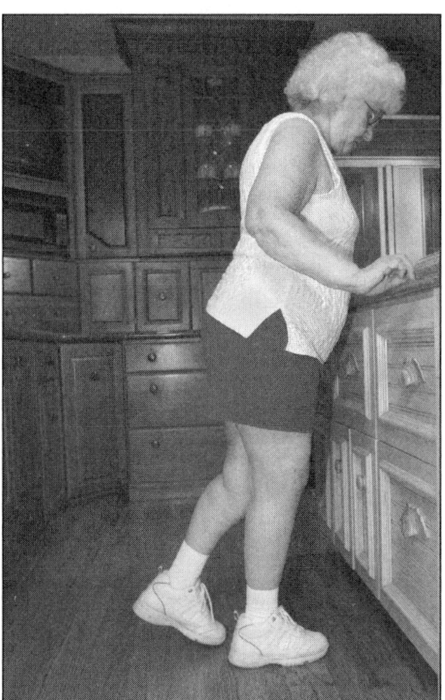

Figure 7.14. Single-leg stance balance exercise

Exercise 45

Single-Leg Heel Raise at Sink

Stand facing the sink, put full weight on your total-knee leg, and try to do a heel raise while standing only on the total-knee leg (Figure 7.15). This exercise is an advancement from last week when you did heel raises with both legs simultaneously (Exercise 29). If you cannot raise your heel as far off the ground as you did when doing the exercise with both legs, wait until next week to do this exercise. Perform 3–5 sets of 10–15 repetitions each, several times per day.

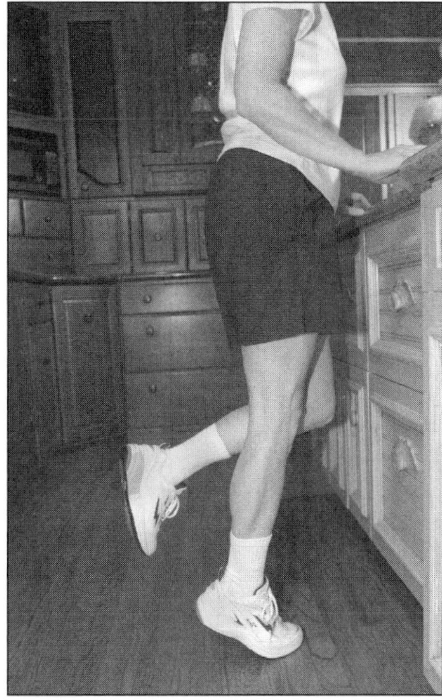

Figure 7.15. Single-leg stance heel-raise exercise

Exercise 46

Straight-Leg Raise Using Nonoperated Leg for Resistance

If you are able to do a straight-leg raise without difficulty, try this modification. Lie on your back or sit in a chair, keep your operative knee straight, and tighten your quadriceps muscle. Place your other foot over the top of your total-knee leg, and then perform the straight-leg raise against the weight of your nonoperated leg (Figure 7.16). Perform 3–5 sets of 10–15 repetitions each, several times per day.

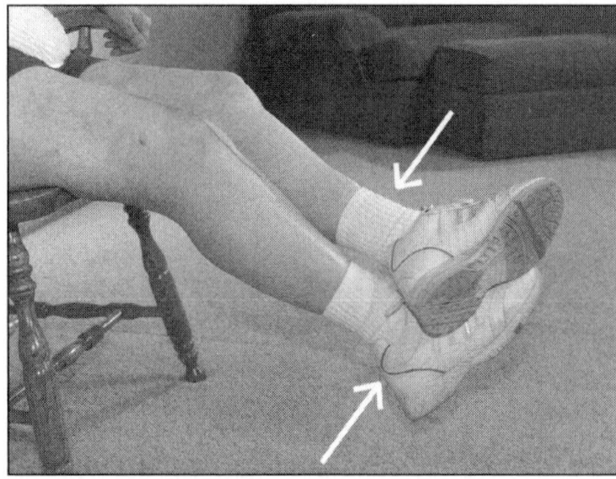

Figure 7.16. Straight-leg raise using nonoperated leg as resistance for TKA leg

■ ■ ■

Thera-Band Exercises

If you have a home physical therapist, ask him or her for approximately six feet of Thera-Band. A Thera-Band is a latex rubber band approximately six inches wide. It comes in different colors, each color representing a different amount of resistance. At one end of the Thera-Band, tie a loop big enough to fit over your foot; at the other end, tie several knots to hold onto with your hands. Here are three simple Thera-Band exercises to start in week two:

Exercise 47

Thera-Band: Ankle-Strengthening Exercise

Sit in a chair, and place the loop around the foot of your operated leg. Be careful to get the loop around as much of your foot as possible to prevent it from slipping off. Holding on to the knotted end of the Thera-Band, straighten your total-knee leg by lifting your foot off the ground. Your leg will be extended directly in front of you (Figure 7.17). Now bend and flex your ankle against the resistance of the Thera-Band to strengthen your calf muscle (the motion will be similar to pressing down on the accelerator of your car). Repeat 3–5 sets of 25 repetitions each, several times per day.

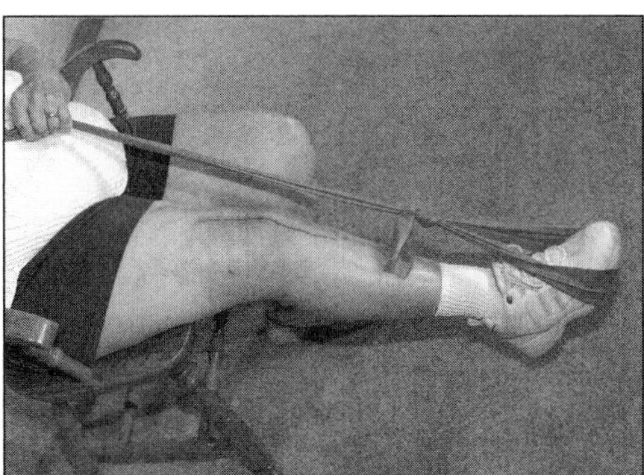

Figure 7.17. Thera-Band ankle-strengthening exercise

Exercise 48

Thera-Band: Knee Flexion and Extension Exercise

Sit in a chair, and place the loop of the Thera-Band around your foot. Bend your total knee as much as possible, and then straighten it as much as you can against the resistance of the Thera-Band (Figure 7.18). Perform 3–5 sets of 10–15 repetitions each, several times per day. This exercise helps the quadriceps and hamstring muscles to start actively contracting again. After surgery, these muscles "forget" how they are supposed to function. The active movement of the quadriceps aids in straightening the TKA knee, while the hamstrings act to bend the knee.

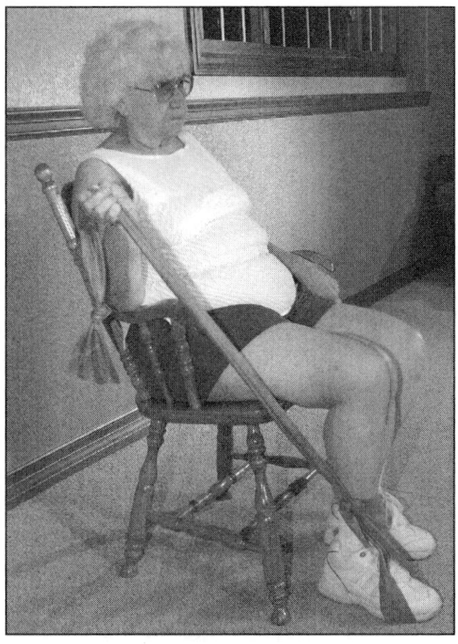

Figure 7.18. Thera-Band knee flexion and extension exercise

Exercise 49

Thera-Band: Hip/Knee Flexion and Extension Exercise

Sit in a chair and place the loop of the Thera-Band around your foot. Bend your hip, bringing your total knee toward your nose. Push the foot down and away from you against the resistance of the Thera-Band, in a motion similar to pushing on the brake of your car (Figure 7.19). This exercise is designed to develop strength, speed of movement, and control in your total-knee leg, all necessary for driving a car. (Your surgeon will tell you when it's okay for you to drive again.) Perform 3–5 sets of 10–15 repetitions each, several times per day.

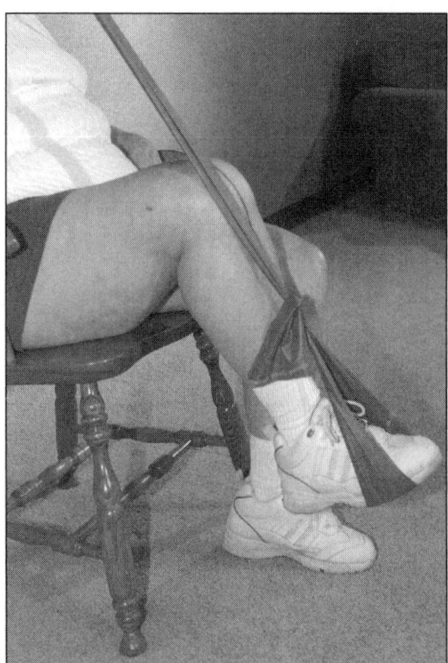

Figure 7.19. Thera-Band hip flexion and extension exercise

Common Questions and Some Answers

- **When will my "normal" appetite return?**

Most patients tell us that once they are able to sleep well and they are exercising vigorously, their appetite begins to return to normal. A well-balanced diet is the best plan for even a poor appetite.

- **How long will my normal sleep pattern be disturbed?**

There is no definitive answer to this question. Some patients experience disrupted sleep patterns for several weeks after surgery, while others are able to sleep relatively normally within a few days. Long after your normal sleep pattern is restored, don't be surprised if for no apparent reason you have an occasional "bad night." This is to be expected.

- **Is it normal that I can't concentrate during activities like reading and watching TV?**

The vast majority of patients report difficulty with concentration for several weeks after surgery. This is a poorly understood phenomenon that may be due to the lingering effects of the anesthesia, a side effect of pain medication, or the sensation of pain. For whatever reason, most patients have this experience. It is a common occurrence that will subside in time.

How long should I wear the T.E.D. stockings?

A majority of surgeons recommend wearing thigh-high (above-the-knee) T.E.D. hose for approximately six weeks postoperatively. They should be worn when you are upright, but they may be taken off while you're sleeping or lying down. The T.E.D. hose help to control swelling and aid in the pumping action of the leg muscles to help prevent blood clots. At approximately six weeks after surgery, most patients have minimal swelling and are active enough that the risk of blood clots is minimal.

Why does my TKA feel like it is going to "give way" at times without warning?

Because the quadriceps muscles are weak after TKA surgery, there may be times when they allow the knee to unexpectedly feel like it is going to collapse. This sensation, in conjunction with your limited balance at this point in the rehabilitation process, may lead you to believe that your knee joint is unstable. This is not the case. The "giving-way" sensation is due to muscle weakness and poor balance, which improve with time and exercise.

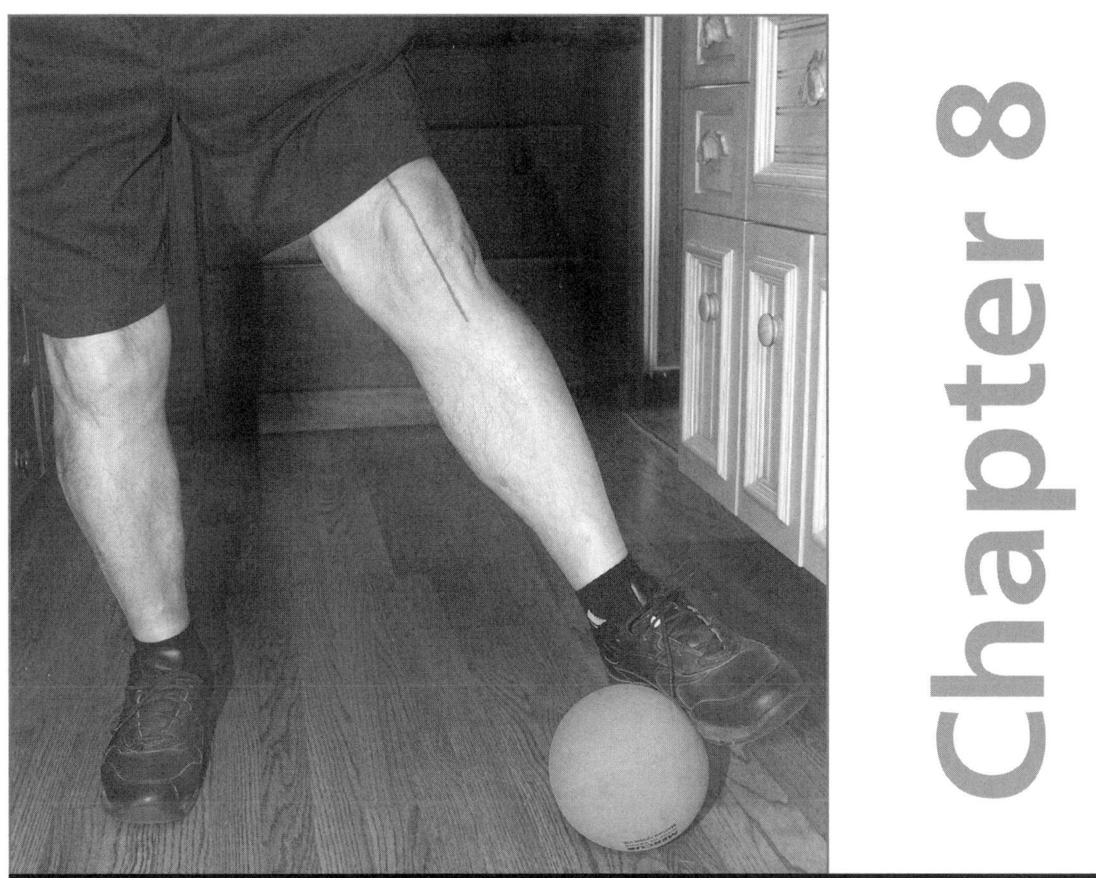

Chapter 8

Week Three

This Isn't As Bad As I Thought It Would Be

By now, your TKA knee is starting to work like it did a long time ago. It is interesting that the vast majority of our patients state that at about week three they begin to notice how other people's knees move. They also wonder if and when their TKA will move "normally" again. There is good news! The good news is that from now on your TKA knee will start moving more freely practically every day and will continue to improve, eventually even moving without pain!

This chapter provides exercises and activities designed to dramatically increase your new knee's mobility, speed of movement, and comfort in movement. Routinely, during week three, friends will remark on how amazed they are with your progress, and/or will comment that they can't believe you had your knee replaced only three weeks ago. You can reply, "You ain't seen nothin' yet!"

Outpatient Physical Therapy

If you arrange for home physical therapy, more than likely it will come to an end during week three. Most insurance companies will only pay for home physical therapy for a limited amount of time. The usual benchmark for discontinuing home physical therapy is when the patient is able to safely and comfortably get out of the house. Once that goal is met, home care is no longer needed, and you are ready to start outpatient physical therapy. By this time, patients are usually ready to take advantage of the equipment that an outpatient PT clinic has to offer. When you visited the surgeon's office last week for removal of the staples or sutures, he or she probably discussed starting outpatient physical therapy. Before making an appointment for outpatient physical therapy, make sure to have a prescription for physical therapy from your surgeon. This is necessary for your insurance company to cover the cost of outpatient physical therapy. When calling to set up your first appointment, ask the outpatient therapy clinic if they take your insurance. It is prudent to have your insurance concerns addressed before scheduling your first appointment.

The first visit to outpatient physical therapy consists of an initial evaluation. Each time you go to therapy, be sure to either wear shorts or bring a pair of shorts to change into. The physical therapist will want to see your knee in order to inspect the incision, monitor healing and soft-tissue changes, determine the amount of swelling, and measure your range of motion in flexion and extension. It is difficult if not impossible to make these initial observations and measurements if the patient is wearing long pants.

Once the initial evaluation is complete, the physical therapist will design an exercise program. One of the major advantages of going to outpatient physical therapy at this stage in your rehabilitation is that the therapist can design and closely monitor a program customized just for you. He or she will modify the exercises as necessary to enable you to gain strength, motion, and function in the most efficient manner possible. A standard outpatient physical-therapy TKA-rehabilitation session might proceed as outlined below.

The PT will probably have you attempt to ride a stationary exercise cycle. Try to make a complete revolution with the pedals. Depending on how much motion there is in your TKA, you may or may not be able to achieve a complete pedal cycle at this time. If you can, great. If you can't, don't worry about it. We will talk more about stationary cycling later in this chapter (Exercise 55), and we will also offer some hints to help you improve your performance on the cycle.

After a period of time to "warm up" on the stationary cycle, the physical therapist will start some mobilization exercises to increase motion in your TKA knee. As we've discussed in several places earlier in the book, it is imperative to communicate your sensations to your therapist! The old adage of "no pain, no gain" does not apply to a TKA when someone is attempting to assist you in mobilizing it. It is our philosophy that forcibly bending the operated knee can actually be detrimental to gaining motion in it. We have achieved excellent results in our patients without using the common practice of "physical torture" that forces the TKA to bend.

A big advantage of going to an outpatient PT clinic is having access to a number of "toys" to play with to help you gain motion, balance, and strength in your TKA—from strengthening machines, to mini-trampolines, to balancing equipment. There are training methods that can be done at home for gaining strength, balance, and functional mobility, and this book will describe them. Still, for most people, it is easier and more convenient to go to a physical-therapy clinic to gain access to specialized exercise devices that are unavailable at home.

The rehabilitation session commonly ends with some soft-tissue massage or mobilization around your TKA. Again, this is a major advantage offered by outpatient physical therapy. Dr. Falkel forgot to do his own soft-tissue mobilization on his TKA until he went to a professional meeting of physical therapists. He was reminded to do so when some of his colleagues asked him if he was doing soft-tissue mobilization on his own knee. (We will discuss this therapy more later in the chapter.)

We highly recommend taking advantage of outpatient physical therapy. Given the confines of managed health care, outpatient physical therapy will last a relatively short time, maybe for only four to six treatment sessions. But the time spent with a rehabilitation professional—who will monitor your progress carefully and adjust your program as needed—will improve the functional result of your TKA. Some people feel they may not need the direction and supervision provided by a physical therapist. This may be especially true for the person who has gone through outpatient physical therapy with a previous TKA surgery. And some exceptional patients are very self-motivated and familiar with the exercises necessary to achieve the best functional result. However, for the average person, it has been our experience that they are mistaken if they think they can do the rehabilitation on their own. For this reason, again, we strongly recommend taking advantage of outpatient physical therapy after TKA surgery.

Continuing Self-Directed Physical Therapy

If you are fortunate enough to get outpatient physical therapy, you will only be there two or three times per week for approximately an hour each session. What are you going to do with the other 165+ hours per week? You need to continue with your self-directed physical therapy at home!

By week three you may be tired of using a walker or crutches to ambulate in and out of the house. In order to walk safely with a cane or without any assistive device, start working on regaining balance in your TKA leg. Balance is a complex activity that involves many different structures located in your brain, eyes, and ears, as well as tiny structures in the muscles, ligaments, and joints called *proprioceptors*. All these structures give your brain feedback about where your body is in space, how fast you are moving, and what needs to happen to help maintain your balance as you move. After TKA surgery, the proprioceptors in your TKA knee "go on vacation" for awhile. They are impaired by swelling and pain, and some of the receptors that were in your "old knee" have been removed by the surgery. Therefore, in order to regain your balance, the proprioceptors need to be retrained. Here are some simple exercises that can be done in the kitchen to regain your balance and proprioception:

Exercise 50

Balancing with Feet Together

Stand in front of the sink, hold on to the sink with both hands, and place both feet together. Slowly let go of the sink with one hand, and then as you feel balanced, let go with the other. Try to stand still, keeping both feet together (Figure 8.1). Note that the Figure shows the patient in a diagonal position so the position of the feet is clearly visible. We recommend performing this exercise facing the sink for better balance.

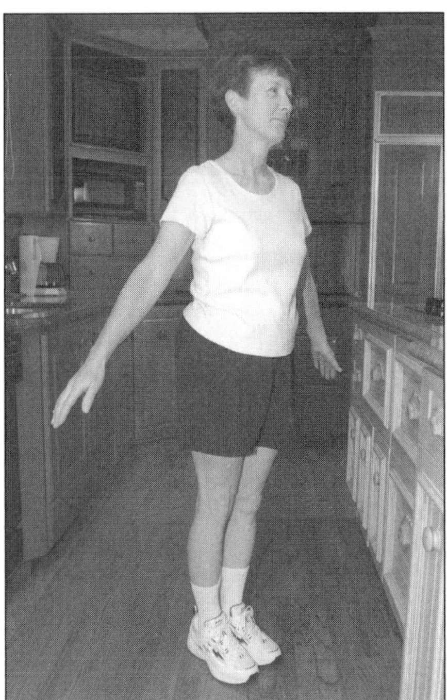

Figure 8.1. Narrow foot-placement balance exercise

Exercise 51

Balancing with Feet Together and Eyes Closed

Repeat Exercise 50, but this time close your eyes before trying to let go with one hand and then the other. This will quickly demonstrate the role that eyesight plays in balance (Figure 8.2). As your balance improves, try standing on only your TKA leg. Be sure to keep your hands near the sink in case you need support.

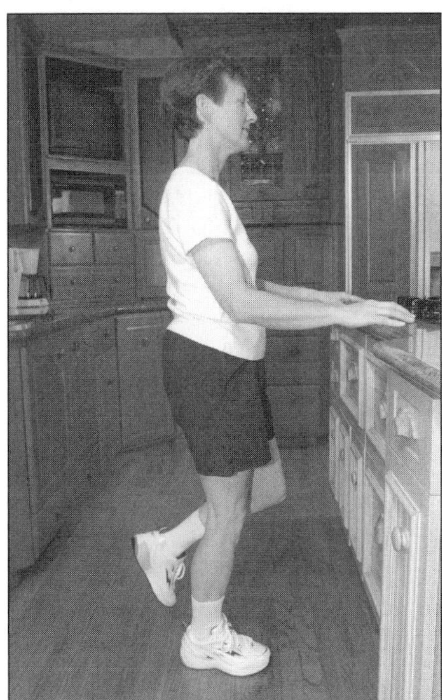

Figure 8.2. Single-leg stand, eyes closed, balance exercise

Exercise 52

Balancing with One Foot in Front of the Other

Stand in front of the sink, and place the heel of your TKA leg just in front of the toes of your other leg. Slowly let go of the sink with one hand and then the other, trying to balance in this position. After several attempts, switch your foot position so that the heel of the "good" leg is in front of the toes of the TKA leg (Figure 8.3).

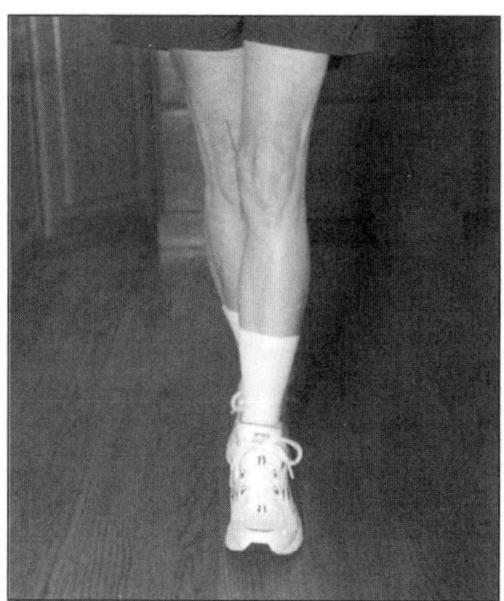

Figure 8.3. Balance exercise with one foot in front of the other

Exercise 53

Balancing with One Foot in Front of the Other and Eyes Closed

Now attempt to do Exercise 52 with your eyes closed.

Exercise 54

Balancing on the TKA Leg

This exercise is critical for walking without an assistive device. Stand with your good side next to the sink, and hold on to the sink with the hand on that side of the body. Shift all of your weight to the TKA leg, and slowly lift and extend the other foot until it is off the ground. Once balanced, let go of the sink and try to balance on the TKA leg alone (Figure 8.4). This can be difficult, so don't get frustrated if you don't succeed at first. Keep trying, and it will happen—sooner rather than later.

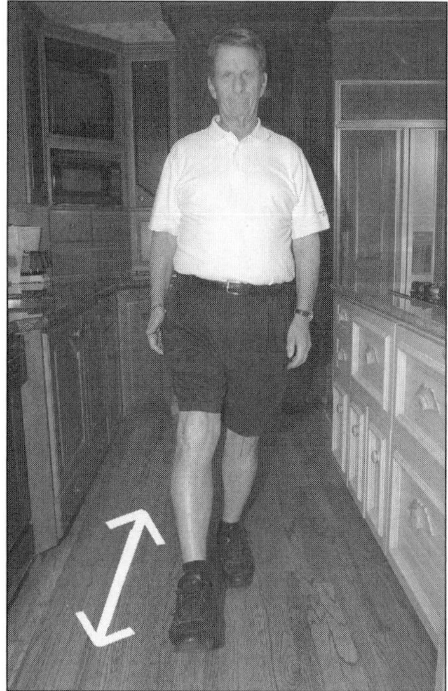

Figure 8.4. Single-leg stance dynamic balance exercise

■ ■ ■

With all of the balance exercises, try to sustain the balance position for 15–30 seconds, and complete 10–15 trials (repetitions) of each balance activity. As your balance improves, attempt to hold the balance position for 60–90 seconds. A good way to time these balance exercises is to do them while watching TV. Practice your balance training each time there is a commercial, performing the exercise throughout the commercial. It seems to make the commercials go by much faster!

Range-of-Motion Exercises

At week three you should be approaching ninety degrees of knee flexion. Your surgeon will tell you how much range of motion she or he expects you to be able to achieve ultimately. Final range of motion depends on the patient's age, the patient's tendency to form excessive scar tissue, and the prosthetic design. Here are several more exercises that can be done independently to help you gain additional range of motion in your TKA knee:

Exercise 55

"Rocking" on Stationary Cycle

As mentioned in Chapter 3, one of the best exercise devices to have at home for TKA rehab is a stationary exercise cycle. You will use it for three primary purposes: (a) to help gain range of motion in your new knee, (b) to help increase your knee's speed of movement, and (c) to help improve your overall muscular and cardiovascular endurance. If you do not have a stationary exercise cycle at home, you probably know someone who has one collecting dust in their garage or basement. Ask them if you can borrow it for a short period of time. If no stationary cycle is available to you, then, as we recommended earlier in the book, consider buying one before surgery so it is readily available. You might be able to find a used one, either in the classified ads of your local paper or at a store that sells used sporting goods. The stationary exercise cycle is an essential part of the TKA rehabilitation program. In addition, it should be used as part of a life-long exercise program. We recommend that your stationary cycle have "toe clips" or straps to prevent the TKA foot from slipping off the pedal while you're exercising.

The first thing to do is adjust the seat height. The higher the seat, the less bend or flexion you need in the TKA knee to allow you to complete a full pedal cycle. However, if you raise the seat too high, you won't be able to pedal at all or to even get on the seat. Through trial and error you will find a seat

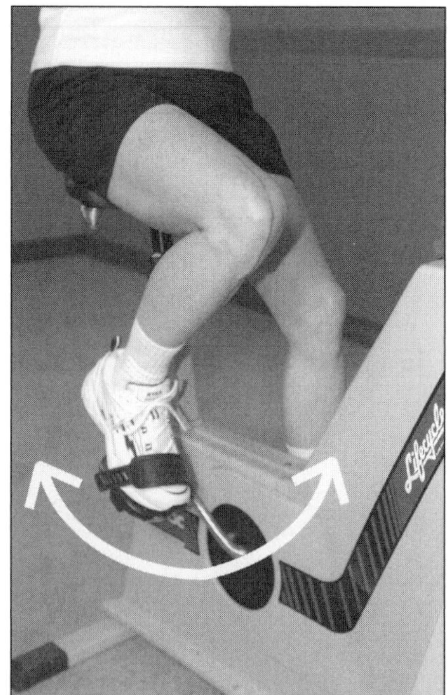

Figure 8.5. Stationary cycle "rocking" for range of motion

height that is comfortable; you can always change it as needed.

To get started, place the pedal of the TKA leg in the down (six o'clock) position. After placing your good foot on the other pedal, slowly start pedaling either forward or backward until your TKA knee can't bend any further. At that point, reverse directions and slowly continue to pedal until you feel the tightness again. Repeat this "rocking motion" back and forth for several minutes to warm up your TKA knee (Figure 8.5).

In order to complete a full revolution with the TKA leg, you need to have approximately 100 to 110 degrees of flexion. If you can't perform a full revolution, then once you're warmed up, push your TKA knee to the position of tightness, and hold that position as long as possible, trying to push it farther and hold it longer each time. This will help stretch the scar tissue that is restricting range of motion. After several attempts at holding the stretch, go back to simply rocking forward and backward. You will be amazed at how much more motion you achieve before reaching the point of tightness. At least 3 times per day, spend about 5–10 minutes "rocking" on the stationary exercise cycle. Consider putting the exercise cycle in a room with a TV, which will serve as a distraction while you're doing the exercise.

Most people are able to reach a full revolution with minimal discomfort in just a few days. Once you can complete the full revolution comfortably, pedaling both forward and backward, lower the seat slightly, and start all over again. It may take a few trials to be able to get all the way around, since lowering the seat requires more knee flexion to complete a revolution. The effort on the stationary exercise cycle is well worth the increase in motion and fitness it will produce in your TKA.

Futebol Exercises

The next several exercises are just plain fun, and they produce tremendous gains in your new knee's range of motion and speed of movement. We recommend using a product called the Brasilian Futebol (pronounced "foo-che-ball") for the ball-rolling exercises described in this and later chapters. The Brasilian Futebol is a small rubber ball that is used by soccer players in Brazil to develop their skill, balance, and ball control. What makes the Brasilian Futebol unique is that it is made of rubber, so it bounces more than a normal soccer ball, basketball, or volleyball. You can use any type of ball for the following exercises, but we have found the Brasilian Futebol to work the best for our patients. And at only about ten bucks, dollar for dollar it may be the best investment you can make for long-term rehabilitation and return of function. The Brasilian Futebol can be purchased online at www.brasilianfutebol.com or by calling (800) 618-3017. The company has agreed to give a discount to readers of this book.

Exercise 56

Rolling *Futebol* Forward and Backward While Seated

Sit in a comfortable chair, place the *futebol* under the TKA foot, and roll it back and forth. Start by rolling the *futebol* forward and backward for several minutes as a warm-up activity (Figure 8.6). After several minutes of rolling the ball back and forth, roll the ball back as far as possible until you feel tightness in your knee. Hold that position for 15–60 seconds. Resume rolling the *futebol* back and forth for several repetitions.

Repeat this rolling/holding sequence several times per day, for 3–5 minutes each session. Using the *futebol* in this way will dramatically improve both your range of motion and your speed of movement.

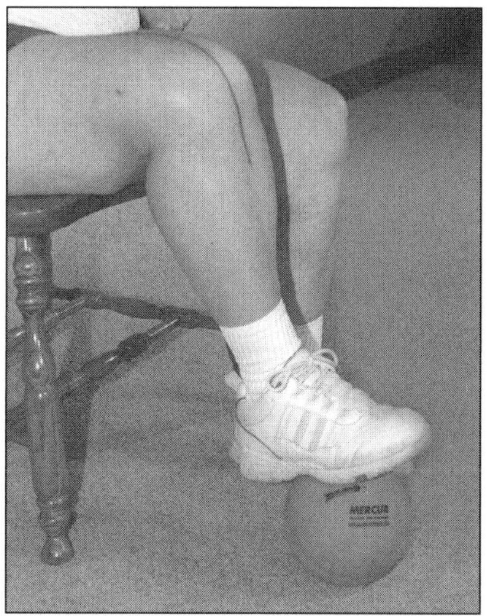

Figure 8.6. *Futebol* rolling exercise for increasing range of motion in TKA knee

Exercise 57

Rolling *Futebol* in Small Circles While Seated

Sit in a comfortable chair, and roll the *futebol* under your TKA foot in small circles, first in a clockwise direction and then in a counterclockwise direction (Figure 8.7). As doing so becomes easier, try rolling the ball in bigger circles. This exercise will not only improve the speed of movement in your TKA knee, but it will also help loosen the scar tissue and reduce swelling around the knee.

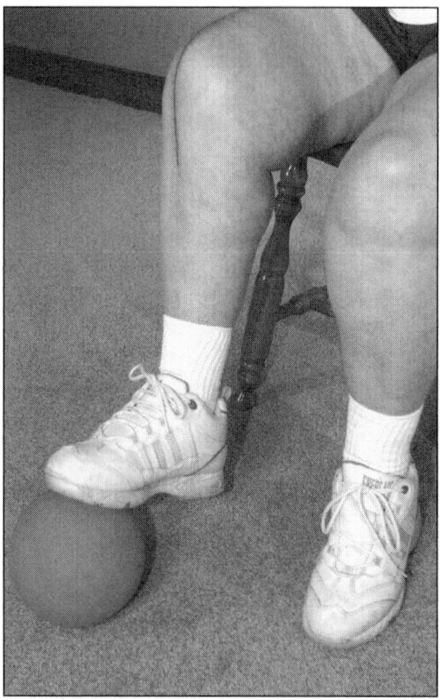

Figure 8.7. *Futebol* rolling while sitting

Exercise 58

Squashing *Futebol* While Seated

Sitting in a chair, place the *futebol* under the TKA foot and try to "squash" the *futebol* into the floor. Hold the foot down on the *futebol* for a count of 5–10 seconds, and repeat 10–15 times (Figure 8.8). This exercise strengthens the hamstring muscles.

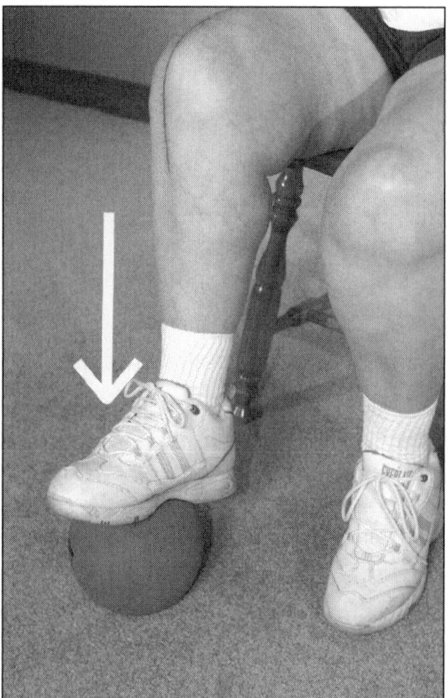

Figure 8.8. *Futebol* strengthening exercise by "squashing" ball into floor

Exercise 59

Strengthening Exercise for Inner Thigh Using *Futebol*

Sitting in a chair, place the *futebol* between your knees and squeeze it as hard as you can for a count of 5–10 seconds; repeat 10–15 times (Figure 8.9). This action may cause some slight discomfort along the inside ligament of your TKA knee, but it will eventually subside, and the pressure and strengthening achieved from performing the exercise are well worth the discomfort. If your knee hurts too much, simply reduce the pressure on the *futebol*. This exercise strengthens the adductor muscles in your inner thigh.

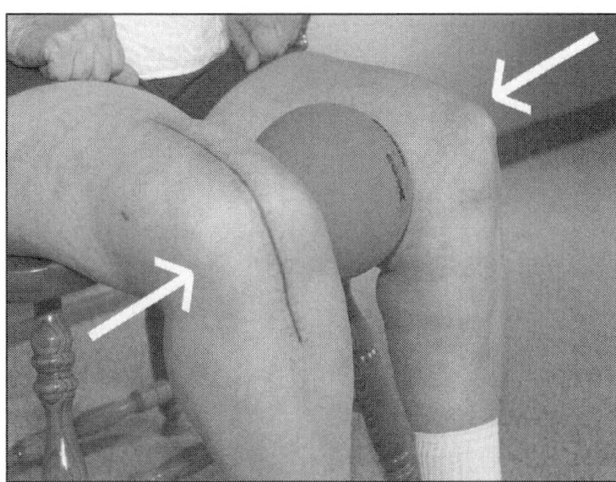

Figure 8.9. *Futebol* strengthening exercise for inner-thigh adductor muscles

Exercise 60

Strengthening/Flexion Exercise Using *Futebol*

Sitting in a chair, place the *futebol* between your feet or ankles. Hold the *futebol* there, and straighten your knees to lift your feet off the floor (Figure 8.10). Keeping the *futebol* between your feet or ankles, bend your knees to bring your feet back to the floor. Repeat 15–25 times. This exercise improves leg strength, knee movement, and coordination.

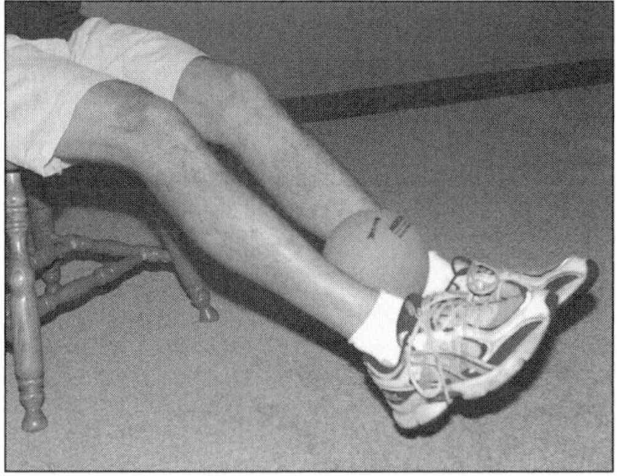

Figure 8.10. *Futebol* strengthening exercise for quadriceps muscles

Exercise 61

Rolling *Futebol* (in Many Directions) While Standing

Standing with your good leg next to the sink, hold on to the sink with that hand, and place the *futebol* on the ground. Place your TKA foot on top of the *futebol*, and roll the *futebol* out to the side as far as possible and then back to the starting position (Figure 8.11). Then roll the *futebol* as far forward as you can, and then as far backward as possible. Repeat the entire sequence 15–25 times. This exercise dramatically improves the coordination and speed of movement in the TKA leg.

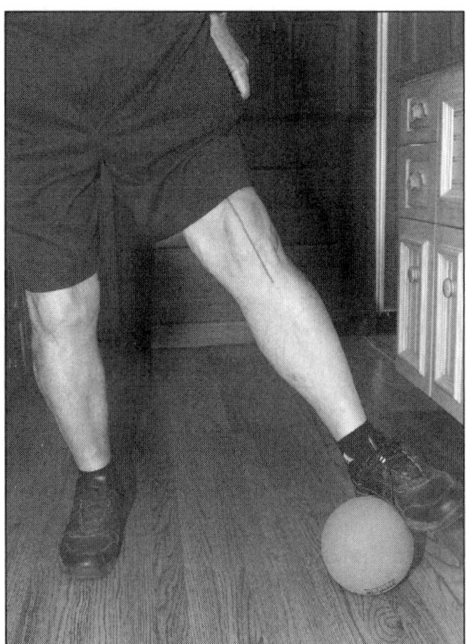

Figure 8.11. *Futebol* "stop" by rolling out to side and stopping under TKA foot

Exercise 62

Rolling *Futebol* in Circles

Standing with your good leg next to the sink, hold on to the sink with that hand, and roll the *futebol* under the TKA foot in small circles in a clockwise direction; repeat 15–25 times. Then make small circles in a counterclockwise direction, repeating 15–25 times. Now extend your TKA leg slightly in front of your body, and repeat both the clockwise and counterclockwise rotations. Next, extend your TKA leg slightly behind your body, and repeat both the clockwise and counterclockwise rotations. In all three positions, gradually make progressively larger circles in each direction. Repeat 15–25 times in each direction and with each leg position. As an advanced variation on Exercise 57 you can also do the exercise while sitting in a chair (Figure 8.12). This exercise improves coordination and speed of movement in the TKA leg.

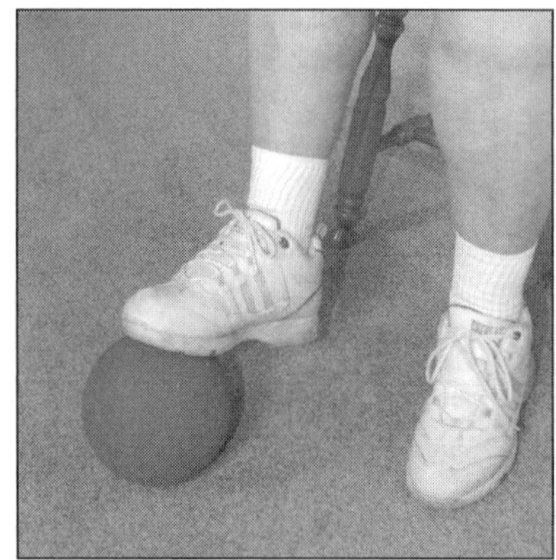

Figure 8.12. *Futebol* clockwise/counterclockwise rolling exercise (advanced variation in chair)

Exercise 63

Rolling *Futebol* Up a Wall

Stand with your TKA leg next to a wall, and hold on to a chair or a counter for balance. Place the *futebol* between the wall and the foot of your TKA leg. Try to roll the *futebol* 6–12 inches up the wall by bending your new knee (Figure 8.13). Lower the *futebol*; repeat 15–25 times. This exercise improves lateral strength, motion, and coordination in the TKA leg.

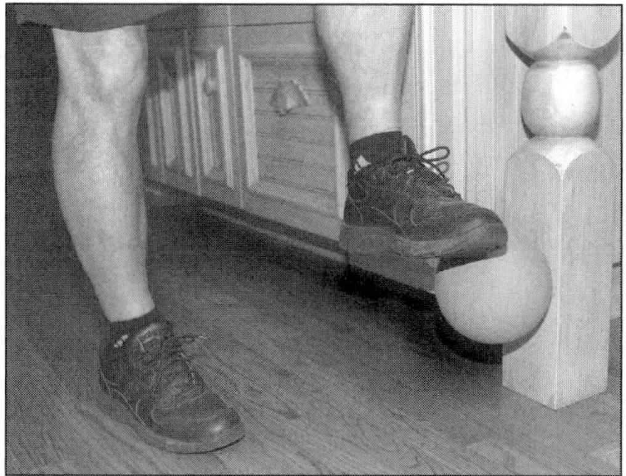

Figure 8.13. *Futebol* wall-rolling exercise

■ ■ ■

Many of our patients keep their *futebol* next to their favorite chair and use it almost like a CPM machine anytime they are sitting. Although the *futebol* exercises may seem overly simple, our experience has proven that they dramatically improve range and speed of motion in the TKA knee. Of all the trials and tribulations of Dr. Falkel's rehabilitation, he was most shocked by the lack of "normal" speed of movement in his two TKAs. For quite some time he was concerned that his TKAs would never move like "normal" knees. However, the *futebol* exercises and the stationary-cycle exercises helped him regain normal speed of motion by the end of week four.

Exercise 64

Using Rolled-up Sheet for Knee Flexion

Roll up a large bath or beach towel lengthwise, and place tape or rubber bands around the towel in several places to keep it rolled up. Sit on a bed, a couch, or the floor with your feet extended in front of you (alternatively, if you're sitting on a bed or couch, the foot of your good leg can rest on the floor). Now bend your TKA knee enough to be able to wrap the towel around the front of your ankle, holding on to each end of the towel. Use the towel to slowly pull your ankle toward your buttocks (Figure 8.14). This works to stretch (flex) your TKA. Hold the stretch as long as possible; then slightly straighten the leg, rest, and repeat, pulling your ankle farther back each time. Repeat 15–25 times.

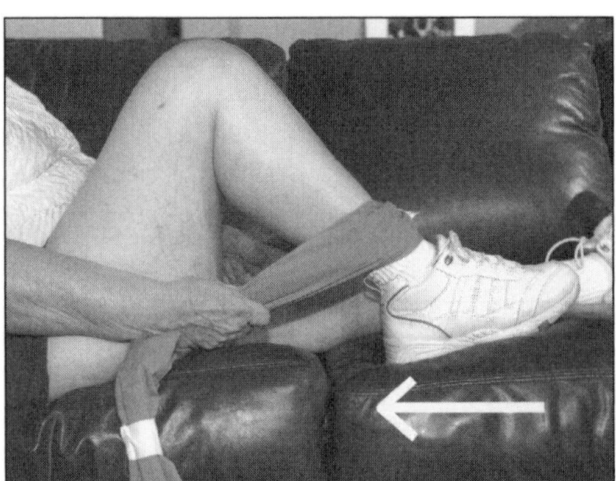

Figure 8.14. Range-of-motion exercise using towel around ankle to gain flexion in TKA knee

Exercise 65

Sitting on Countertop for Knee Flexion

If you can, sit on a countertop. Place a towel roll under your TKA for comfort (so the back of the TKA knee doesn't become irritated by the edge of the counter), and bend your knee as much as possible. Swing your knee out to full extension and then back down again into flexion. If you can open a cabinet door below where you are sitting, you will be able to swing into more flexion (Figure 8.15). Repeat 15–25 times.

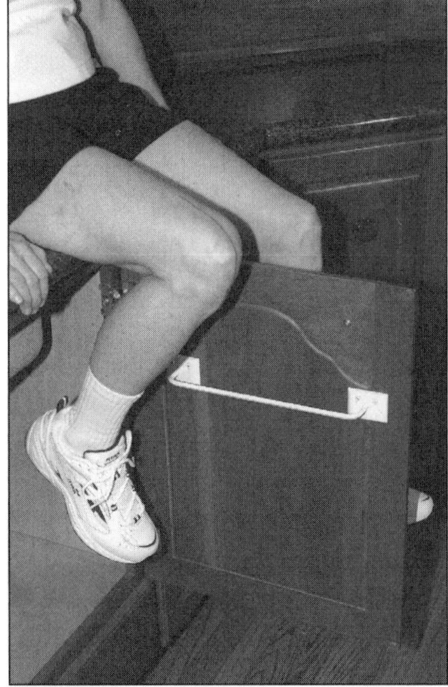

Figure 8.15. Range-of-motion exercise sitting on countertop swinging TKA knee

Exercise 66

Thera-Band: Hamstring Strengthening Exercise

Sit in a chair, and place the loop end of the Thera-Band around the foot of your TKA leg. Tie the other end of the Thera-Band around an immovable object located in front of you, or have someone hold the other end of the Thera-Band while sitting or standing in front of you. Straighten your leg as far as possible, and then with gentle tension on the Thera-Band, bend your knee as much as you can against the resistance of the Thera-Band (Figure 8.16). Hold the flexed position for 5–10 seconds. Complete 3–5 sets of 15–25 repetitions. This exercise will improve speed of movement in bending your knee, something you need to be able to do quickly while driving in order to operate the clutch or to move your foot from the accelerator to the brake.

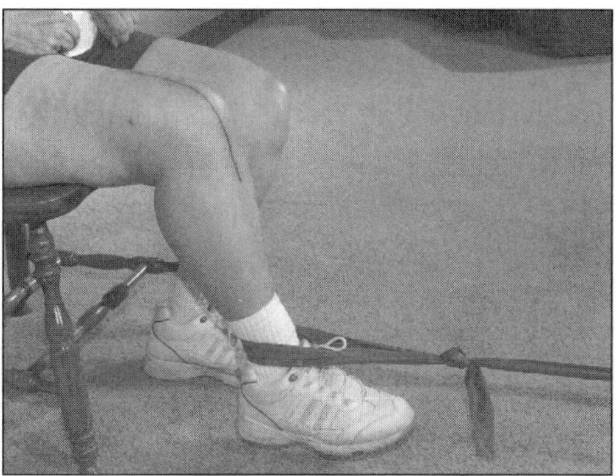

Figure 8.16. Thera-Band hamstring strengthening exercise

Walking With or Without a Cane

By week three there has probably been at least one occasion when you have stood up and walked, then stopped after a few steps and realized that you did not have your walker or crutches. This is a sure sign of improvement, because two weeks ago you would not have even considered trying to walk without your walker or crutches! As you gain confidence with your TKA, you will attempt to walk without any assistive device. During walking, there is a point in time when all of your weight is on one foot (the *stance phase*) while the other foot is swinging through the air to start the next step (the *swing phase*). Until you have the confidence and strength to put full weight on your TKA leg during the stance phase, you can't walk without an assistive device. In order to walk "normally" you need both strength and balance in your TKA leg to support you during the swing phase of your good leg. This is why it is so important to work on the balance exercises described in this chapter, and why we will provide additional balance exercises in the next few chapters.

Once you're able to perform Exercise 54, and once you feel confident with just finger-touch support while balancing on your TKA leg, you may be ready to start walking with a cane. A cane needs to be the correct height for you. To determine the correct height for the cane, put it in the

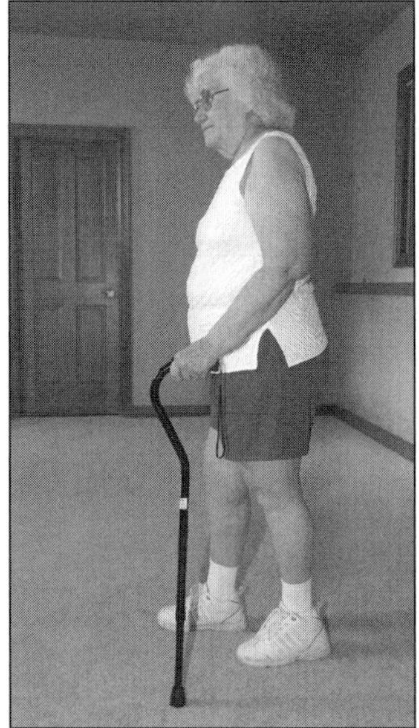

Figure 8.17. Determining the proper length for a cane

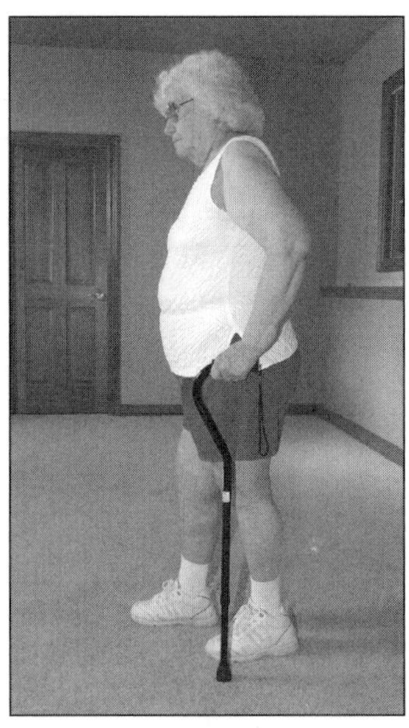

Figure 8.18. Alternative method for determining cane length

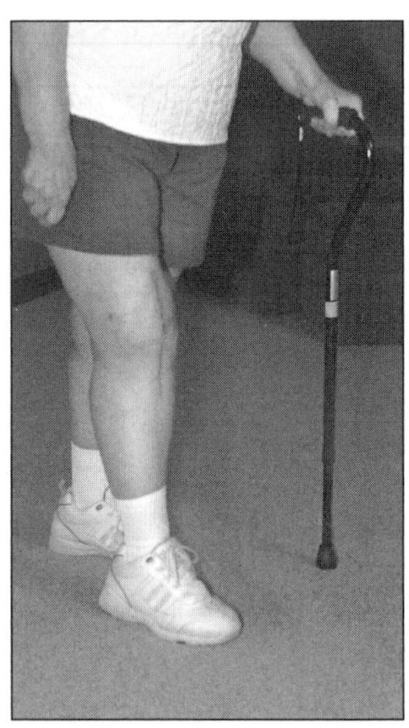

Figure 8.19. Using a cane for walking after TKA surgery

hand on the side opposite your TKA knee, with the tip about six inches in front and to the outside of your good foot (Figure 8.17). In this position, you should have a slight bend in your elbow, and as you put your weight onto the TKA leg, you should feel stable with the cane in this position. Another technique to determine your optimal cane height is to place the cane against the outside of your good leg. Feel the "bump" on the outside of your hip; this bump is called the *greater trochanter* of the hip. The top of your cane should come to approximately the height of the greater trochanter (Figure 8.18).

The best method for walking with a cane is to use it on the side of the good leg. The reason for this is that during walking, having the cane on the side opposite the TKA knee will allow you to shift a small amount of weight onto the cane, thus allowing you to put less weight on the TKA leg. Moving the cane and TKA leg forward simultaneously gives you a better base of support for balance. While it may seem unnatural to use the cane on your good side, it really is the best way.

Practice using your cane in a kitchen or hallway that has few obstacles to maneuver around. When walking with the cane you need to move the cane when you move the TKA leg (Figure 8.19). As you bring your TKA leg forward, bring the cane forward with the opposite hand so that cane and TKA leg are both moving during the swing phase at the same time. Once you begin to put weight on the TKA foot, shift a small amount of weight to the cane, thus placing the TKA leg and cane in the stance phase together. Then, as you bring your good foot through the swing phase and start putting weight on it, release the pressure on the cane and TKA leg, and move them both forward during the swing phase of the TKA leg.

A cane is primarily used for balance during walking. If you don't feel balanced while walking with a cane or if you sense that you are putting "too much weight" on the cane, then you are not quite ready for the cane. During week three, as you gain confidence in your TKA, practice walking with a cane in the house but use your walker or crutches while walking outdoors. There are many obstacles, uneven surfaces, and other people walking around you when you are out of the house, and you may need the added stability of a walker or crutches to prevent falling. So at least for this week, be sure to use your walker and/or crutches when going out of the house.

Soft-Tissue and Scar Management

By week three the incision should be completely healed, with no open areas or scabs remaining. Most of the Steri-Strips should have fallen off as well. Now is the time to start working with the quadriceps muscle and the structures around the knee to make them as pliable as possible. The best way to accomplish this is with soft-tissue mobilization techniques. These techniques are designed to place the scar tissue under a "positive" stress to help soften the scar and make it move more like normal tissue. After surgery, scarring of both the incision and the soft tissues around the knee (i.e., ligaments, tendons, muscles) is inevitable as a part of the normal healing process. In order to help "train" the scar tissue to become more like "normal" tissue, here are a few activities you can do:

1. Last week, we recommended performing massage along the incision by moving your thumb in a small circular motion. Continue doing that massage technique, and also add the following new technique. Using both thumbs—one on each side of the incision—find the tissue in your quadriceps muscle that feels much harder than the rest of the muscle. This hardened area is where the quadriceps muscle was cut and repaired during surgery. It has developed its own scar tissue and is one of the factors limiting flexion in your TKA knee. Rather than moving your thumbs in circles, simply rub your thumbs up and down or back and forth over the area where your quadriceps is tight (Figure 8.20). Put as much pressure on the scarred area as you can tolerate, and continue moving your thumbs back and forth for several minutes. Rest, and then repeat several times. This soft-tissue massage technique should be performed as much as possible throughout the

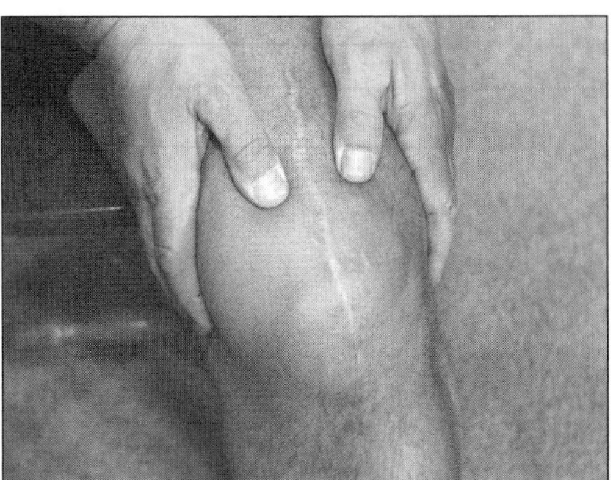

Figure 8.20. Soft-tissue mobilization along scar tissue in quadriceps

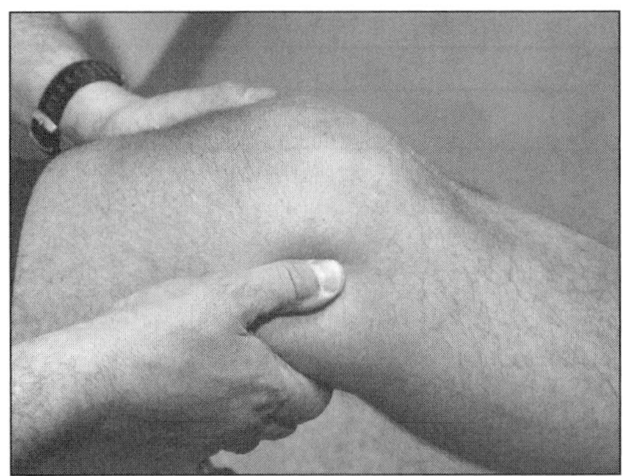

Figure 8.21. Mobilization of knee's collateral ligament soft tissue after TKA surgery

day; there is no danger of doing it "too much."

2. The next step in soft-tissue mobilization is to concentrate on the collateral ligaments located on the side of your TKA (Figure 8.21). These ligaments were stressed and stretched during the TKA surgery, and may even have been surgically reconstructed. Therefore, they, too, need soft-tissue mobilization to facilitate their return to normal function and to permit more movement in the TKA. If you had severe bony deformity due to your arthritis, your surgeon may have found it necessary to reconstruct one or both of the two collateral ligaments to enhance the stability of the knee joint. If this is the case, extra attention needs to be focused on soft-tissue mobilization of these ligaments.

   Soft-tissue massage over the collateral ligaments is similar to the technique used over the scar tissue in the quadriceps muscle. Simply place your thumb over the area of the collateral ligament, and then, using as much pressure as you can tolerate, run your thumb up and down the area of the collateral ligament. Continue massaging the ligament for 3–5 minutes, and then repeat on the other collateral ligament. Performing this massage will dramatically loosen the tightness many patients feel on the sides of their TKA.

3. The last type of soft-tissue mobilization you will do this week is patellar mobilization. This involves moving the patella, or kneecap, in all four directions: up, down, and side to side (Figure 8.22). Because the surgical incision was made around the patella, scar tissue has a tendency to encase the patella. In addition, the patella is everted (flipped over) during surgery to gain exposure to the undersurface, thus stressing the entire patellar mechanism. As a result of these surgical manipulations, the patella scars down, thus lim-

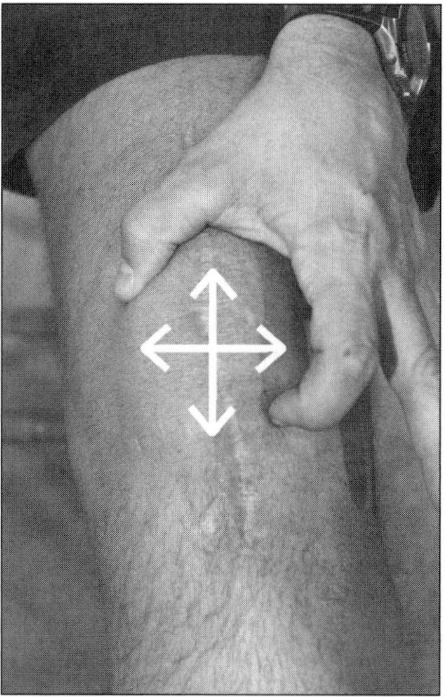

Figure 8.22. Patella mobilization after TKA surgery

iting knee motion. Therefore, it is important to move the patella as early as possible with your hand to minimize scarring and maximize knee motion. While sitting in a chair with your knee extended and your leg completely relaxed (heel resting on the floor), take the patella between your thumb and index finger, and slowly and gently move it in all directions. Move the patella in one direction as far as possible, and then hold that position for 15–30 seconds. Repeat in all four directions, eventually holding each position for 90–120 seconds. This will aid in "remodeling" the scar tissue around the patella.

■ ■ ■

This has been a big week, and one in which you have seen dramatic changes in movement, range of motion, confidence, and comfort level in living with your new TKA. The good news is that it only gets better! Each day you will gain more confidence and comfort with your TKA. There may still be an occasional day when you feel stiff or sore. If this happens, take the day off from your exercise routine. Remember that knowing when to take time off is an important component of your recovery. Even a world-class athlete needs to rest at times in order to improve. The same holds true with TKA rehabilitation. If you find yourself resistant to taking needed time off from your rehab program, review our discussion of rest and its role in your recovery in Chapter 6.

Common Questions and Some Answers

How do I know when I am overdoing it with my TKA?

Good question! Our general rule is that if you experience increased pain immediately after exercise, later that night, or the next morning, you probably overdid it. Conversely, if the pain is not significantly increased immediately after exercise, later that night, or the next day, you have probably done an appropriate amount of exercise and can "push" your TKA harder the next day. This is a retrospective method of judging how much exercise to perform, and it will differ for every person.

What should I do if my insurance company limits the number of outpatient physical-therapy visits?

Although we feel outpatient physical therapy is very important, it is possible, although more difficult, to rehabilitate your TKA with a self-directed program. This book is the only guide available for a comprehensive rehabilitation program specifically designed for patients who have had TKA surgery. By paying close attention to the guidelines outlined in this book and with strong personal motivation it is possible to achieve a successful outcome with a self-directed rehabilitation program. Therefore, if you know that you will have only a limited number of physical-therapy visits—home or outpatient—notify your therapist of this restriction. The limited number of visits will need to be used judiciously to obtain the most benefit from the expertise of the therapist. By knowing the number of visits allowed by the insurance company, the therapist can design your rehabilitation program most effectively.

When will I feel stable using my cane?

The cane is used primarily for balance during walking. If you can't put full weight on your TKA, you are not quite ready to use a cane. In fact, if it is necessary to lean on the cane to support part of your weight during walking, this is unsafe and may result in loss of balance or even falling. Use a walker or crutches and continue with the balance exercises until you gain the confidence to use the cane only for balance while walking.

Will my balance ever return to normal?

Yes, for the majority of patients, balance will eventually return to normal. It commonly takes over a year for balance to completely return. It also takes practice and patience with the exercises. The harder you work at the balance exercises, the earlier your balance will return to normal.

Why is my thigh muscle so hard just above my kneecap?

The quadriceps muscle is divided during the surgery so the surgeon can gain exposure to the joint, and then it is repaired. This results in a significant amount of scar tissue forming in the quadriceps muscle. Scar tissue is inherently harder than muscle tissue; some patients say it feels almost like a piece of wood. As you continue with your exercises for mobilizing the scar tissue and increase your overall level of daily activity, this area will soften and feel more like normal.

Why do my hamstrings hurt?

There are two main reasons why your hamstring muscles (muscles in the back of the thigh) might hurt. First, they have probably not had as much exercise in years as they are getting now through your rehab efforts. Second, for a significant number of patients, knee arthritis slowly causes a flexion contracture of the joint before surgery. That is, because of the pain and cartilage destruction, it becomes impossible to fully extend, or straighten, the knee. After surgery, the knee is able to fully extend, placing a great deal of stress on the tight hamstring muscles and tendons behind the knee. With stretching, over time, this pain should subside.

What is the "clicking" sound I hear and/or feel, and is it bad?

One common cause of "clicking" in the artificial knee is the plastic patella (kneecap) component tapping on the metal femoral (thigh-bone) component. Another reason for clicking is the newly formed scar tissue in the joint. This hard, gristle-like tissue often snaps over the edge of bone or prosthetic components, causing a click. It usually subsides as the scar tissue matures and loosens. Painless clicking is nothing to worry about. Even occasional painful clicking should be ignored. However, if you develop a persistent, painful clicking sensation, notify your surgeon.

How long should I continue to use ice on my TKA?

Another good question. Ice is a good anti-inflammatory agent. It also works to numb some of the postoperative discomfort in the TKA. As long as there is any swelling, pain, or inflammation, ice is the treatment of choice. Some patients get so much relief from ice that they continue to use it on their TKA regularly.

When can I start using heat on my TKA?

Once the staples or stitches are removed from the incision and the incision is completely healed, heat can safely be applied to the knee. Heat is a very effective method of increasing blood flow to an area and can work well to help relax tightness around the knee. The most convenient and effective form of heat we have found is a heating pad. There are numerous other microwaveable products available that contain gel or some other substance to retain the heat. Using a heating pad or other heat source for fifteen or twenty minutes prior to performing range-of-motion exercises can be very effective.

When will my TKA knee move "normally" again?

The reason why most patients undergo TKA surgery is to relieve pain. It is not to allow their knee to move "normally" again. After TKA surgery, your knee will never move "normally" again, but it will move better than it did before the surgery. It will take several months to reach maximal range of motion in your TKA. Until this happens, the speed of movement in the TKA will be diminished. We have provided several exercises in the next few chapters that will help you work specifically on gaining speed of movement in your TKA.

What does it mean when my PT says I have "95 degrees" in my TKA?

The amount of flexion (bending) and extension (straightening) in the TKA are measured in degrees using a flexible ruler called a *goniometer*. When the knee is completely straight, or fully extended, that is called zero degrees. As you bend your knee, the angle of bend is recorded on the goniometer, so when the TKA is bent to 90 degrees, it is at a right angle between the top of your thigh and the front of the shin bone. Ninety-five degrees is five degrees past 90 degrees. Most TKAs will bend or flex to between 110 and 130 degrees, depending on the type of prosthesis used, the amount of scar tissue, and the tightness of the muscles and ligaments around the knee. Ask your surgeon how much flexion or bend you should achieve with your TKA.

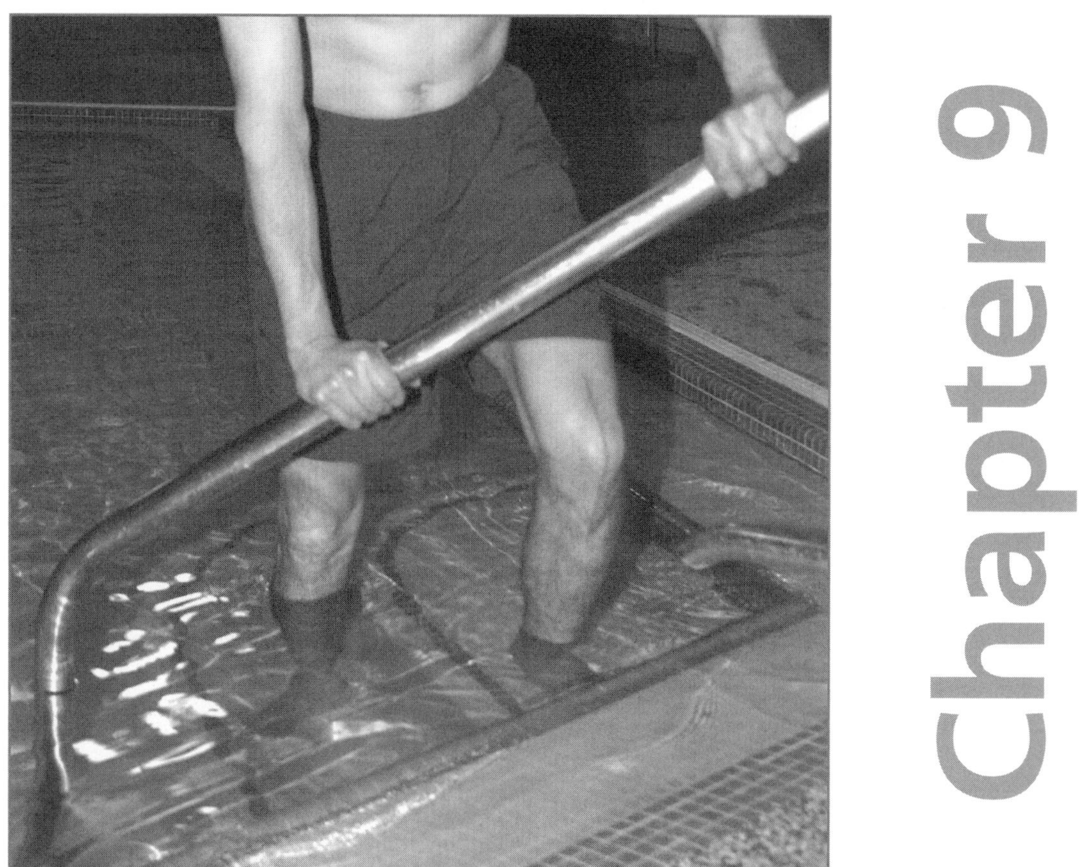

Chapter 9

Pool Therapy

The TKA's Best Friend

For many people who suffer from arthritis in their knees, one of the few places they can exercise without much pain is in the water. The buoyancy of the water takes most of the weight off the knees during walking and other aquatic exercises, and if the water temperature is warm, it helps reduce pain in the knees. Additionally, the water produces a massaging action on the joint when the joint is put through a range of motion, which feels soothing to the patient. All in all, water therapy works very well after total knee replacement. This chapter offers exercises and activities that can be done in a hot tub, a whirlpool, or a lap pool. Find your swimsuit; your new knee is going to love the water!

When to Start Pool Therapy

The general rule of thumb about starting pool therapy revolves around the complete healing of the incision. While it is safe to take a shower after the staples or sutures are removed, as we mentioned in Chapter 7, the incision should not be immersed in water, such as a bath or a pool, until all the scabs are completely gone from the incision. This usually takes two to three weeks after surgery.

Once the incision is completely healed, we recommend that you wait an additional week before starting pool therapy. Unfortunately, Dr. Falkel did not heed his own advice after he had a Baker's cyst removed, and the incision on the back of his knee got infected because it was not completely healed when he got in the water. We will discuss the seriousness of infections in Appendix A; meanwhile, suffice it to say that you do not want your TKA incision or any part of the TKA to get infected. That is why we suggest waiting at least one week after the last of the scabs fall off the incision before getting into a pool.

Finally, ask your surgeon for approval before starting pool therapy. Normally the surgeon will see a TKA patient approximately six weeks after surgery for a checkup and X ray. While some patients will wait until this visit to start pool therapy, if your incision is healed you may want to start exercising in the water before your six-week visit. Obtain permission from your surgeon before getting in the water.

Finding a Pool

The most common location for pool therapy is at a local park-district recreation center. Typically, this type of facility will have both a lap pool and a large hot-tub whirlpool. If such a facility is unavailable in your community, many private health clubs also offer pool therapy. Call your local chapter of the Arthritis Foundation; they should be able to direct you to pools in your area that are set up specifically for treating patients.

Many patients enjoy the hot tub so much that they have one installed at their home. While there is more expense involved with owning your own hot tub, it does provide more freedom and privacy, easier access, and unlimited availability.

Hot vs. Cool Water—or Both?

So what temperature is best for pool therapy for a TKA? Unfortunately, unless you have a hot tub at your home, the temperature of the water will be regulated by the facility where the pool is located. Not to worry. As long as the temperature is not too hot (in excess of 106 degrees Fahrenheit) or too cold (below 70 degrees Fahrenheit), the temperature of the water is not a problem. However, you will find that hot water works better for some exercises and that cool water is ideal for others. The best-case scenario would be to do your pool therapy at a recreational facility or health club that has a large hot tub or whirlpool as well as a lap pool. Range-of-motion exercises work best in hot water, and conditioning and walking exercises should be done in cool water. However, if the pool facility only has one or the other, all the exercises suggested in this chapter can be done in either hot or cool water.

Getting Into and Out of the Water

For many patients, getting in and out of the pool is the biggest obstacle. Some pools lack stairs with a railing. The only way to enter or exit is via a ladder at the side of the pool. Until a patient has more than 115 degrees of motion in their TKA, this type of ladder is too difficult to use to get into and out of the water. Many pools that lack stairs and railings will have a hydraulic-lift apparatus that attaches to the pool deck and safely transfers you in and out of the water until you gain enough knee motion to use the ladder on the side of the pool. Ask the facility attendant or lifeguard if they have one of these lifts available for your use.

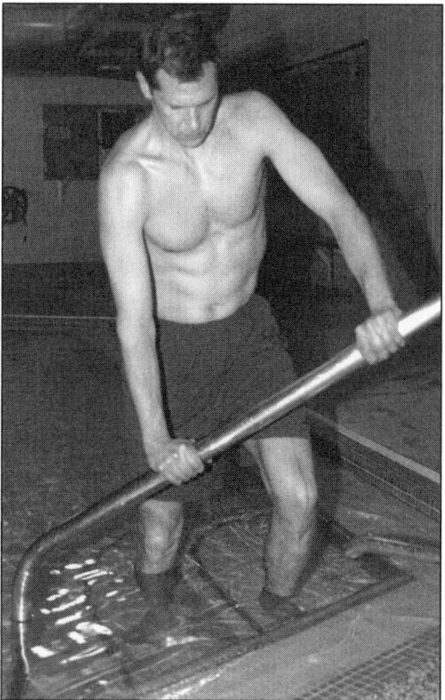

Figure 9.1. Getting into pool using side-step method

At some pools with stairs and railings, the steps have a very high rise that may be difficult to negotiate due to the limited motion in your TKA. If this is the case, the easiest way to get into the water is to turn and face the railing, then "side step" down the stairs into the water, leading with the TKA leg and controlling your weight and descent by holding onto the railing (Figure 9.1).

Even with bilateral TKAs, Dr. Falkel was able to use this technique safely and successfully with very limited range of motion.

How Long and How Often?

Once you try pool therapy, you may want to do it every day! Why not? At this stage of rehabilitation, there is no reason not to use the hot tub every day. The major concern about using a hot tub is staying in too long. The higher the temperature of the water, the harder the heart has to work to help dissipate the heat the body absorbs from the water. That is why it is difficult and even exhausting to exercise or swim vigorously in extremely warm water.

For the hot-tub range-of-motion exercises outlined below, we recommend no more than twenty minutes at a time in the warm water. More vigorous, aerobic exercises should not be performed in warm water. *If you have any form of cardiovascular medical condition, before starting pool therapy you must discuss it with your primary-care physician, internist, or cardiologist as well as with your orthopedic surgeon.*

For cool-water therapy, the duration of exercise is limited by the temperature of the water and the level of activity of the exercise. With more vigorous walking and swimming exercises, the body will heat up so that the coolness of the water is not a concern. However, when performing less intense range-of-motion exercises in a cool pool, ten to fifteen minutes may be all that is tolerable. The duration of exercise in cool water is determined by your endurance as well as by your tolerance to the colder water.

The best of both worlds would be to use a facility that has a hot tub and a lap pool in the same area. In this case, we recommend starting with fifteen to twenty minutes in the hot tub to warm up the TKA with range-of-motion exercises, then twenty to thirty minutes in the lap pool for walking and conditioning exercises, followed by ten to fifteen minutes in the hot tub. It will be the best hour of your day, and your TKA will love it!

Range-of-Motion Exercises

We have divided pool-therapy exercises into four sections: self-directed range-of-motion exercises, water-walking exercises, water plyometric exercises, and swimming for exercise.

Although a TKA may be stiff on dry land, it will seem much "looser" in the water. In fact, for some patients, the water is where the most range of motion is gained. Dr. Falkel's experience serves as a case in point. At four weeks post-op, he had very limited motion in both TKAs—88 degrees flexion on the left, and 72 degrees on the right. He was convinced that something was wrong and went back to one of his surgeons for an evaluation. The X ray showed no blockage or anything wrong with the TKA, and it was determined that his knees were just tight. The surgeon was concerned as well, and he gave Dr. Falkel two weeks to get to at least 90 degrees of flexion in both knees or he would have to have his TKAs manipulated (more on TKA manipulation in Appendix A). So Dr. Falkel headed straight to the pool. He spent thirty minutes in the hot tub, sixty minutes in the lap pool, and another thirty minutes back in the hot tub. By the end of his third day of pool therapy he had 105 degrees of flexion in both TKAs! After two more weeks of pool therapy he was able to reach his goal of 120 degrees of flexion in both knees; and after a month of pool therapy his knee stiffness was gone for good!

Here are some simple yet very effective self-directed range-of-motion exercises that can be done in a hot tub.

First, sit on the bench in the hot tub for approximately five minutes to warm up your TKA. If the bench is too low for you to comfortably sit on, see about having a plastic chair placed in the hot tub for you to use instead.

Exercise 67

Sliding on Chair in Hot Tub

Sitting on the bench, move the foot of your TKA leg back as far as possible. Then slide your bottom forward on the bench while keeping the TKA foot still (Figure 9.2). Hold this position as long as possible. (This is similar to Exercise 23.)

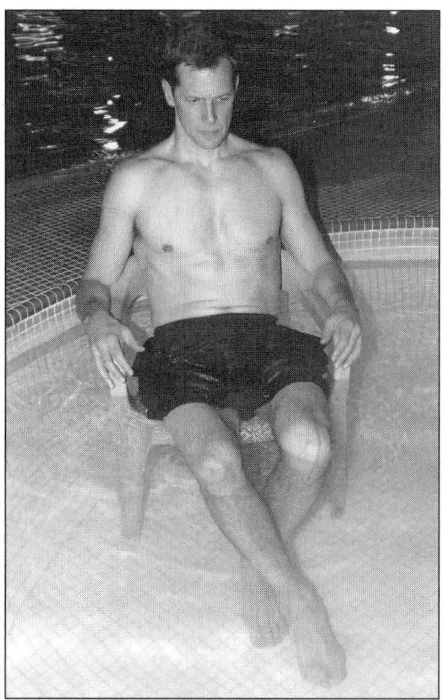

Figure 9.2. Range-of-motion exercise in hot tub, sliding back and forth while sitting on bench or chair

Exercise 68

Sitting Down with Heels Against Chair in Hot Tub

Stand in front of the bench with your heels against the riser of the bench. If you're using a chair, place your heels against the legs of the chair. Try to sit down without letting your TKA foot slip forward from the riser of the bench (Figure 9.3).

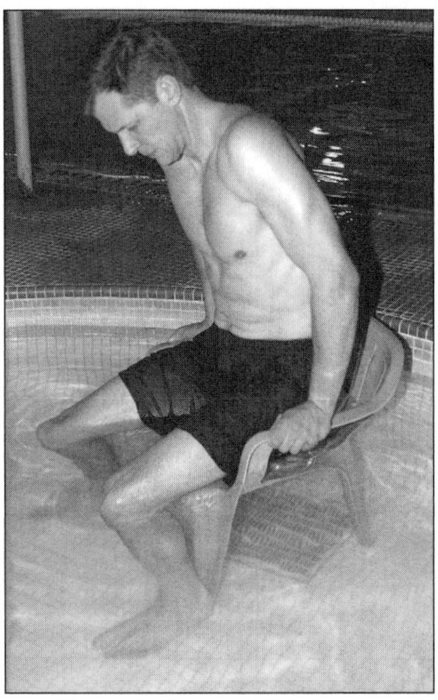

Figure 9.3. Range-of-motion exercise in hot tub, placing heels of both feet against bench or chair and sitting down without moving heels

Exercise 69

Knee-Rocking Exercise in Hot Tub

Stand next to the railing, and while facing the step or bench, place the foot of your TKA leg on the stair step or bench with your toes against the riser of the stair or bench.

1. Rock back and forth, working on getting as much flexion as you can in the TKA (Figure 9.4).
2. Rock back and forth for 10–15 repetitions; then flex the TKA as much as possible, and hold the flexed position for 2–5 minutes.

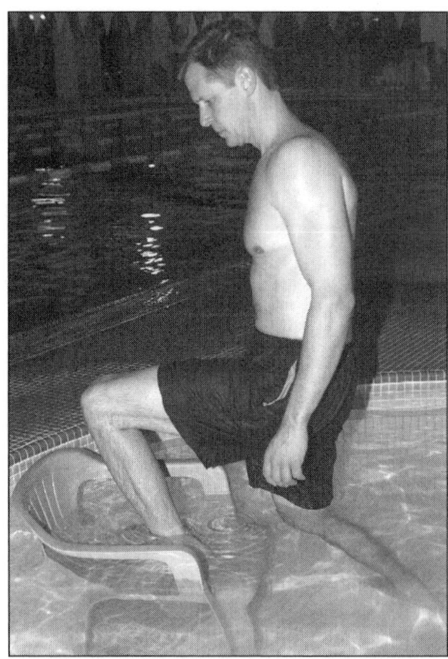

Figure 9.4. Range-of-motion exercise in hot tub, placing foot of TKA leg on bench or chair and rocking forward and backward to increase flexion

3. Rock back and forth for 10–15 repetitions; then lower your bottom to get as much flexion as possible in your TKA (Figure 9.5). Hold this position for 2–5 minutes.

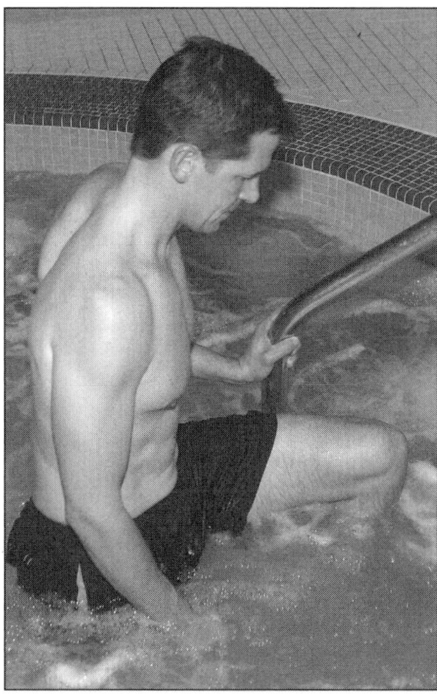

Figure 9.5. Range-of-motion exercise in hot tub, lowering hips with TKA foot on stair step to increase flexion

Exercise 70

Active Knee Motion in Hot Tub

Sitting on a chair or bench in the water, try to kick yourself in the buttocks with the heel of your TKA leg (Figure 9.6). This adds the resistance of the water to your attempts at knee flexion.

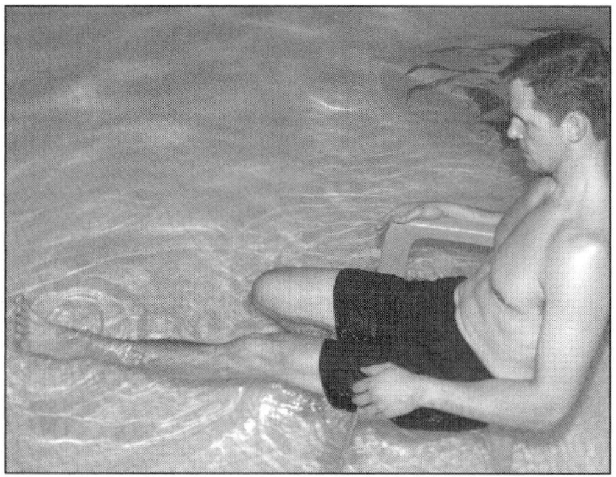

Figure 9.6. Range-of-motion exercise in hot tub with active knee motion of TKA leg

Exercise 71

Active Flexion and Extension Against Water Resistance

Sit on the edge of the hot tub with your TKA knee flexed as much as possible. Straighten your TKA leg using the resistance of the water. Then once again bend the TKA knee against the resistance of the water (Figure 9.7). Complete 3–5 sets of 5–10 repetitions each.

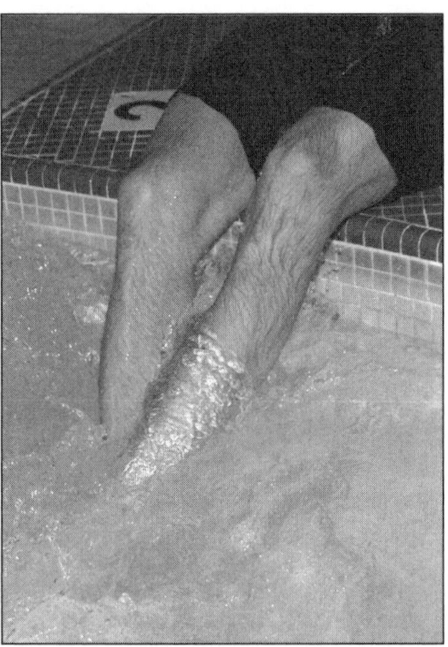

Figure 9.7. Active flexion and extension against resistance of water

Exercise 72

Sit-to-Stand Exercise in Hot Tub

Sit on the edge of the bench, and practice going from sitting to standing and then back to sitting (Figure 9.8). Hold on to a handrail only if necessary.

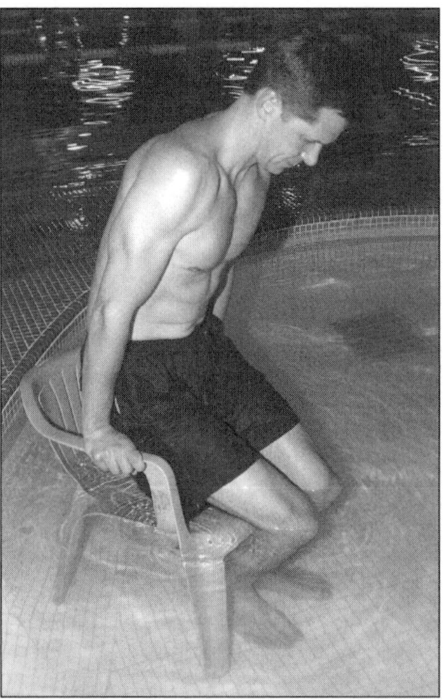

Figure 9.8. Sit-to-stand strengthening and range-of-motion exercise in hot tub

Exercise 73

Hamstring Stretch in Hot Tub

Standing, hold on to the railing, and face the bench or stair with the heel of the TKA leg resting on the bench or stair and the leg nearly straight (Figure 9.9).

1. Bend the TKA knee slightly.
2. Bend forward at the waist.
3. Try to straighten the TKA knee while maintaining position 2.
4. Hold the stretch in the hamstrings for 60–90 seconds, and repeat 5–10 times.

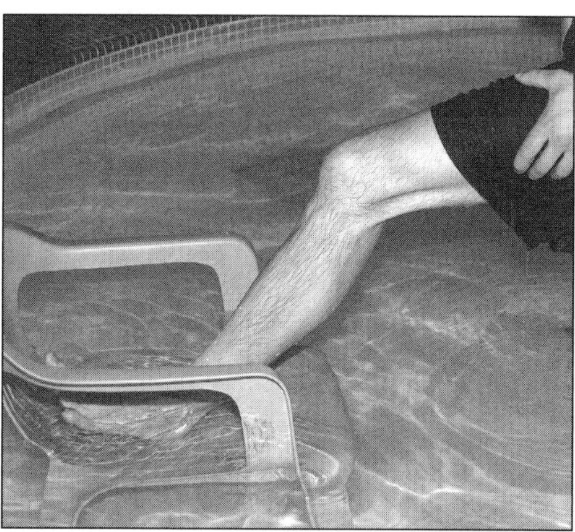

Figure 9.9. Hamstring stretching exercise in hot tub

Exercise 74

Soft-Tissue Massage in Hot Tub

Sit on the bench, and perform soft-tissue massage over the incision and along the side of the incision over the tight area in the quadriceps (Figure 9.10). Soft-tissue massage should also be done along the inside and outside of the lateral knee ligaments, as discussed in Chapter 8. The warm water enhances soft-tissue massage.

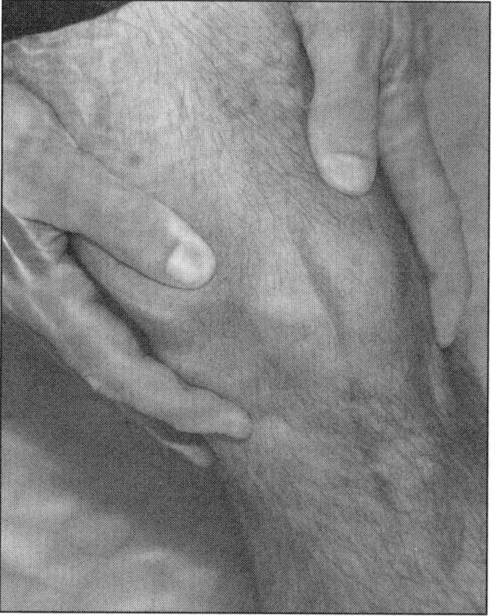

Figure 9.10. Soft-tissue mobilization while in hot tub

Exercise 75

Walking in Hot Tub

If possible, walk around in the hot tub for 5–10 minutes trying to walk as "normally" as possible.

Exercise 76

Balancing on TKA Leg in Hot Tub

Stand on the floor of the hot tub, holding on to the rail for support. Stand on the TKA foot, and lift the opposite foot to balance on just the TKA leg (Figure 9.11).

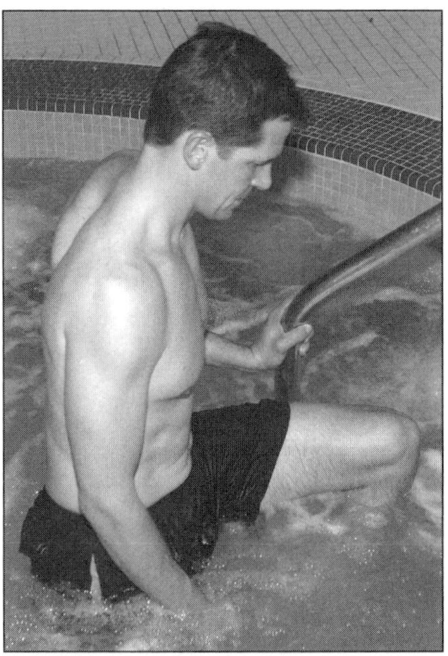

Figure 9.11. Single-leg stance balance training in hot tub

Exercise 77

Balancing on TKA Leg in Hot Tub While Swinging Other Leg

Stand on the TKA foot, and swing the opposite leg against the resistance of the water.

Exercise 78

Mini-Squat on TKA Leg in Hot Tub

Stand on the TKA foot, lift the opposite foot off the bottom of the hot tub, and do mini-squats on just the TKA leg. Let go of the railing as your balance improves.

■ ■ ■

The first few times most patients participate in pool therapy they achieve more range of motion than they had previously during the rehab process. What a glorious feeling! However, as a result, most patients also experience some additional soreness in their quadriceps muscles and around their TKA after pool therapy. This is perfectly normal and will subside after several pool-therapy sessions. As long as you follow the guidelines discussed in the question-and-answer section of the last chapter, you don't need to worry about whether you're overdoing it. The gains you will reap from water therapy far outweigh the pain!

Water-Walking Exercises

After twenty minutes or so in the hot tub, go to the lap pool for water-walking exercises. When was the last time you can remember walking "normally" and without a limp? For a majority of TKA patients, years of knee pain and dysfunction have produced an abnormal gait. Part of the goal of rehabilitation from here forward is to relearn to walk normally. A lap pool is a perfect place to practice. In waist-deep water the buoyancy of the water eliminates almost 50 percent of your body weight, and in chest-deep water almost 75 percent of your weight. Therefore, little stress is placed on your TKA during water walking. In addition, the water will help with balance, enabling you to walk in the water without assistance from a cane, crutches, or a walker. (If you still have problems with balance, most pools have various floatation devices that you can use to make you feel more secure in the water.) There are several different types of walking exercises that will help you regain both a more normal walking pattern and strength and conditioning after your TKA surgery.

Exercise 79

Walking Forward in Pool

Concentrate on spending the same amount of time on each foot. Counting to yourself or "marching" in time to music will help you do this. (Part of the reason for your preoperative limp was because you spent more time on your "good" foot and less time on your "bad" foot.)

Exercise 80

Walking Backward in Pool

This is a great exercise for strengthening and conditioning the hamstrings. Be careful to avoid running into anyone or anything.

Exercise 81

Walking Sideways in Pool

Move one hip and leg out to the side (Figure 9.12), and then bring the other toward the first. Alternate leading with both the right and the left side.

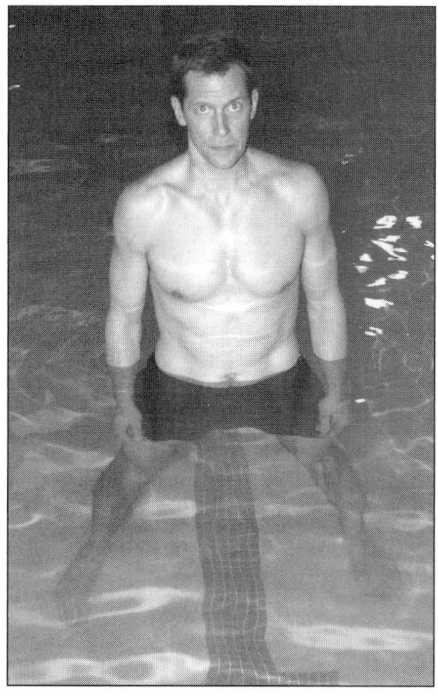

Figure 9.12. Walking sideways in pool

Exercise 82

High-Knee Walking in Pool

Walk forward by lifting your knees as high as possible against the resistance of the water with each step (Figure 9.13).

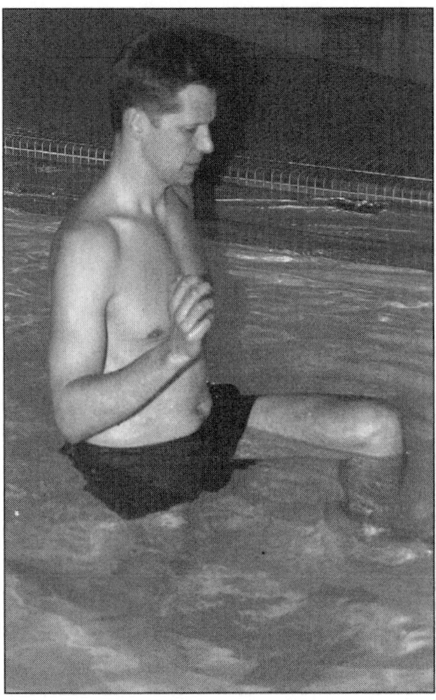

Figure 9.13. High-knee walking in pool

Exercise 83

Lunge Walking in Pool

Walk forward by taking progressively larger and longer steps (Figure 9.14). This works best in the shallow end of the pool so you can lower your bottom and get more knee flexion with each step.

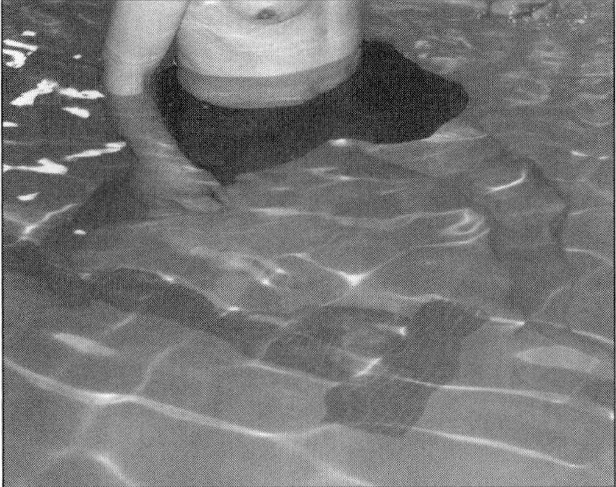

Figure 9.14. Lunge walking in pool

Exercise 84

Toe Walking in Pool

On your toes, walk forward, backward, and sideways.

Exercise 85

Swinging Nonoperated Leg While Balancing on TKA Leg in Pool

Stand on the TKA leg in chest-deep water, and swing the opposite leg forward and backward against the resistance of the water (Figure 9.15).

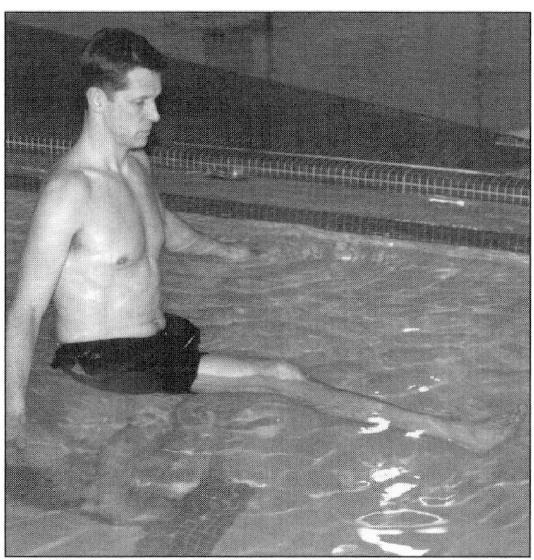

Figure 9.15. Dynamic single-leg stance balance exercise in pool

■ ■ ■

With each of these exercises, start slowly and deliberately, concentrating on trying to walk with good form. Then progressively walk faster against the resistance of the water to increase your strength and conditioning.

Water Plyometric Exercises

Plyometric exercises are used primarily with athletes to teach them how to change directions quickly. Although your "athletic career" may be a thing of the past, you still need to be able to stop and change directions quickly while walking. The water is the easiest and best place to practice this skill. Eventually we will recommend doing these types of movement on land—it makes going to the store or mall a lot safer.

Note: *The pictures of the aquatic exercises are taken in shallow water to better illustrate the legs while performing the exercises. The descriptions of the exercises frequently state that the patient should start in chest-deep water. The deeper the water, the less effect gravity has on the patient. Unfortunately it is more difficult to show the exercise in deeper water. Therefore, we recommend that while actually performing these exercises, the patient should start in chest-deep water.*

Exercise 86

Exaggerated Marching in Place in Pool

Stand in chest-deep water. Practice marching in place, but exaggerate bringing your knees up as high as you can against the resistance of the water (Figure 9.16).

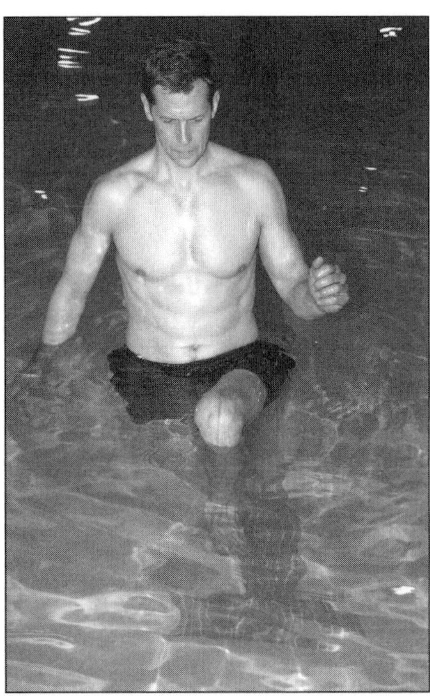

Figure 9.16. Marching in place in pool

Exercise 87

Jumping Up and Down in Pool

Stand in chest-deep water. Practice "jumping" up and down (Figure 9.17).

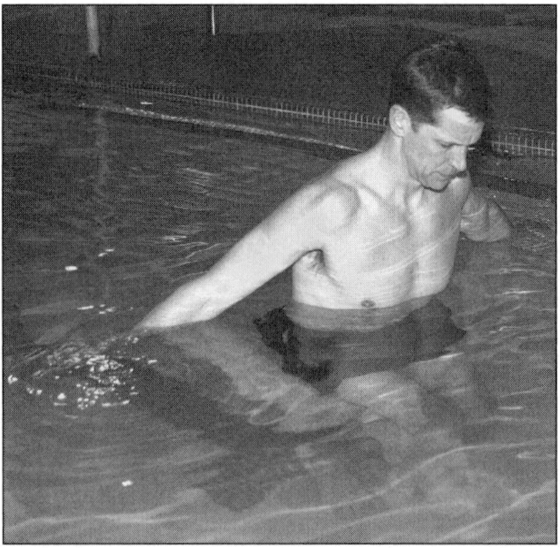

Figure 9.17. Standing jumps in pool

Exercise 88

Crunch Jumps in Pool

Stand in chest-deep water. Practice "jumping" up and down, but this time bring your knees up as high as possible with each jump (Figure 9.18).

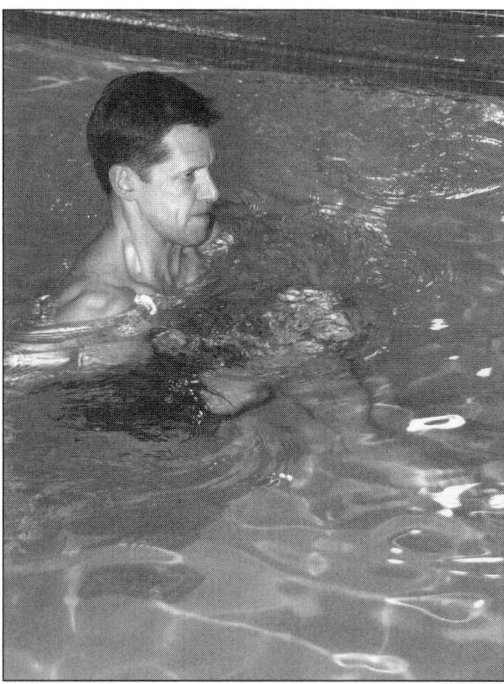

Figure 9.18. Crunch jumps in pool

Exercise 89

Running in Place in Pool

Stand in chest-deep water. "Run" in place.

Exercises 90 and 91

Hopping Side-to-Side on Both Legs or TKA Leg in Pool

Stand in chest-deep water. "Hop" from side to side over the lane line on the bottom of the pool (Figure 9.19).

1. Start with both legs.
2. Progress to hopping on just the TKA leg.

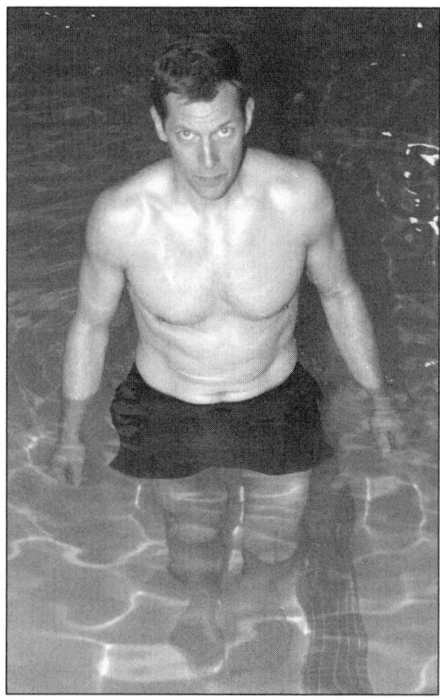

Figure 9.19. Side-to-side hops over lane line in pool

Exercises 92 and 93

Hopping Forward and Backward on Both Legs or TKA Leg in Pool

Stand in chest-deep water. "Hop" forward and backward over the line on the bottom of the pool (Figure 9.20).

1. Start with both legs.
2. Progress to hopping on just the TKA leg.

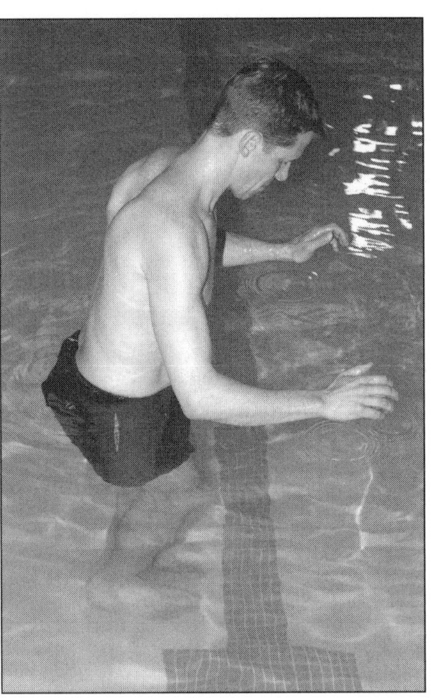

Figure 9.20. Forward and backward hops over lane line in pool

Exercise 94

Kicking an Imaginary Ball in Pool

Stand in waist-deep water. Stand on your nonoperated leg and "kick" an imaginary ball with your TKA leg (Figure 9.21). Exaggerate the forward and backward motion of the kick.

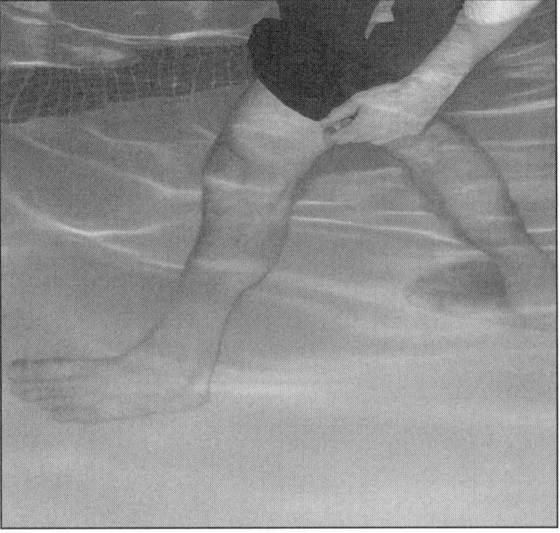

Figure 9.21. Kicking against the resistance of the water

Exercise 95

Jumping Jacks in Pool Against Water Resistance

Stand in waist-deep water. Jump up and then land with both feet apart, and then jump up and land with both feet together, like you're doing jumping jacks (Figure 9.22).

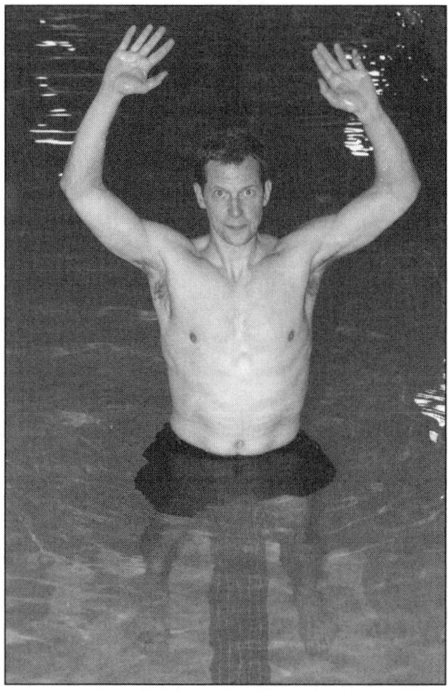

Figure 9.22. Jumping jacks against the resistance of the water

Exercise 96

Scissor Kicks in Pool Against Water Resistance

Stand in waist-deep water. Scissor kick one leg forward while the other leg goes backward. Repeat in the opposite direction.

Exercise 97

Running in the Deep End Wearing Life Vest

Using a life vest, "run" in place in the deep end so your feet cannot touch the bottom of the pool. If you are not a good swimmer and/or if you are not comfortable and confident in the water, we would suggest that you not attempt this exercise.

Swimming for Exercise

If you were a good or proficient swimmer before your TKA surgery, then swimming is a great rehabilitation exercise. However, if you are not a good swimmer, or if you do not have a great deal of confidence in the water, the exercises described above can be done safely in the shallow end of the pool, with or without floatation devices, to allow you to be as comfortable as possible. If you do not know how to swim, don't let this prevent you from doing pool exercises. The water is too good a medium for rehabilitation to avoid using it just because you don't know how to swim. The previous exercises can be done by most patients regardless of their swimming ability.

For patients who can swim, here is a progression that will help get you back to swimming laps again. It will take some time before you are able to swim effectively because your TKA leg will be weaker than the other leg when you first return to the pool.

Exercise 98

Kicking While Holding On to Side of Pool

Hold on to the side of the pool, let your legs float up to the surface, and practice kicking (Figure 9.23).

Exercises 99, 100, and 101

Flutter, Dolphin, and Frog Kicks Using Kickboard

Grab a kickboard. Using it to help with floatation, practice kicking in the following patterns:

1. Flutter kicks
2. Dolphin kicks (as for the butterfly stroke)
3. Frog kicks (as for the breaststroke)

Being able to do the frog kick may take some time due to soreness in the collateral ligaments on the sides of the knee.

Exercise 102

Strengthening Upper Body Using Flotation Device

Swim with a floatation device (pull buoy) between your legs. This will help get your arm and torso muscles in shape for swimming laps.

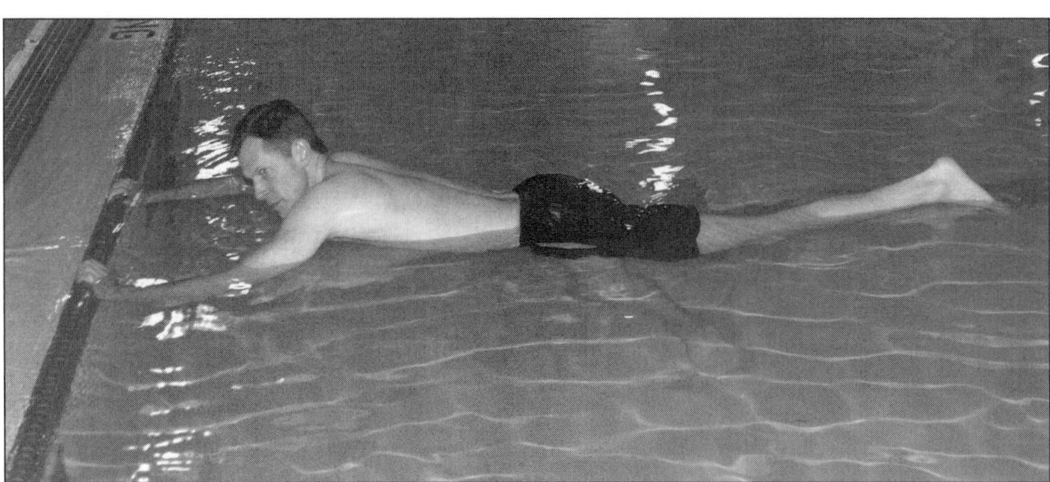

Figure 9.23. Flutter kicks holding on to side of pool

■ ■ ■

Start with three to five minutes of swimming or swim exercises, and gradually progress to twenty or thirty minutes per training session. Swimming is an outstanding exercise for patients who have undergone total knee replacement. It confers many benefits (described throughout this chapter) while producing none of the weight-bearing stresses of other types of exercises.

Pool Therapy with Other Exercises

We have one last suggestion. If there is a hot tub or pool at the facility where you will be doing your other TKA rehabilitation exercises (i.e., a health club or recreation facility), consider starting your exercise session by warming up in the hot tub. The hot tub will loosen up your TKA, allowing more range of motion and comfort while doing the other exercises. Some people also find that using the hot tub after a general exercise program helps to relax their TKA, allowing them to leave the training facility with their knees feeling loose and relaxed. Whether you use the hot tub before or after your exercise program is up to your individual preference; both ways offer benefits. Experiment by trying either way, and do what works best for you.

? Common Questions and Some Answers

Where can I find a pool or hot tub near my house?

In addition to checking with the local Arthritis Foundation chapter, your surgeon or physical therapist can be a good resource for finding a nearby pool facility. You can also call the local park and recreation district for more information.

Will my insurance pay for pool rehabilitation?

It is possible that your insurance company might pay for pool therapy as part of an overall outpatient physical-therapy program, as long as it is prescribed by your surgeon. Some insurance companies may even pay for part of a health-club membership, if prescribed by a physician. Check with your specific insurance company to see if you have this benefit.

How long should I continue pool therapy?

Pool therapy is extremely beneficial for all aspects of TKA rehabilitation for the first three to six months after surgery. After six months of rehabilitation, pool therapy is a great modality for a long-term exercise program because of the low-impact nature of the water. Some form of exercise is needed for long-term maintenance of the TKA as well as for cardiovascular health and weight control. If pool therapy is convenient and enjoyable, it is highly recommended as a form of exercise.

- **Is pool therapy used as part of an outpatient physical-therapy program?**

Pool therapy is often used in the overall treatment of the TKA patient in outpatient physical-therapy clinics that have easy access to a pool or hot tub. Although it's not absolutely essential, we feel it is worth the effort to attend an outpatient physical-therapy clinic that routinely uses pool therapy in their rehabilitation program. Since pool therapy is not available in all outpatient physical-therapy clinics, we suggest checking into this before starting your rehabilitation program.

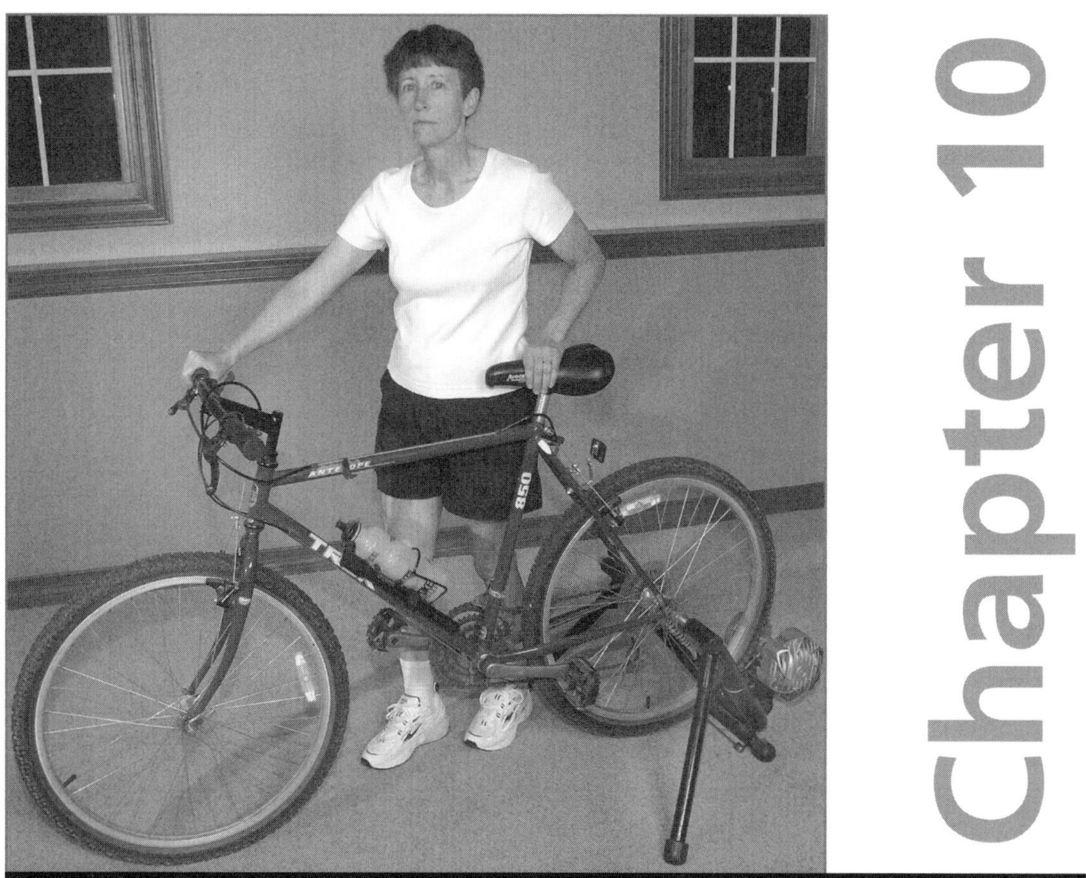

Chapter 10

Week Four

I Made It to My "Olympics"!

An orthopedic nurse working with one of our colleagues tells all of her total-knee-replacement patients that they need to approach the first month of their rehabilitation as though they were Olympic athletes preparing for the biggest competition of their lives. While there are few, if any, TKA patients who go on to compete in an Olympic event, all TKA patients need to have the same dedication and commitment to their rehabilitation that Olympic athletes have to their sport. At week four most patients have good range of motion, fair strength, and moderate endurance, and they are ideally sleeping through the night. In this chapter we will address these issues as well as the topic of getting back to a "more normal" life.

The Transition from Outpatient to Self-Directed Physical Therapy

If you receive outpatient physical therapy, your time there may be coming to an end due to insurance restrictions. Not to worry. There are many exercises and activities you can do on your own that will allow you to progress by building on the gains you made while in outpatient physical therapy.

At this point in your recovery you have several options for the continuation of rehabilitation. We will provide a number of exercises and activities that can be done at home, and we suggest you at least try each of them to find the ones that you enjoy and that seem to be most beneficial. However, many people who start pool therapy would rather continue their rehabilitation at a recreational facility or health club. This alternative is highly recommended as well. The advantage of using a health club or similar facility is that it will offer equipment comparable to that which most patients use during their outpatient physical therapy. Therefore, it is relatively easy to make the transition to a recreation center or health club. If you are going to utilize one of these facilities for your continued rehabilitation, we have a few suggestions:

1. Let your physical therapist know which facility you plan to attend. Many PTs will go with their patients one time to a health club to demonstrate which machines and equipment are "right" for them and how to adjust or modify the equipment to meet the needs of a TKA patient.
2. If your PT is unavailable to show you how to use the equipment at your facility, be sure to ask the facility manager if there is anyone on staff who might be able to demonstrate how to use the equipment safely, given the restrictions of having undergone TKA surgery a little over a month before. Most recreation centers and health clubs have professionals on staff who are certified in personal training or strength and conditioning. They should be able to assist you with any questions or concerns you might have.

Picking and Choosing from the Exercise "Smorgasbord"

By now we have described a multitude of different exercises that can be done at home to gain range of motion, strength, and endurance. If a patient were to do all of these exercises every day there would be no time left for a life! Therefore, at this point in your rehabilitation you should start picking and choosing which exercises work best for you.

In the last chapter we discussed pool therapy. If you have already started a pool-therapy program, we suggest continuing this form of training. The water provides both a great buoyant medium for exercise and an accommodating form of resistance. Increase the duration of your water walking, and increase your speed of movement in the water to gain more strength and muscular endurance.

The remainder of this chapter provides additional exercises that can be done at home using specialized equipment. It is important that patients do not limit their exercise program to one modality. Pool therapy and/or swimming is an excellent modality for cross-training. We recommend balancing your exercise program between pool therapy and home exercise.

If you are unable to continue your rehabilitation at a recreation facility or health club, we suggest that you obtain some exercise equipment for home use that will maximize the functional outcome of your TKA. The first piece of equipment we recommend is a stationary cycle. Dr. Falkel used one for most for his rehabilitation and continues using it on a daily basis for fitness and conditioning. As we discussed in Chapter 8, using a stationary cycle for gaining range of motion and speed of motion in the TKA is one of the best things a patient can do for his or her knee replacement. Using the stationary cycle at this point in your recovery will facilitate even greater range of motion, more speed of movement, and increased muscular and cardiovascular (heart) endurance for fitness and weight control. It is common for people who start using a stationary cycle at the PT clinic to find that their knee just doesn't feel as good when they don't get to use a stationary cycle every day. So get one! We suggest making an investment in a good stationary cycle, one that has an adjustable seat and adjustable braking tension that allows you to increase the resistance as you progress. Patients who enjoy riding a conventional bicycle outdoors can "create" their own custom stationary cycle by purchasing a bicycle stand from a specialized bicycle shop. The stand fits on the rear tire axle and allows for "riding" the bike indoors while developing range of motion and conditioning (see Figure 10.1 on the next page). Then when the patient is ready to start riding outside, all he needs to do is remove the bicycle stand and off he goes. A track stand also permits indoor riding when the weather is bad. The only drawback is that some of the bicycle stands lack a means to increase resistance while cycling. If this option is appealing, take your bicycle to the bike shop to discuss

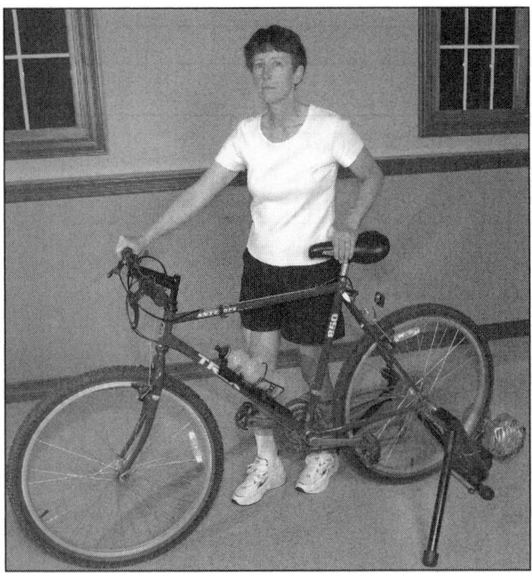

Figure 10.1. Track stand to allow for "riding" a regular bicycle after TKA surgery

your needs for rehabilitating and conditioning your TKA with the professionals. They should be able to get you set up and riding in no time!

Stationary-Cycling Exercises

Starting about one month following your surgery we recommend doing the following exercises while you're stationary cycling:

1. Lower the seat gradually to increase your knees' range of motion. Some patients ride for 10–15 minutes with the seat up high, and then after their TKA has gotten warmed up they ride for 10–15 minutes with the seat set lower. Other patients will lower the seat a little more each week to gain additional motion.
2. Try to pedal at a faster rate. When using a stationary cycle in the initial stages of rehabilitation you normally keep your movements very slow and controlled to avoid stressing the TKA and creating stiffness. Once you can easily pedal a full cycle, increase your rate of pedaling to improve speed of movement in your new knee. Aim for 50–100 revolutions per minute.
3. Increase the length of time you spend on the stationary cycle. Start with 5 minutes twice a day, and progress to 20–30 minutes twice a day. For optimal fitness and assistance in weight control, we recommend 30–45 minutes of stationary cycling at least four days per week. This will not only dramatically improve the muscular endurance in your legs, but it will also improve your heart and lung endurance.

Futebol Exercises

It is now time to include some advanced *futebol* exercises to help gain range of motion and speed in your TKA leg. These exercises are also a lot of fun—if TKA rehabilitation can be considered fun!

Exercise 103

Futebol "Catching" Exercise

Stand with your nonoperated leg next to the sink, and hold on to the sink with the hand on that same side of your body. Place the *futebol* under the bottom of your TKA foot, and then roll it gently away in front of you. Once the *futebol* starts rolling, lift your TKA foot and try to stop or catch the *futebol* while it's rolling. Then roll the *futebol* backward away from you, and, again, lift your TKA foot and try to catch the *futebol* behind you. Repeat, rolling the ball out to the side and then again in front of your standing leg (Figure 10.2). Complete 10–15 movements in each direction.

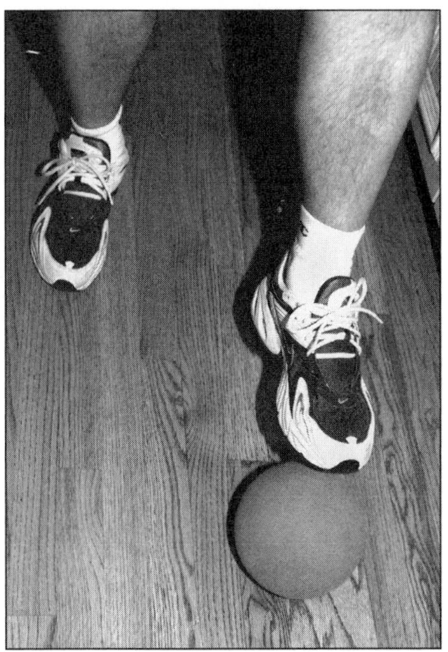

Figure 10.2. *Futebol* "catch" exercise with TKA leg

Exercise 104

Futebol "Scooping" Exercise

Stand with your nonoperated leg next to the sink, and hold on to the sink with the hand on that same side of your body. Place the *futebol* under your TKA foot, about 12–18 inches in front of you. Roll the *futebol* back with the bottom of your foot, then quickly bring the toes of your TKA foot behind and under the *futebol*, and try to scoop the ball up in the air. If the *futebol* bounces, place your TKA foot on top of the *futebol* to stop it from bouncing and try again (Figure 10.3). Complete 15–25 trials.

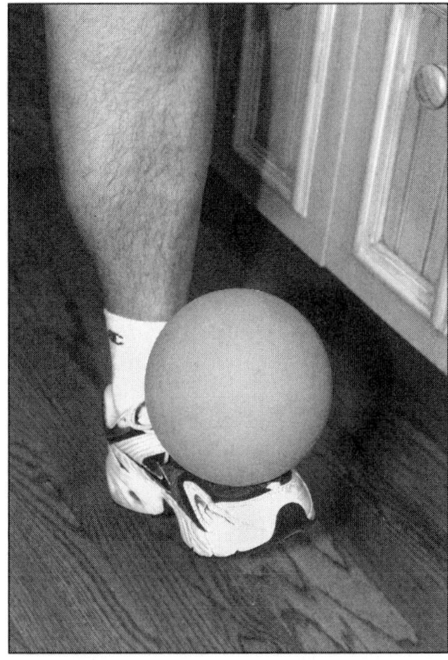

Figure 10.3. *Futebol* "scoop" exercise with TKA leg

Exercise 105

Futebol "Bounce-and-Stop Exercise

Stand with your nonoperated leg next to the sink, and hold on to the sink with the hand on that same side of your body. Hold the *futebol* with the other hand. Drop the *futebol* near the foot of your TKA leg. After the first or second bounce, lift your TKA foot and stop the ball's bouncing by placing the sole of your foot over the *futebol* (Figure 10.4). After the ball stops bouncing, pick it up and repeat the exercise 15–25 times.

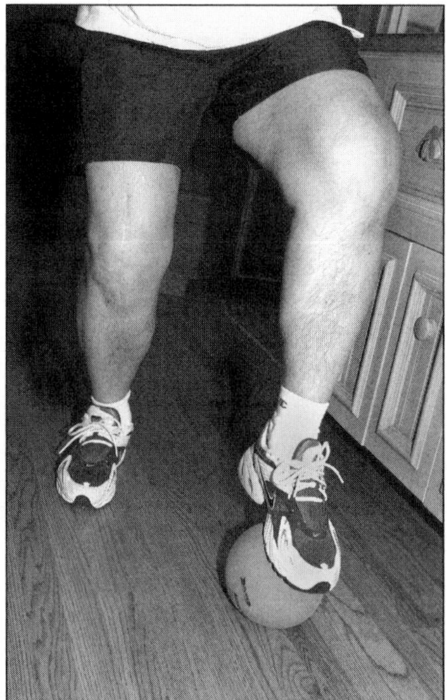

Figure 10.4. *Futebol* "bounce-and-stop" exercise with TKA leg

Exercise 106

Futebol "Bounce-and-Slap" Exercise

Stand with your nonoperated leg next to the sink, and hold on to the sink with the hand on that same side of your body. Hold the *futebol* with the other hand. Drop the *futebol* near the foot of your TKA leg. After the first or second bounce, lift your TKA foot, and try to keep the *futebol* bouncing by slapping it with the sole of your foot. Continue to slap the *futebol* with your foot to keep it bouncing, like a basketball player would dribble a basketball (Figure 10.5). After the *futebol* stops bouncing, pick it up and repeat the exercise 15–25 times.

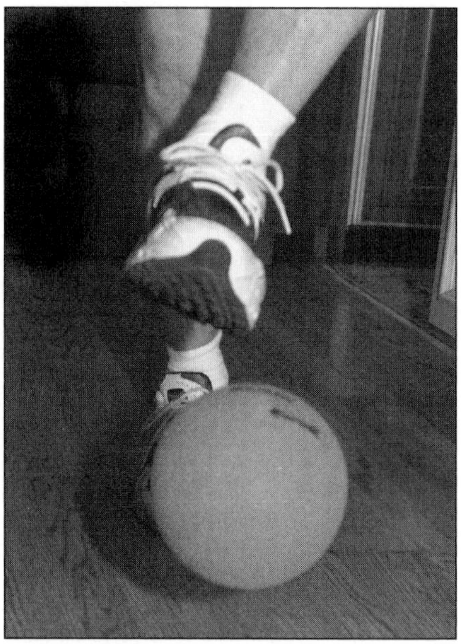

Figure 10.5. *Futebol* "bounce-and-slap" exercise with TKA leg

Exercises Using the Total Gym

An exercise apparatus used by many patients in outpatient rehabilitation is a Total Gym, described in Chapter 3. The Total Gym is an ingenious exercise machine that allows control of the resistance of the exercise based on movement of your body weight. By changing the height of the platform, you change the resistance created by the machine. The resistance can be as low as 10 percent of your body weight or as high as more than 70 percent of your body weight. And if you want even more, a weight bar can be added to increase the resistance for any exercise.

Other features of the Total Gym that make it ideal for home use by TKA patients are its portability, its silence, and its relatively low cost (when compared to memberships at health clubs). It can be used at any time of the day, by anyone in the family. But best of all, it provides a great workout for TKA patients.

For patients who do not want to join a health club or who for some other reason simply want to do their TKA rehabilitation at home, a Total Gym may be the answer. It allows gradual range-of-motion increases with each exercise, and it provides whole-body strength and conditioning exercises with minor adjustments. The setup for hamstring exercises is the best available for TKA patients. In Chapter 3 we described some overall conditioning exercises using a Total Gym. In this chapter we present several specific exercises for TKA rehabilitation. If you are interested in purchasing a Total Gym for home use, we recommend visiting their website for special patient discounts: www.totalgym.com.

The first several exercises are variations on squats. Lying on your back on the glideboard, place your feet on the squat stand in the various positions described below. (Imagine that the face of a clock appears on the squat stand. We will describe placement of the feet in terms of their position on the imaginary clock face.)

For each position, complete 3–5 sets of 10–15 repetitions each, and squat as much as your TKA will allow. Alternatively, for a great variation to improve muscular endurance, perform 10 repetitions of each exercise, one right after the other.

Exercise 107

Total Gym: Squat Variation, Feet at 9 o'clock and 3 o'clock

Place your feet in the wide position, with one foot at 9 o'clock and the other at 3 o'clock (Figure 10.6).

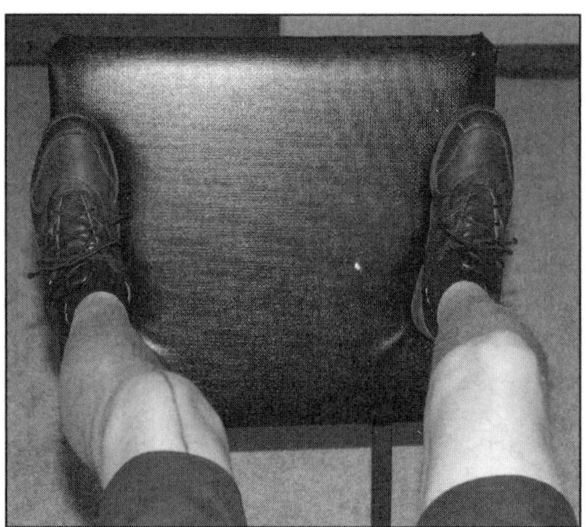

Figure 10.6. Total Gym squat-exercise variation: wide position

Exercise 108

Total Gym: Squat Variation, Feet Together

Place your feet together in the middle of the squat stand (Figure 10.7).

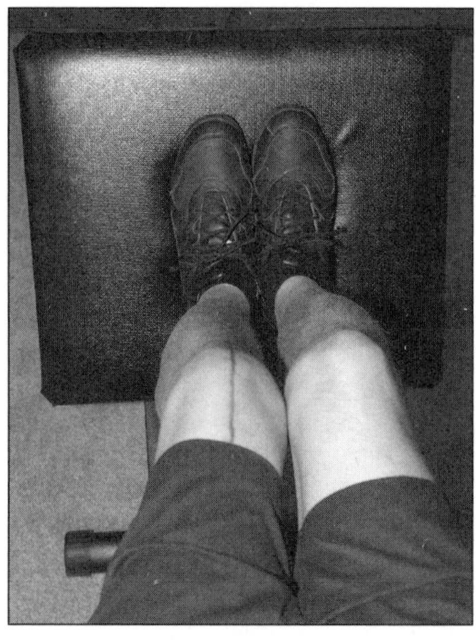

Figure 10.7. Total Gym squat-exercise variation: middle position

Exercise 109

Total Gym: Squat Variation, One Foot in Front of the Other

Place one foot at 12 o'clock and the other at 6 o'clock, so that one foot is in front of the other. Keep your toes pointing forward (Figure 10.8). Reverse the position of your legs, and repeat.

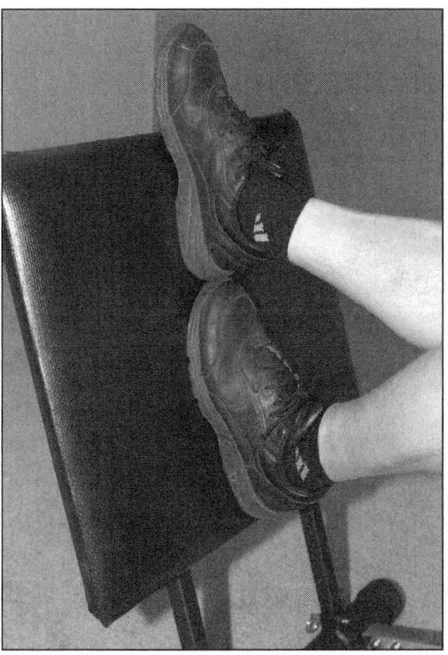

Figure 10.8. Total Gym squat-exercise variation: slalom ski position

Exercise 110

Total Gym: Squat Variation, Diagonal Foot Positions

Place your feet at 8 and 2 o'clock (Figure 10.9), and then at 10 and 4 o'clock.

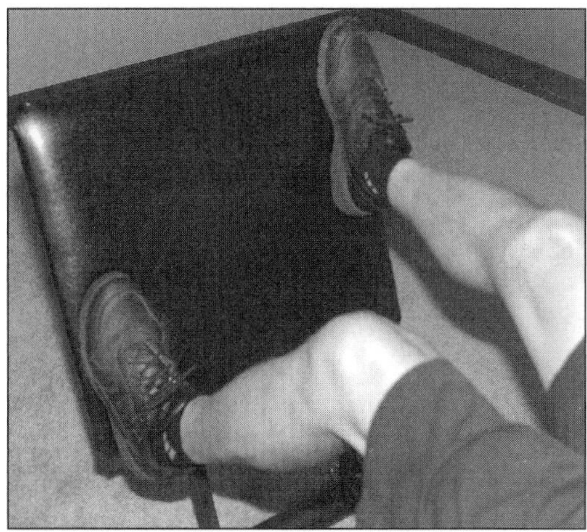

Figure 10.9. Total Gym squat-exercise variation: diagonal position

Exercise 111

Total Gym: Squat Variation, Heels Raised

A variation on Exercise 107 is to place your feet in the wide position, with one foot at 9 o'clock and the other at 3 o'clock. Then raise your heels and perform the squat movement while staying on your toes (Figure 10.10).

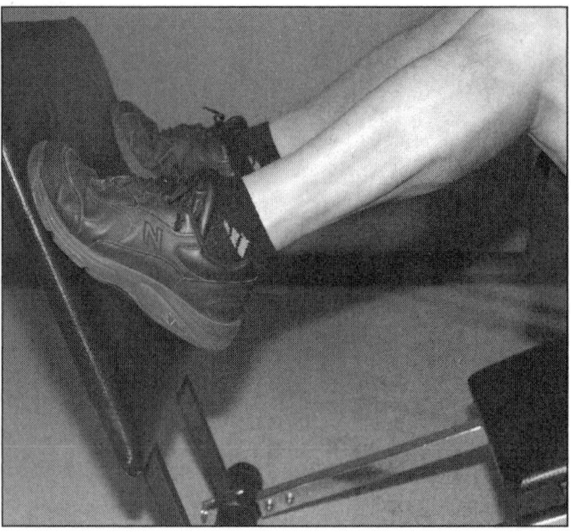

Figure 10.10. Total Gym squat-exercise variation: on-toes position

Exercise 112

Total Gym: Squat Variation, Single Leg

Stand on one leg in the center of the squat stand (Figure 10.11). Repeat on the other leg.

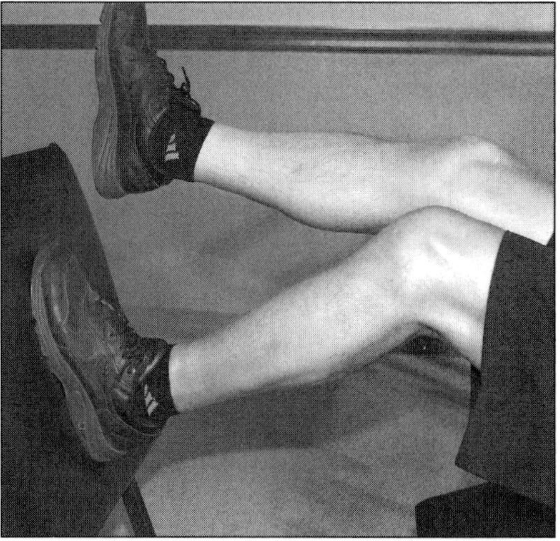

Figure 10.11. Total Gym squat-exercise variation: single leg in center position

Exercise 10

Total Gym: Hamstring Pull

(Also Described in Chapter 3)

Secure your feet in the wing. Lie on your back with your legs straight and your buttocks near the top of the glideboard. Point your toes toward the ceiling. Pull the glideboard toward your feet until it nearly reaches your heels. Lower the glideboard slowly. Next, try an advanced variation using one leg at a time. Rest the foot of the nonworking leg on the glideboard (Figure 10.12). This exercise is fantastic because it strengthens the hamstrings while avoiding any aggravation of the incision that normally occurs with most hamstring-exercise machines. Perform 3–5 sets of 10–15 repetitions each.

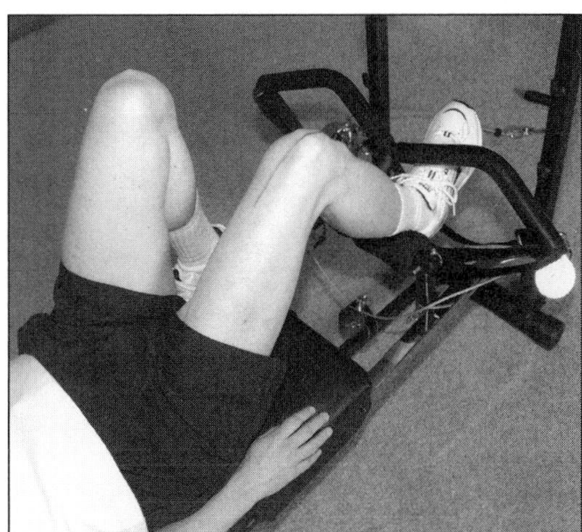

Figure 10.12. Total Gym hamstring-pull exercise (single leg)

Exercise 113

Total Gym: Incline Lunge

Remove the squat stand. Stand at the rear of the Total Gym, facing toward the ladder. Place the foot of the TKA leg on the lower part of the glideboard. Push the glideboard up the rails with the TKA foot, performing a partial squat (Figure 10.13). Slowly lower the glideboard to the end of the rails, and repeat. Perform the same exercise with the TKA foot on the ground and the foot of the nonoperated leg on the glideboard. Perform 3–5 sets of 10–15 repetitions each.

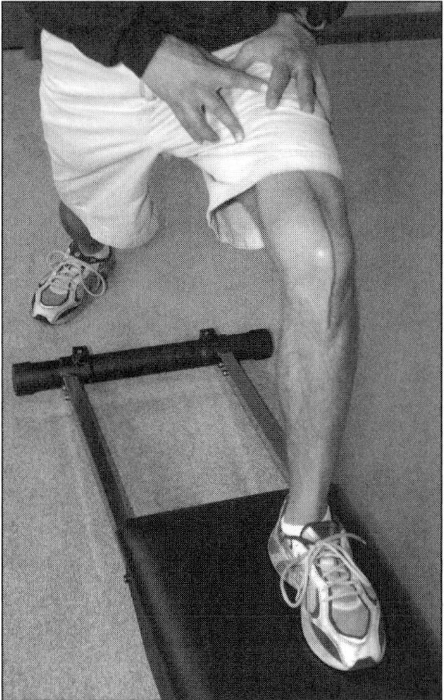

Figure 10.13. Total Gym incline lunge exercise

Exercise 114

Total Gym: Decline Lunge

Remove the squat stand. Stand at the rear of the Total Gym, facing away from the ladder. Place the foot of the TKA leg on the lower part of the glideboard. Push the glideboard up the rails with the TKA foot, performing a partial squat (Figure 10.14). Slowly lower the glideboard to the end of the rails, and repeat. Perform the same exercise with the TKA foot on the ground and the foot of the nonoperated leg on the glideboard. Perform 3–5 sets of 10–15 repetitions each.

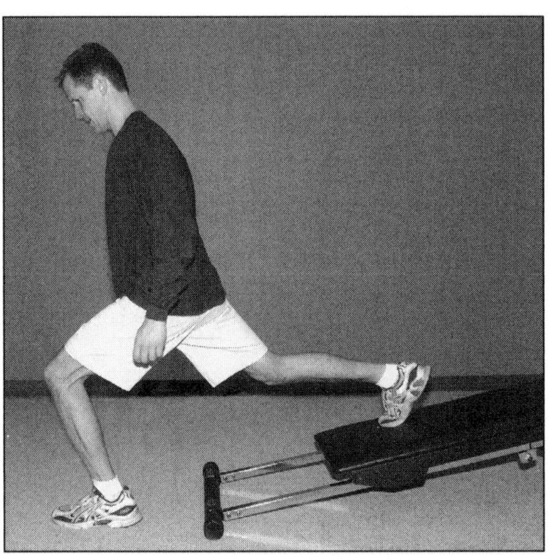

Figure 10.14. Total Gym decline lunge exercise

Exercise 9

Total Gym: Heel Raise

(Also Described in Chapter 3)

Lie on your back on the glideboard, facing away from the ladder. Place your toes on the bottom edge of the squat stand. Push your heels off the squat stand by rising up on your toes, lifting the heels as high as you can. Return to the starting position and repeat. Next, try an advanced variation in which you raise the heel of each leg one heel at a time (Figure 10.15). Perform 3–5 sets of 10–15 repetitions each.

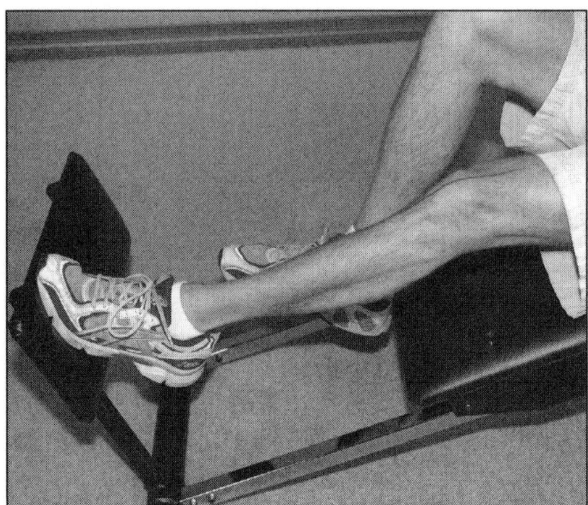

Figure 10.15. Total Gym heel-raise exercise (single leg)

Stationary Rowing

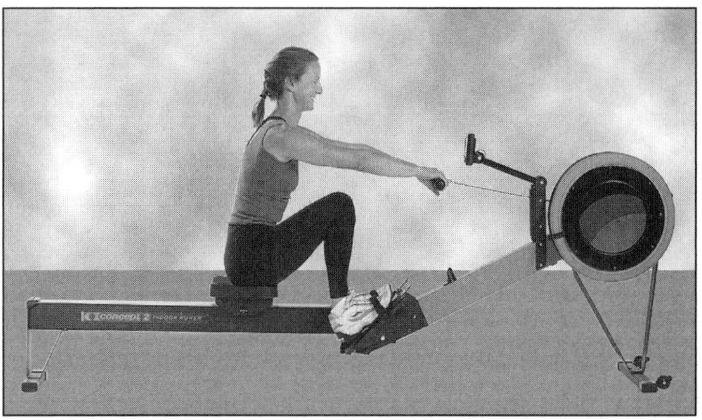

Another type of exercise apparatus that works very well for TKA patients is the stationary rowing machine. Stationary rowing enhances the knee's range of motion and increases overall conditioning. While there are many stationary rowing machines on the market today, the best and only model we can recommend is the Concept2 Indoor Rower (Figures 10.16 a and b). This rowing machine is unique because it uses a variable-air-resistance flywheel that allows for rowing as hard or as easily as the user chooses. It can be used for rehabilitation by people of all ages and fitness levels. It has a sliding seat that works extremely well for gaining dynamic range of motion after TKA. Because the resistance varies as a function of how hard the user pulls, when working on range of motion the user does not have to use any resistance to get a good training effect. Once your range of motion has improved, the Concept2 Indoor Rower is an excellent device for strength and endurance training of the lower body and cardiovascular system. Rowing is one of the best means of burning calories; therefore, the Concept2 Indoor Rower will also help the TKA patient with weight control. It is an excellent training apparatus, and one that we highly recommend.

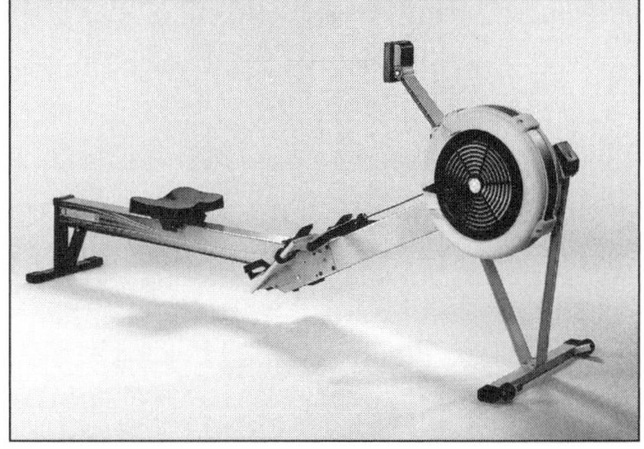

Figure 10.16a/b. Concept2 Rowing Ergometer Concept2 Indoor Rower. (Photos courtesy of Concept2 Indoor Rower)

For more information or to order a Concept2 Indoor Rower, contact Concept2 Inc., 105 Industrial Park Dr., Morrisville VT 05661. Call toll-free at (800) 245-5676, or visit their website at www.rowing@concept2.com.

Ice vs. Heat

At this time in the rehabilitation program, the use of ice or heat before or after exercise is really up to each individual patient. As long as there is no swelling after exercise, either ice or heat will work to make the TKA feel less painful and more relaxed. If there is swelling after exercise, many patients find that they respond better to using ice rather than heat. However, this is not true for all patients. Although ice and heat work via different mechanisms to reduce pain and stiffness in your TKA, they are both effective methods to relieve postexercise swelling and stiffness. Many patients use both—heat before exercise to warm up the TKA and ice after exercise to cool it down and reduce potential swelling. This is a very good option that works for a lot of patients. However, there is nothing that says ice before exercise or heat afterward cannot also be effective. Some patients prefer ice only, others, heat only. It is really up to each patient, and sometimes each knee. Although Dr. Falkel personally prefers heat, he has had four bilateral TKA patients in the past year who used ice on one of their TKAs and heat on the other. Whatever works, works!

Starting to Live Again!

After four weeks of rehabilitation it is time to start venturing out into the world. Although every TKA patient gets cabin fever from staying at home after surgery, be careful as you start leaving the house and returning to a more normal life. A wise physical-therapist colleague and friend of Dr. Falkel used to constantly remind him, "The bad news about feeling good is you get careless, so be careful!" And that PT is right. As your TKA feels better and you gain more confidence, you become less protective of your knee than you were just two weeks ago. As you begin interacting with people outside of your home, you should be extremely cautious. Just because you are walking with a cane in the grocery store or mall does not mean that other people are going to be watching out for you. In fact, many patients tell us that when they walk in public with their cane, they feel like it is invisible. We recommend that for at least the next few weeks you use a cane for balance when walking in public, especially in a crowd. We also suggest that you keep a cane in the car for the next several months so that you have it if you need it. Dr. Falkel kept a cane in his vehicle to use whenever there was snow or ice on the ground. Just having that extra stability when walking on slippery surfaces gave him confidence and security that he would not fall.

Standing Still

One of the biggest complaints of our patients at this stage is that they have a hard time standing still. For example, standing in a line at the grocery store can be problematic. It seems as if it takes only a few minutes for their knee to get stiff and perhaps even start to swell. This is perfectly natural, and it happens to everyone who has a TKA.

So what can be done to correct this problem? Practice standing! Although this suggestion may seem incredibly simplistic, it is the only way to develop the tolerance necessary to allow you to be comfortable with prolonged standing. Start with standing still in one spot for sixty to ninety seconds at a time, and slowly increase the time. You can practice while you're watching TV, doing the dishes, or even carrying on a conversation with friends or family. However, without practice to increase your standing tolerance, the next time you have to stand for a long time, such as in a line, your TKA will tell you loud and clear that you *should* have been practicing your standing tolerance! Typically, by three to six months after surgery, most TKA patients can comfortably stand still in one spot for a prolonged time without experiencing any residual stiffness in their TKA.

Sitting Tolerance

Starting this month you should also work on increasing your sitting tolerance. Even though there is no weight placed on your TKA when you're sitting, it can be difficult to sit in one place—such as in a car or movie theater—for any length of time. Just as with learning to stand in one place, you need to practice in order to develop your sitting tolerance.

Try to sit in chairs that allow you to move your legs comfortably without disturbing other people. Sitting in a car usually presents the most difficulty for TKA patients because the legroom is limited. If you are traveling any significant distance this month, we suggest that you stop every sixty to ninety minutes to get out and stretch your legs to minimize the stiffness in your TKA. This also improves the circulation in your legs, minimizing the chance of blood clots.

Before trying to go to a movie, practice sitting still at home. Depending on the number of people that are attending the show, it may be difficult or impossible to sit in an aisle seat, or to have extra room around your seat. It is quite common for TKA patients attending a movie to experience discomfort midway through the movie, affecting their concentration and sometimes forcing them to leave.

Driving

By this time in the rehabilitation process many TKA patients feel like they are ready to drive again. For most patients, when they *feel* ready to drive, they probably *are* ready to drive. A general guideline is that you should be able to support your full body weight on the operated leg and be able to quickly move your feet. To be safe while driving it is necessary to be able to move your foot quickly and to apply force to the pedals. Before you get behind the wheel, here are some suggestions:

1. Contact your surgeon for his or her approval.
2. It is critical to be off all narcotic pain medication.

3. If you have a left TKA and have a vehicle with manual transmission, practice working the clutch in your driveway before getting out on the road.
4. If you have a right TKA, practice moving your foot quickly from the accelerator to the brake. You must also be able to generate enough force to step hard on the brake.
5. Practice driving in an open area, such as a parking lot, where there will be fewer cars to worry about.
6. Go out for short trips at first, preferably with someone else who can drive if you are unable to complete the trip.
7. Avoid congested traffic as much as possible until you feel your speed of movement in the TKA leg is normal.
8. And as Dr. Falkel likes to joke with all of his TKA patients when they are first starting to drive again, "Please call me ahead of time so I can get off the road!"

Returning to Work

During your visits with your surgeon, the subject of returning to work usually comes up. The date when you can return to work is influenced by your overall health, the type of prosthesis used in your TKA, and the demands of your job. Because every job is different, and the physical and mental requirements of each job vary significantly, it may take four to six weeks after surgery to even start to think about returning to work. When you feel ready, discuss a return to work with your surgeon.

Working part-time at first, if possible, seems to be the ideal situation. Even though you might practice being up all day at home, the mental demands of many jobs can be extremely exhausting. It is amazing how easily and how quickly you tend to lose concentration upon first returning to work. We suggest working only two to four hours for the first few days (maybe for as long as a week) and then gradually increasing from there. Patients have found it helpful to return to work on a Thursday or Friday in order to have the weekend to rest before beginning a full week.

Many people are able to work from home for several weeks on their computer. It is our experience that these patients are able to make the transition back to full-time work more easily. If you have any questions, be sure to discuss them with your surgeon; he or she can probably authorize work modifications to make your transition to full-time work more tolerable.

Sleeping Through the Night

By this time you are hopefully able to sleep through the night. If you are not sleeping, be sure to ask your surgeon or primary-care physician for some prescription sleep medications that will allow you to get a good night's rest. Many TKA patients find that sleeping on their side with a pillow between the knees is the most comfortable position for them. A small pillow, similar to the size used on airliners, works extremely well. It is large enough to disperse the pressure of the top leg on the bottom leg, but small enough so that it will not interrupt your sleep if it falls out from between the knees when you turn over. Other people find that they get the best rest in a recliner; they might alternate between sleeping in bed and sleeping in the recliner.

Adequate sleep is of critical importance. Sleep encourages proper healing and prepares you to cope with postoperative pain. Proper rest is essential if you want to get the most out of your rehabilitation exercises.

Daily Activities

You and your TKA will know when it is time to begin a gradual return to your normal activities of daily living. Cooking, cleaning the house, going to the store, watching the kids' sporting activities, and other such endeavors can all be attempted without damaging the knee. Hopefully your knee is now only minimally painful or even pain free. Any residual pain typically fades with time. Many patients state that one of the main reasons why they elected to have surgery was to return to their normal daily activities without pain. Our suggestion is to try to do whatever you *think* you can do at this point in your rehabilitation. Don't get frustrated if you are unable to complete the task you are trying to accomplish. Remember, you underwent major surgery just over a month ago; therefore, you need to allow more time to finish any activity you start.

One task most patients cannot do at this time is to kneel on their TKA. Although you will not hurt the prosthetic components by kneeling on your TKA, for the majority of patients it is just too uncomfortable to kneel, particularly on the incision. Dr. Falkel still cannot comfortably kneel on either of his TKAs, and his surgery was in October 2000. So what? Other than trying to tie a five-year-old's soccer shoe one time, he has not had any occasion to have to kneel. He has learned how to avoid kneeling, and you will too. At the same time, some patients are able to kneel on their TKA as soon as the staples are removed. Everyone is different, and every TKA is different.

Going for a Walk

Part of venturing out of the house and getting back to normal is the need to walk longer distances. Many health-care professionals believe there is no better exercise than walking, and we agree. While many patients may at this point find an assistive device unnecessary, we highly encourage patients to use a cane while walking out in public, especially during the first few outings.

Before you can safely start walking longer distances, it is important to gradually build your stamina and endurance in both the TKA leg and your cardiovascular system. The best way to safely increase your stamina is to walk only the distance of one or two houses away from your home, using a cane or a walker. Then turn around and walk back to your home. If you are tired, you are back where you need to be. If you are not fatigued, you can walk one or two houses in the other direction and then return. It is a helpless feeling to start walking and then to experience overwhelming fatigue so far away from home that you can't make it back. Gradually increase the distance of your walks from home by adding three or five houses in each direction, as tolerated. Another alternative is to walk with someone else who can carry a chair for you to rest in if necessary.

Many patients walk around the local mall when pedestrian traffic is minimal, where it is warm and dry, with a smooth surface free of ice and snow. Have someone scout the mall before beginning a walking program. If there are no places to stop and rest in the mall, wait a few more weeks before walking there so you will have a little more time to improve your endurance beforehand. In the next chapter we discuss walking in greater detail, and we present some exercises and activities to help you start walking "normally" again.

? Common Questions and Some Answers

- **How much can I push myself with the activities of daily living?**

The patient is the one who best knows how much to push. We tell our patients to use the "retrospectoscope." Following activity, if they experience an increase in pain later that night or the next morning, they have probably pushed themselves too hard. If there is no significant increase in pain following activity, it is safe to increase your activity level.

- **When can I discontinue using the cane?**

The primary reason for using a cane is to provide some extra stability and balance while walking. As your balance improves, you will find you put less and less weight on the cane while you are walking. The first indication that the cane is no longer necessary is when you begin to forget it and start walking without it. As you continually leave your cane behind, it is time to put it in the closet and start walking without it. However, you may need to use it when you're walking on uneven surfaces or in inclement weather such as ice, snow, or rain. The best rule to follow is if you think you should use your cane for safety, then use it. We recommend to all of our patients that they keep their cane in their vehicle for several months, just in case.

Why is the skin still numb near my TKA incision, and how long will that last?

When the skin incision is made during surgery, small, almost microscopic sensory nerves near the skin are cut. This is unavoidable. Once these sensory nerves are damaged, the result is skin numbness around the incision. The numbness will resolve with time. The rate and degree of improvement varies with each individual and can even be different for each TKA in the same patient. It may take a year or two for the sensation to reach maximal improvement, and some patients will always have a small area that remains numb. Any residual numbness will not affect the overall function of the TKA.

Why is it easier to pedal backwards on the stationary cycle?

When you pedal forward, the quadriceps muscle in the front of your thigh has to be stretched at both ends in order to bend your knee. Because of the surgical cutting of the quadriceps, this stretching can be very painful. However, when you pedal backwards, the lower end of the quadriceps is stretched while the upper end, attached to the pelvis, goes "slack"; therefore, it is initially easier to pedal the stationary cycle backwards. After a few backwards revolutions, it becomes easier to pedal forward.

How long will my TKA look swollen?

The amount and duration of swelling is different for every patient. The majority of swelling is gone between six and twelve months after surgery. However, there may be occasions when the TKA will swell in response to a change in activity level or even a change in weather. If this occurs, the swelling is usually gone within a day or two.

How long do I have to sleep with a pillow between my knees?

As long as it is comfortable. Some patients sleep with a pillow between their knees forever. The pillow has nothing to do with the healing of the TKA; it is just for comfort while sleeping.

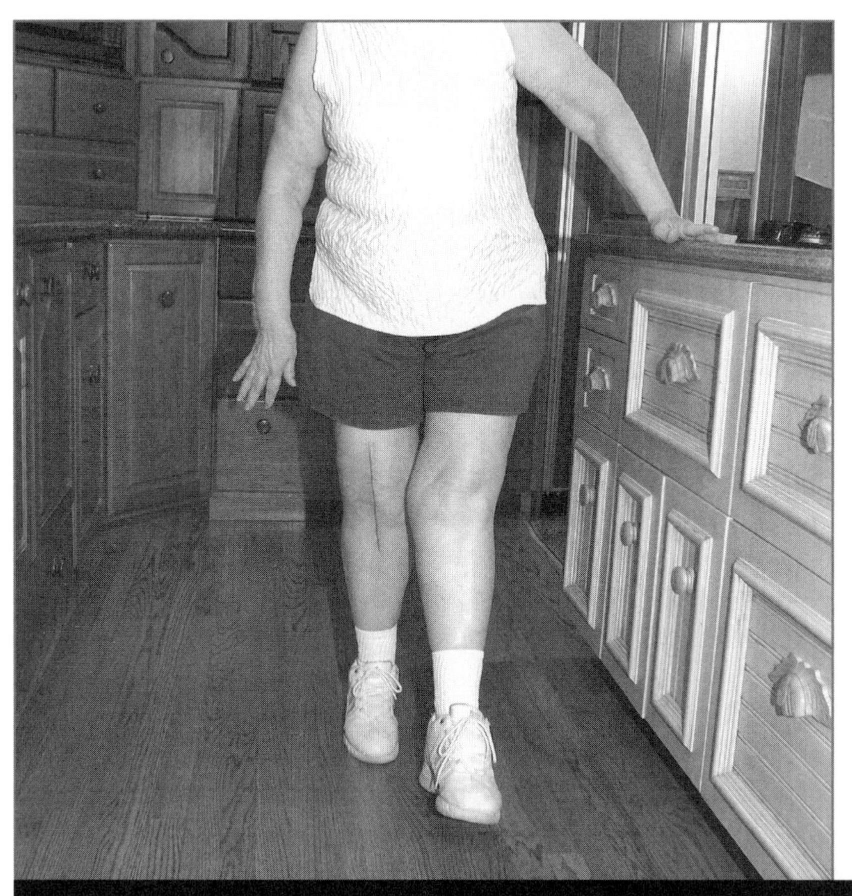

Chapter 11

One to Three Months

Don't Stop Now!

You've made it past the first month. Congratulations! The worst is behind you. In fact, in a couple of weeks you won't even be able to see it in the rearview mirror! But your work is not yet over. In the next two months you will make even more amazing strides in your recovery—as long as you remain as focused on your rehabilitation as you have been for the last four weeks.

By this time most of the postoperative pain is gone (with the exception of the occasional tightness, to be discussed later in the chapter). Most patients have good range of motion and are actually very glad they had their knee replaced. In fact, some patients with arthritis in their other, nonoperated knee begin to seriously consider replacing it as well, because *it* now becomes "the bad knee." Most patients at this stage experience so much less pain than they did for years before surgery that they are happy with the level of function they have achieved so far in their new TKA. But don't get complacent. With more work your level of function can continue to improve significantly. Diligently doing the work now will yield many years of benefits. So let's get back to it!

Reversing Muscular Atrophy

As you have perhaps realized, the strength in your TKA leg was declining for many years prior to your surgery. Arthritis in the knee tends to limit a person's daily activities and level of exercise—even how much walking she or he does. In addition to the preoperative decline in strength, the muscles are traumatized in the process of taking out the old knee and putting in the new TKA. The combination of reduction in activity over the years and recent surgical trauma to the muscles renders them extremely weak. Well, they have been "on vacation" long enough.

When a muscle is not exercised, it loses its size and strength. This phenomenon is called *atrophy*. If you have ever seen someone's arm or leg that had spent several weeks in a cast, you probably noticed how small it appeared compared to the other arm or leg. This is caused by atrophy of the muscles in the limb. The muscles still contain the same number of muscle fibers; however, each individual fiber has become smaller in diameter. Thus the entire muscle appears smaller. The postsurgical swelling around your knee may have given you the impression that the size of the thigh and calf muscles were the same as on the nonoperated leg. But as the swelling subsides in the next two months, you will probably notice the atrophy in your leg muscles. Dr. Falkel's youngest son used to refer to his legs as "Jell-O Jigglers" because they had atrophied so much. There was a whole lot of shaking going on whenever he walked or exercised!

Muscle atrophy is a reversible effect of lack of muscle use. In order to regain the strength and size of the muscle—to rebuild the muscle's bulk—it must be gradually overloaded and made to work harder. To get stronger, you need to progressively increase the intensity, resistance, and duration of your exercise sessions.

To regain the strength in your legs, we recommend that you adopt the following progression in your exercise program over the next two months:

1. If you are using a Total Gym for your home rehabilitation, keep performing the same exercises as described earlier in the book, but for each exercise try to work up to 3 sets of 25 repetitions each. Once you reach this goal, raise the level on the Total Gym so that you are exercising against a higher percentage of your body weight. With the increased resistance, you will probably need to initially reduce the number of repetitions to 5–10, and that is fine. Gradually work up to 3 sets of 25 reps each, and then raise the height of the Total Gym to the next level.
2. If you are exercising at a health club or recreation facility, you can follow the same procedure: For each exercise, work up to 3 sets of 25 repetitions each, and then add more resistance or weight to the exercise device. With the newly added resistance or weight, initially drop back to doing sets of 5–10 repetitions, and progressively increase to 3 sets of 25 repetitions each. When you feel comfortable, increase the weight and start the progression all over again.

The progression may take several weeks, and it may vary with each exercise. No problem. We suggest keeping a logbook of your exercise sessions, listing the number of repetitions, the number of sets, and the amount of weight/resistance for each exercise. With this record, each time you start an exercise you can see what you did in the last training session, and you will have a reference point from which to gradually increase your efforts.

Preventing Injury

We want to emphasize that the best way to decrease the amount of atrophy and increase a muscle's size and function is to *gradually* progress the work that the muscle must train against. If too much is done too fast, the muscle may become overstressed and actually be slightly damaged. The treatment for an injured muscle is rest. However, if the muscle is slowly and gradually strengthened, it will not become damaged, and increased size, strength, and function will soon follow.

What about the muscle soreness that you feel *after* exercising? It is critical at this point in your rehabilitation that you be able to distinguish between acceptable muscle soreness from exercise and pain or soreness due to muscle injury from too much exercise. As we mentioned in earlier chapters, the use of your "retrospectoscope" is the key to determining muscle soreness versus muscle injury. Following exercise, if you experience more pain later that night or the next morning, you have probably pushed too hard and may have injured some muscles. If you experience no significant increase in pain following an activity, it is safe to increase the difficulty of the exercise.

The muscle soreness that typically occurs a day or two *after* exercise is a sign that you are working the muscle in a constructive way. It is called *postexercise muscle soreness* and is a natural result of slightly overstressing a muscle. Note that this type of soreness does not occur until sometime the next day. Almost everyone has done some form of exercise that caused them to feel the residual effects of muscle soreness the next day. The muscles are letting you know loud and clear that it has been a long time since they performed that particular movement. Some microscopic swelling around the muscle fibers occurs when a muscle is used in a new or unfamiliar way, and it is probably this swelling that causes the pain when the muscle is contracted. The muscle is not damaged, and in several days the soreness is gone. Postexercise muscle soreness is normal and happens to everyone.

What can be done to relieve postexercise muscle soreness? Local remedies such as anti-inflammatory medications, ice, and/or heat will help significantly. However, the best medicine is actually more exercise, but at a much reduced level. Stationary cycling at a slow speed or even slow walking seems to work well to aid in the reduction of the microscopic swelling. Some TKA patients have found that walking backwards for short distances—twenty-five to thirty yards at a time, for five to ten minutes, several times a day—can speed up the recovery from postexercise muscle soreness.

Muscle soreness or pain that occurs during an exercise or immediately after completion of the exercise is another story. When a muscle is overstressed too quickly or with too much resistance, the individual fibers develop microscopic tears. This can cause significant swelling around each muscle fiber, requiring more time for the torn fibers to heal. During TKA rehabilitation, subjecting the muscles to too much resistance or too many repetitions can potentially cause muscle injury. If this happens, allow the injured muscle to heal by resting it. Avoid contracting the affected muscle for several days. If the injured muscle is the quadriceps or hamstrings, it will be stressed with any and all rehabilitation exercises; therefore, rehabilitation must come to a screeching halt.

So how can you prevent muscle injury? We repeat: With *gradual* and *progressive* increases in the number of exercises, in the number of repetitions and sets of exercises, and in the intensity or resistance used with each exercise.

Another aspect of the rehabilitation process that will affect muscle soreness and the potential for muscle injury is the amount of time you allow between exercise sessions. Since the beginning of your rehabilitation, it has been 60-60-24-7-4 (see Chapter 5). Everything you did was rehabilitation! Now, however, in order to progressively gain strength in your muscles, you must deliberately incorporate rest and recovery into your overall rehabilitation and exercise program. Believe it or not, a muscle actually increases in size and strength during the recovery period between exercise sessions rather than during the actual training itself. This is why athletes vary their training and exercise sessions: to allow for recovery and the rebuilding of the muscle between workouts. Our recommendation is to limit strength-training exercises to three or four days per week. If you want to exercise more than that, you can supplement your rehabilitation with fifteen to thirty minutes of stationary cycling, pool therapy, or walking on days when you are not doing strength training.

Range-of-Motion Exercises

At this point in the rehabilitation process it is still critical to continue to work on range of motion in your new knee. Until you can effortlessly achieve 120–125 degrees of flexion and zero degrees of extension (i.e., you can fully straighten your leg), you need to perform range-of-motion exercises daily.

We have already described many different range-of-motion exercises. You will be relieved to learn that we are not going to present any new ones here. However, it is very important to find several range-of-motion exercises that work well for you and continue to spend time every day doing them. Many of our patients like to roll the *futebol* around with their TKA leg whenever they are watching TV. They feel it loosens up their TKA better than any other form of exercise. By this time you know which exercises work well for you, so concentrate on those. Find the four or five exercises that help you obtain the maximum range of motion possible. We recommend performing range-of-motion exercises at least twice a day, preferably in the morning and again at night. Dr. Falkel still performs his favorite range-of-motion exercises several times each day, as well as performing them when he is treating his TKA patients. Occasionally, to help loosen up his knees if they are tight he performs a few prior to riding his stationary cycle. After three to five minutes of range-of-motion exercises, his TKAs are ready to roll.

Many patients find it helpful to use some form of heat on their knee prior to starting their range-of-motion exercises. The heat warms up the muscles and the scar tissue, and makes stretching them and gaining additional range of motion somewhat more comfortable. By now you should not experience any pain when performing range-of-motion exercises. It should feel more like a stretching sensation than a pain. In other words, it should "hurt so good"!

Endurance Training

"Why am I so tired?" is one of the most common questions asked by our patients during the second and third months following TKA surgery. There are several answers to the question:

1. Recovery from major surgery is extremely demanding on the body. The number of calories burned is significantly higher in an individual recovering

from surgery than in one who has not undergone surgery. Depending on the patient's age, health, and level of fitness going into TKA surgery, it may be several months before he or she feels back to normal.

2. Many patients at this point still have difficulty sleeping through the night. Sleep patterns will hopefully improve during this phase of rehabilitation, but until they do, the lack of sleep, or even the lack of quality sleep, will result in excessive fatigue.
3. Most patients suffered greatly reduced muscular and cardiovascular conditioning in the months and years prior to surgery because the arthritis pain in their knee forced them to limit their daily activities. They lose even more conditioning during the first few weeks after TKA surgery when it is difficult to move.
4. Many patients report losing their appetite for several weeks after surgery. Although eating less can help with weight control, the body needs good nutrition to assist in its recovery from surgery. In addition, with all the exercise required during rehabilitation, it is paramount that good nutrition become a part of the recovery equation. Until patients are eating normally again, a less than adequate diet can be a source of fatigue.
5. Prolonged pain can be a significant cause of fatigue. Being in pain results in less sleep, less ability to focus on other activities, and more anxiety about achieving pain relief.
6. Returning to normal daily activities—including work and social life—can be mentally, physically, and emotionally draining.
7. Finally, the patient probably has been exercising much more since surgery than she or he did for many years prior to surgery. In addition, the fact that recovery until now has absorbed every minute of the patient's life has put significant demands on all facets of her or his endurance: mental, physical, and emotional. (Remember the 60-60-24-7-4 syndrome from Chapter 5?)

What can be done to improve endurance and eliminate the feeling of fatigue? The good news is that time not only heals all wounds; it also improves endurance and reduces fatigue.

To improve muscular endurance in your legs, we have the following specific recommendations:

1. Increase the duration of your stationary cycling to thirty minutes daily over the course of the next two months.
2. Increase the duration of your walks to thirty minutes over the course of the next two months. (We will discuss getting rid of the limp later in this chapter.)
3. Alternate endurance-training exercises on different days. For example, do stationary cycling on Monday, Wednesday, and Friday, and take long walks on Tuesday, Thursday, and Saturday. (Sunday is a day for rest, and you deserve it!) If you are still doing pool therapy, you

could alternate between two days of stationary cycling, two days of walking, and two days of pool therapy. The combinations are totally up to you.

4. On some days the best way to increase endurance and fight fatigue is to do *nothing!* Sometimes one step back allows for two or three steps forward. Listen to your body; it will tell you if it needs to take a day off from exercise. If it does, then just enjoy relaxing. You will not lose ground on your rehabilitation, and you may actually gain some ground by resting rather than training!

As you progress through the next two months, you will find that your energy level will gradually increase and the feelings of fatigue will slowly diminish.

Soft-Tissue Mobilization

One of the most important tasks at this stage in your recovery is mobilization of the soft tissue over the incision and in the surrounding muscles and ligaments. It is during the second and third months after surgery that much of the scar tissue matures. During maturation, if the scar tissue is kept soft and pliable, function and movement of your TKA will be dramatically improved.

Let's review the soft-tissue mobilization techniques we discussed in Chapters 7 and 8:

1. Perform cross-friction massage over the incision area by pressing with your thumb or fingers on the incision and making small circles the size of a quarter all along the sides of the incision (Figure 11.1). Spend approximately 5–10 minutes 3 or 4 times a day performing cross-friction massage over the incision.

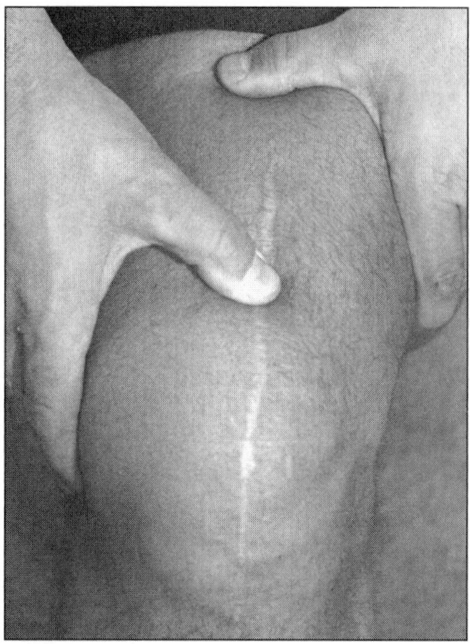

Figure 11.1. Cross-friction massage over TKA incision

2. Soft-tissue mobilization over the quadriceps muscle, which was cut and repaired during surgery, is very important during these two months. You should be able to clearly feel where the scar tissue meets the normal muscle tissue. Many patients describe this area as having a woodlike texture because it is so

much harder than the normal quadriceps tissue. Massage lengthwise with your thumbs and/or index fingers along either side of the incision throughout this area (Figure 11.2).

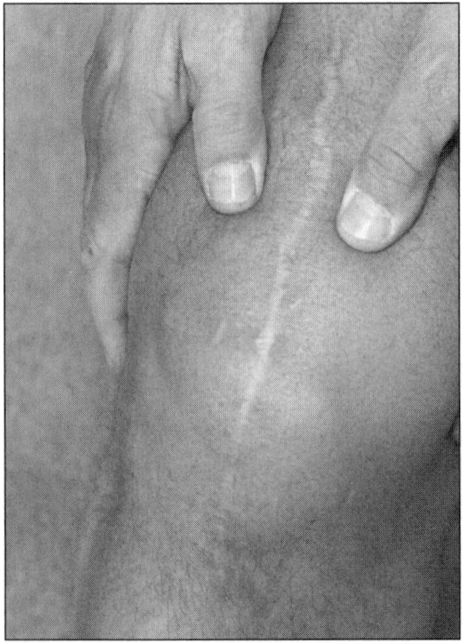

Figure 11.2. Lengthwise friction massage over TKA incision

When Will I Walk Normally Again?

Prior to your surgery, when was the last time you were able to walk without a limp? Or when was the last time you were able to walk as fast as other people? For most patients, it has been years since they walked normally. There is no time like the present to learn to walk normally again!

Patients who have been utilizing pool therapy—and specifically water walking—as part of their rehabilitation program may be walking almost normally by the second or third month after surgery. We highly recommend that all patients who have access to a pool perform water-walking exercises. In the water, your limp will simply disappear! The buoyancy of the water allows for a more normal, fluid walking pattern. If you have not tried pool therapy and water walking, you don't know what you're missing—and you *really* should find out.

Patients limp before surgery because arthritic pain prevents them from placing full weight on their knee. Postoperatively, the limp is caused by surgical pain, but it is exacerbated by the patient's lack of confidence in his or her ability to put full weight on the TKA leg. Therefore, many TKA patients spend as little time as possible on the TKA leg in single-leg stance (standing on one leg only). This means when they're walking they move their non-TKA leg as fast as they can through the swing phase so they can transfer their weight onto it quickly. Another factor contributing to the limp is the different length of each step. The step length of the TKA leg is shorter than the step length of the other leg. A combination of these factors produces the classic limp that almost all patients with knee arthritis and/or TKA surgery develop at some point. So what can be done to get rid of the limp?

Exercises to Improve Walking

Exercise 115

Marching in Place at Sink

Stand facing the sink and hold on to it. Practice marching in place. Count to yourself, or even out loud if necessary, to help you concentrate on spending an equal amount of time on each foot. Ask a family member or friend to watch you march in place and to provide feedback about whether you're spending an equal amount of time on each foot.

Exercise 116

Changing Pace While Marching in Place

Once you have become proficient at marching, try marching at different paces—that is, march as slowly as possible, and then increase your speed in increments until you're marching as fast as possible. As you change speeds, the time you spend on each foot will vary, so, as in Exercise 115, have someone watch you march at different speeds and provide feedback to help you keep a steady cadence between the TKA leg and the nonoperated leg.

Exercise 117

Swinging the Nonoperated Leg to Simulate Single-Leg-Stance Phase

Stand with the hip of your nonoperated leg next to the sink, holding on to the sink if necessary. Place all your weight on the TKA leg, pick up the foot of the nonoperated leg, and swing it back and forth without touching the ground (Figure 11.3). This simulates the single-leg-stance phase of walking. As your balance improves while doing this exercise, your walking will also improve.

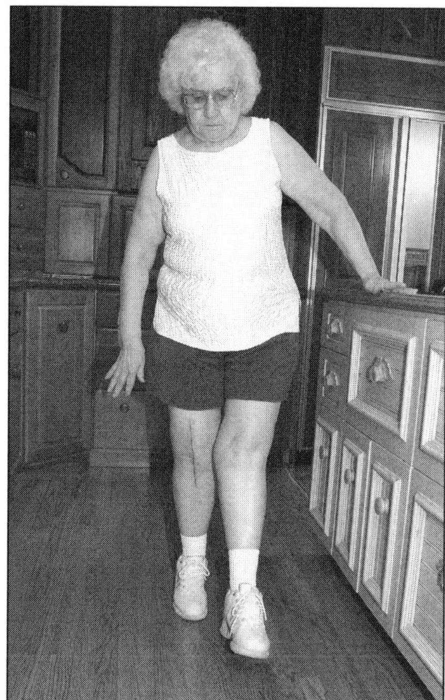

Figure 11.3. Stance-phase simulation on TKA

Exercise 118

Stride-Length Training

To work on developing an equal step length, find a concrete surface with a small puddle of water. Step in the water, and then walk on the concrete. This will leave several footprints on the ground that can be examined to determine which leg produces the longest step. To equalize the step lengths, try to lengthen the shorter stride (usually the TKA leg) and/or to decrease the other one. This will take practice, and again, if you have a friend or relative who can walk behind you, they should be able to coach you to achieve equal step lengths even without the water and footprints.

Exercise 119

Arm-Swing Training

Another factor that affects a patient's gait is his or her arm swing. While using assistive devices such as a walker, crutches, and/or a cane, the normal arm swing is eliminated. Once the assistive devices are discontinued, most patients "forget" to swing their arms normally when they walk. In normal walking, the right arm swings forward as the left leg comes forward, and the left arm swings forward as the right leg swings forward. As you practice walking, make a conscious effort to work on the arm swing. Dr. Falkel teaches his patients to exaggerate the arm swing initially, simply to get back in the habit of using their arms while walking.

Exercise 120

Crutch/Cane Training

Practice all the walking exercises in this chapter using a single crutch and then a cane. The assistive devices are there for just that purpose: They *assist* you with walking by taking some of the weight off the TKA leg, allowing for more stability while the TKA leg is in the single-leg-stance phase. As your confidence and balance improve, the crutch or cane begins to take less and less of the weight from the TKA leg, and eventually you no longer need it. As suggested before, continue to keep a cane in your vehicle so that you have it if needed. It can be very frightening to be without your cane when you really need it, such as on snow, ice, wet leaves, sand, or uneven surfaces.

Be careful when walking in public with a cane. Although almost everyone will see someone who is walking with a walker, there is a unique "invisibility" to a person walking with a cane. Don't assume that people will give you room to maneuver or will even hold a door open for you. Be careful, and walk defensively.

Exercise 121

Singing While Walking to Improve Gait

One patient told Dr. Falkel that her best technique to improve her gait was to sing a song to herself while practicing her walking. She would sing a song that had a suitable beat and would walk in rhythm to the beat. Doing so helped her develop more equal stance times, step lengths, and a more normal cadence.

Exercise 122

Shadow Walking

Another technique is to walk with the sun at your back, viewing your shadow on the ground in front of you. This allows you to see if your arms are swinging, if your head is keeping relatively still (rather than bobbing from side to side due to your limp), and how your trunk is moving. Assuming there's enough sunshine available, watching your shadow is an effective method of gauging your own progress.

■ ■ ■

Most orthopedic surgeons want their TKA patients to walk as much as they can. However, they do not recommend that their patients run, and we concur. Running places an excessive amount of stress on each knee, which may result in premature damage or wear to the components of the TKA. This does not mean that you cannot run across the street to avoid being hit by a car! We suggest that patients with TKAs do not run or even jog for fitness purposes. Save any form of running for emergencies only. Walking, cycling, and swimming are much better and safer modes of exercise after TKA surgery.

Don't be frustrated if it takes several days or even weeks for you to develop a more normal walking pattern. Remember, it took a long time to "perfect" your limp, and likewise it will take some time to relearn how to walk again. But one of the goals of every TKA patient should be having the ability to walk normally, whenever and wherever they choose. In the next chapter we will talk about walking on uneven surfaces.

"How much should I walk?" Great question! As with all of the exercises we have discussed, start gradually, and slowly increase the distance you walk. Start by walking for five minutes at a time, and progress to walking for thirty or forty-five minutes. It can be very frightening to start walking and then to realize that you don't know how you are going to return to where you started. Follow the suggestions offered in the section "Going for a Walk," in Chapter 10. By the sixth month postoperatively, many patients are able to walk for nine holes of golf, something they probably have been unable to do for years.

Preventive Antibiotics

At one to three months postoperatively you will begin to realize that you can live with this new piece of equipment, hopefully for a long time. Up until this point we have discussed rehabilitation efforts to achieve optimal function in your new joint for a long time to come. Another important issue concerns the prevention of infection. As you begin to live life after TKA surgery in a world full of bacteria, there are some precautionary measures to be taken to help prevent your TKA from becoming infected.

As the owner of a new artificial knee, you now have a permanent foreign object inside your joint. This is important as it relates to infection. Foreign material anywhere in the body has a greater risk of becoming infected than "normal" tissue does. This is mostly due to blood circulation. There is no blood supply running through metal or plastic, and the circulation around this foreign material is altered by the scar tissue resulting from surgery.

If for some reason bacteria get into a person's circulation, they can travel in the bloodstream and potentially "land" on the foreign object. We rely on our circulatory system to transport infection-fighting cells (white blood cells) to wage war on bacteria anywhere in our body. If the circulation is altered in an area of the body, such as around the knee following TKA surgery, it may hamper our ability to deliver white blood cells to fight infection in the affected region. This may lead to an infection of the artificial knee joint, which can cause serious problems (discussed in Appendix A).

Since there is a risk of infection in the knee joint following TKA, any time there is the potential for bacteria to be released into the circulatory system, prophylactic (preventive) antibiotics should be strongly considered. Bacteria can be released into the bloodstream during any type of major or minor surgery. This is particularly true during oral surgery or even routine teeth cleaning. Bacteria can also gain entry into the circulation if there is an infection anywhere in the body. Some common examples include sinus infection, bronchitis, pneumonia, a tooth abscess, a bladder infection, skin boils, or even infected skin lacerations. Infection is an even greater risk in individuals with a comprised immune system, such as the elderly, people taking immunosuppressive drugs, those with a chronic debilitating illness, and patients with a history of frequent infections.

It is our recommendation that anyone who has undergone a TKA be placed on prophylactic antibiotics prior to any surgery, routine teeth cleaning, or whenever a significant infection is detected. The most common antibiotics used are oral amoxicillin, cefazolin, or clindamycin. They are inexpensive and have a low incidence of adverse reactions. The subject of antibiotic prophylaxis is currently somewhat controversial. Some surgeons believe that prophylactic antibiotics are unnecessary in patients who are relatively young and healthy or in those who have had an artificial knee in place for longer than two years. There is general agreement that preventive antibiotics are needed in any patient with a compromised immune system. The dosage and type of each antibiotic are still debated. Most experts recommend dosing before any proposed surgery or teeth cleaning, but the number of doses afterwards can vary. As a TKA patient, it is essential that you discuss the use of preventive antibiotics with your surgeon and your dentist and follow their recommendations.

■ ■ ■

In this chapter we have tried to illustrate the most common obstacles that patients encounter during the first three months following TKA surgery. TKAs do not come with an owner's manual, because every TKA is different and thus cannot be approached with one set of hard and fast rules. Every patient is different, too, with a unique set of experiences. However, we have seen common trends throughout our patients' recovery efforts. Our suggested exercises should serve as general guidelines for your rehabilitation program. Still, remember that the *most important* exercise is the exercise of common sense.

Common Questions and Some Answers

When can I start driving again?

Before you can safely drive again, you need to be able to put your full weight on the TKA leg and have sufficient leg strength and control to be able to move your TKA leg on and off the pedals rapidly. For most patients, this happens about six weeks after surgery. However, if you have an automatic transmission and underwent a left TKA, your surgeon may permit you to drive sooner than six weeks postoperatively. The size of your vehicle and the amount of flexion in your TKA may also influence when it is safe for you to drive again. Whether your prosthesis is cemented or cementless also affects the timetable for returning to driving. Most surgeons will not let you put full weight on a cementless prosthesis for six weeks postoperatively; therefore, driving will not be considered safe until some time after this point. The decision to resume driving is part of the "art of medicine" and needs to be shared by patient and surgeon.

When will my TKA knee move as fast as my other knee or like a normal knee?

Eventually, the TKA knee will move as fast as a normal knee can move. However, as with so many variables after TKA surgery, each patient will gain speed in their TKA at a different rate. Some patients regain normal speed of movement in six to twelve weeks; for others, it may take up to a year.

When will my TKA knee look normal again?

Following surgery the knee may remain swollen for six to twelve months, making it look huge. Eventually the swelling will subside. After that, there may be subtle changes in the TKA knee that make it permanently look different from how it looked before surgery. Such changes can include the following: (a) the bony architecture is altered when bone spurs are removed from around the joint; (b) the shape of the artificial components may be slightly different from the contours of the original bone; and (c) soft-tissue scarring may slightly change the outline of the surrounding soft tissue. Any change in how the TKA knee looks is usually slight and has no effect on function.

When can I change from my prescription pain medications to Tylenol or Advil?

Pain control is important so the patient can get adequate sleep and participate in therapy. However, one must be sensitive to the side effects of prolonged narcotic use, particularly addiction. The use of narcotics can be tapered off and replaced with acetaminophen (Tylenol) or ibuprofen (Motrin, Advil) to assist with pain control. We recommend that patients taper off their narcotic pain medications as soon as they feel comfortable doing so. Some orthopedic surgeons hold the opinion that in the cementless TKA, anti-inflammatory medications may slow bone growth into the prosthesis. Therefore, ask your surgeon before taking any anti-inflammatory medications (such as ibuprofen or naproxen) postoperatively for pain control.

Should I continue taking Vioxx or Celebrex?

If you were taking Vioxx or Celebrex only for your arthritic knee, you probably no longer need it. If you were taking it for other arthritic joints, it is safe to resume taking it after six weeks. Because of the variables with each patient, be sure to discuss the matter with your surgeon before resuming either of these medications.

When will my TKA stop feeling warm to the touch?

Assuming there are no signs of infection, the TKA feels warm to the touch because of inflammation. This is a normal healing response and can be aggravated by range-of-motion exercises. As the swelling and inflammation subside with time, the warmth will eventually disappear.

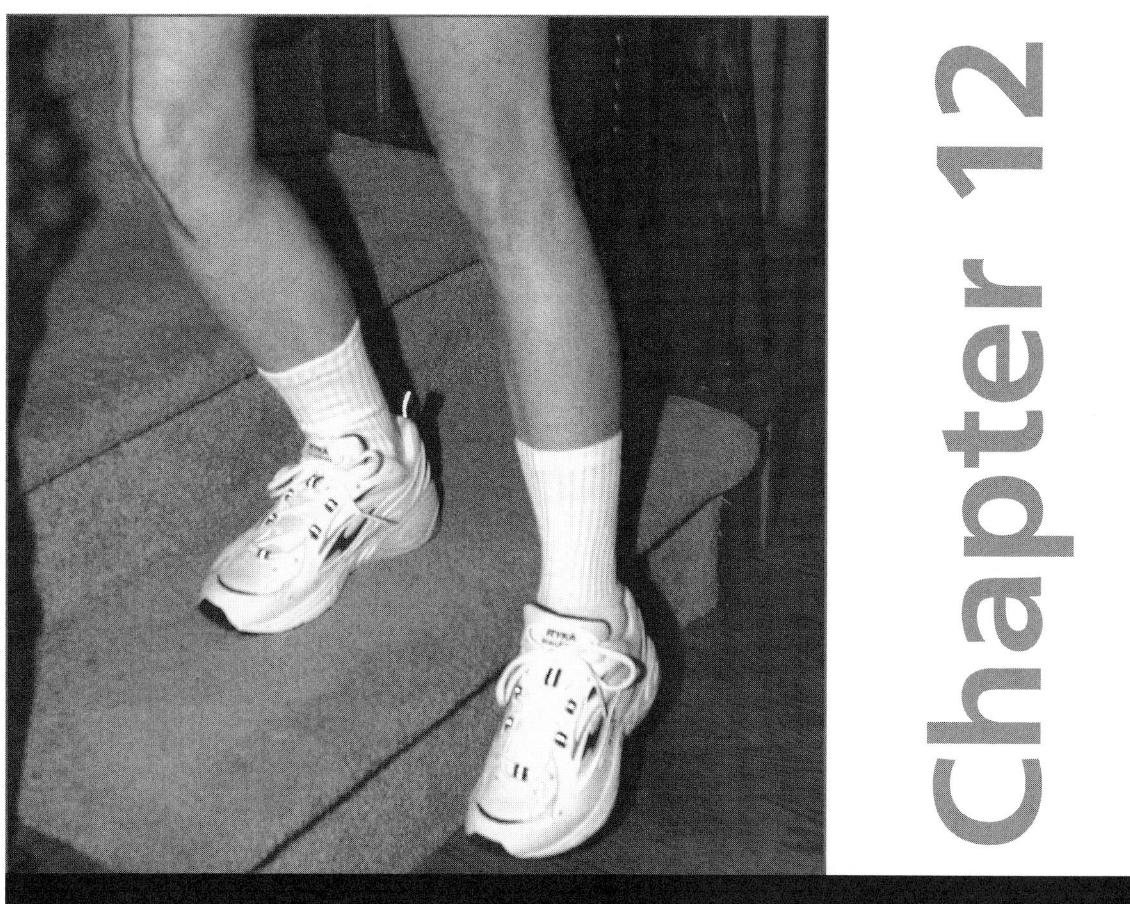

Chapter 12

Three Months to Six Months

I Think I Need a Vacation

Did you ever think you would get to this point in your recovery? The vast majority of our patients experience the three months immediately following surgery as some of the hardest, yet most rewarding, months of their lives. We are sure your family is very proud of your accomplishments, and you should be too! At this point you can see that your hard work has paid off, and for many patients their new TKA is now their best knee (more about that topic later in the chapter). So where do we go from here?

Many surgeons routinely see their TKA patients approximately three months postoperatively. During this visit, they may X-ray the TKA to make sure the prosthetic components look good, but most importantly they want to see how the patient is doing from a functional viewpoint. Based on the surgeon's evaluation, the TKA patient may get the green light to begin doing what they can in terms of activities of daily living, without restrictions. The surgeon may discuss some precautions about living with a TKA, but more often than not the recommendation is to get back to a normal existence.

At three months, Dr. Falkel got the green light from his surgeons to do whatever he wanted. So the first thing he did that evening when he got home from the appointment was to climb up and down the two sets of stairs in his home thirty times. Why? Because he could. After completing the exercise he was very excited because (a) he could do it and (b) he had no pain in his TKAs. However, the next evening, his quadriceps, hamstrings, and calf muscles were ready to catch the first plane out of Denver because those muscles had not climbed that many stairs in years! It took three days for the muscles to recover from their postexercise muscle soreness. The only bright spot in those three days was that his TKAs felt great! So a word to the wise about the green light: Proceed with caution as you step into your life with your new TKA.

This chapter will discuss the transition period from rehabilitation to your return to a normal life. Although at this stage you can approach your rehab exercises with a little less intensity, the importance of exercise is just as critical now as it was during the previous phases of your rehabilitation. Take time now to enjoy life and to "smell the roses." Even professional athletes cannot train hard all year long; however, when the professional athlete is not competing, he or she is still active, preparing for the next season. This three- to six-month period of the rehabilitation process is the time to prepare for the next "season": a lifelong enjoyment of living without pain in your new knee.

Precautions for Living with Your TKA

One of the things that most surgeons and other health-care practitioners discuss with their TKA patients several times throughout the entire recovery and rehabilitation process is what sort of activities should be limited or perhaps prohibited with a TKA.

If this has not been addressed, make it a priority at the three- to six-month office visit/evaluation. For example, as discussed in Chapter 11, most surgeons do not want their TKA patients to jog for exercise. This does not mean you can't run in case of emergency. It refers to regular running for exercise and fitness. Many surgeons will allow their TKA patients to run enough to play doubles tennis. The thought here is that in doubles tennis a player covers only about half of the court, resulting in less running and less weight-bearing stress on the TKA. Dr. Brugioni uses the analogy of a tire on a car that is particularly difficult to change. The more miles that are put on the car, the earlier the tire will wear out. Same with a TKA. Although the TKA can be replaced, it requires an operation that is usually more involved than the first knee-replacement surgery. If a patient has her or his heart set on a particular activity that may be hard on the knee, she or he needs to weigh the risks and benefits. Discuss playing tennis with your surgeon.

Another daily activity that may be difficult is kneeling. Dr. Falkel has treated several patients who could kneel after only a few weeks of rehabilitation. However, as mentioned earlier in the book, it's more than two years after his surgery and he still cannot kneel. Some TKA patients are never able to kneel comfortably. Kneeling will not cause any damage to the prosthetic components of the TKA, but it may be uncomfortable. The pressure from kneeling tends to irritate the incision below the kneecap, making it too uncomfortable or painful. Patients may kneel as much as they can tolerate, depending on their level of pain. They are encouraged to use their own judgment.

Weight control is a major concern for patients with TKA. In a number of patients, the arthritis pain in their knees was so severe for so many years that they were unable to exercise prior to their surgery. Consequently, that reduction in activity level contributed to their being overweight. Some surgeons ask their patients to lose as much weight as they can prior to receiving the TKA, but many patients simply cannot do so because they are unable to exercise. For the past three months you have done a tremendous amount of exercise. Many patients report that their increased level of physical activity during the months after surgery causes them to lose a significant amount of weight. If that is the case for you, then that's terrific! Very simply put: The less body weight the TKA has to carry with each step, the longer it will last and the "happier" it will be. We again use the motor-vehicle analogy. The more weight you carry in the trunk of your car, the faster the tires will wear out. Same with your TKA. It should be your goal to make these "tires" last as long as possible. Now that you have entered this phase of your rehabilitation, it is time to seriously commit to losing those extra pounds and keeping them off through diet and regular exercise. For patients who need help with weight control, we recommend discussing the matter with your primary-care physician to find a safe and effective method of losing weight that will suit your individual needs.

The last obstacle our patients face is knowing when is the "right" time to try a new activity. There are no hard and fast rules in the art of medicine for when is the right time to return to a particular activity. It has been years since most patients have enjoyed their desired activity level. They've missed out on activities of daily living that most of us take for granted. One of the main reasons for having their knee replaced was to return to a normal life and enjoy participating in activities with family and friends. We emphasize a simple precaution: If you think you shouldn't try a particular activity, then don't try it. Listen to your built-in defense mechanisms. Over the past three months there were many times when you *knew* there was no way you were going to be able to walk down the hall without your walker or sit down and get up from a very low chair. Right? However, with persistence, you have been able to obtain your goals on a weekly basis. Over time you have developed a confidence in your TKA that should be tested consistently. However, don't take unnecessary chances with daily activities. If you don't think you can do a particular activity, you probably can't, and you definitely shouldn't try. Use your good judgment. You will know when you are ready to try something new. For example, Dr. Falkel loves to ski, and both his surgeons said he could ski with certain precautions one year after surgery (see Chapter 13 for a discussion of the precautions). However, after a year, even though he was strong enough and fit enough to ski, he felt that his balance was inadequate for him to be able to ski safely. So he worked on balance for a whole year. Two years and two weeks after his surgery he was back on skis for the first time in eight years. It was especially wonderful because he had the confidence to ski safely. If you've waited this long to try a particular activity and are still hesitant, why not wait slightly longer until you are confident in your ability so that you can truly enjoy yourself with minimal risk of injury to your TKA?

Range-of-Motion Exercises

By this time, you probably have obtained as much range of motion as you need for most everyday activities. How do you maintain this mobility? We have presented a number of range-of-motion exercises throughout the book, and you have found some that work better for you than others. We recommend selecting three to five of your favorite exercises and continuing to perform them for the next three months of your rehabilitation. You do not need to spend nearly as much time every day working on range of motion as you did earlier. But it is still important to devote at least thirty minutes per day to keeping the range of motion in your TKA at an optimal level.

One suggestion is to incorporate range-of-motion exercises into normal activities. Below are two exercises that will help you do so. These exercises can be done almost anywhere at any time and are just as effective as the other range-of-motion exercises we've presented. However, they only work if you work at doing them.

Exercise 123

Knee Flexion While Sitting

While working at your desk, watching TV, or at any other time when you're sitting for a prolonged period, pull the TKA foot back as far as possible under the chair and try to hold that position for several minutes (Figure 12.1). Then let it rest, and repeat the exercise again later.

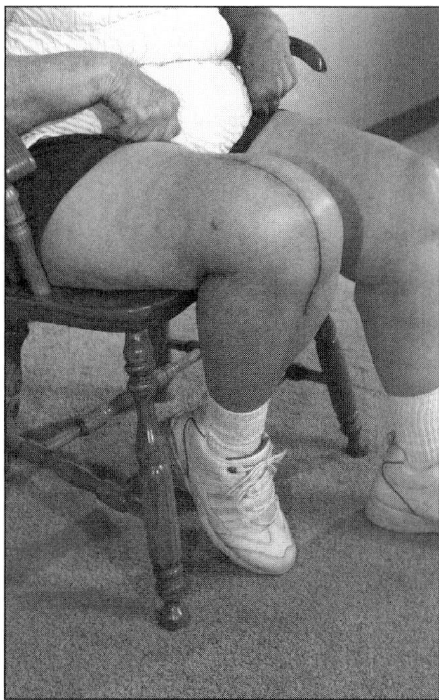

Figure 12.1. Range-of-motion exercise sitting in chair

Exercise 124

Knee Flexion While Standing with Foot on Chair

Another exercise to improve range of motion can be performed while standing. Put the TKA foot on a chair or stair step, and rock forward to hold the stretch for several minutes (Figure 12.2). Relax and repeat several times.

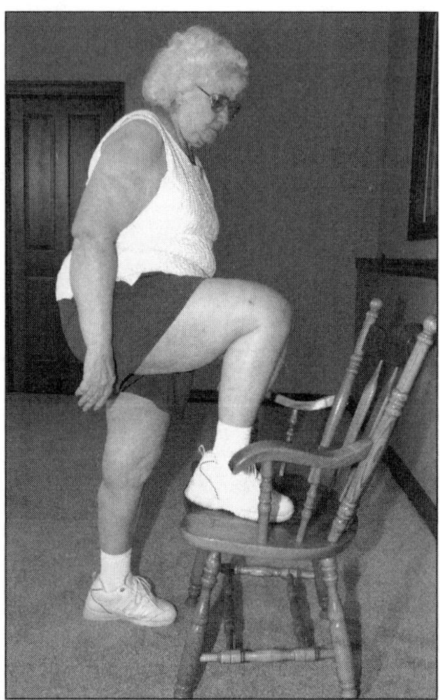

Figure 12.2. Range-of-motion exercise standing with TKA foot on chair

Strength and Endurance Exercises

The last thing most patients want to think about at this stage is more exercise. They are tired of exercise and simply want to do the things that "normal" people do. After three months of rehabilitation and many repetitions of the same exercises, they are bored with the routine. One way to keep the exercises interesting yet still effective is to alternate the types of exercises you do, as we suggested in earlier chapters. After about three months of rehab, it was extremely hard for Dr. Falkel to make himself go downstairs to his basement and exercise. He found all kinds of excuses to avoid the stationary cycle, rowing machine, and Total Gym. So he alternated days of exercise. He did stationary cycling on Monday, Wednesday, and Friday; Total Gym on Tuesday and Saturday; and rowing on Thursday and Sunday.

Just as maintaining range of motion is important, strength training is also necessary during these three months. We recommend that patients who want to take a break from the rigors of rehabilitation decrease their strength-training exercises to three days per week. This will allow for strength to slowly improve while still allowing the patient to have a life other than in the weight room.

Another suggestion for adding strength and endurance training to normal activities is stair training. For most patients with arthritic knees, the stairs were their worst nightmare. In the year before his surgery, Dr. Falkel went to great lengths to avoid stairs at any cost. However, at this point you can use stairs to gain range of motion, strength, and muscular endurance. They also provide an excellent form of cardiovascular exercise. Here are a few suggestions for exercises using stairs:

Exercise 125

Stair Walking

Use the stairs whenever possible rather than taking the elevator. Be sure the stairwell has handrails, and if you have to carry anything in your hands, use caution when climbing stairs. Taking the stairs rather than the elevator during your workday will significantly improve muscular strength, endurance, and overall fitness.

Exercise 126

Stair-Walking Variation

If your workplace is on an upper floor, take the elevator to a floor a few levels below your floor, and then walk up the last few flights to your office. If you have to go between floors during the workday, use the stairs rather than the elevator.

Exercise 127

Home Stair Training

Climb the stairs at home as part of your exercise program. Walking up and down a flight of stairs three to five times daily, several days a week, is a great way to improve strength and endurance.

Exercise 128

Lifting Body Weight Two Steps at a Time

Place the foot of your TKA leg on the second step of a stairway and the foot of the other leg on the ground floor. Straighten your TKA leg as though you were going to climb the stairs two at a time, and then slowly bend the TKA leg to lower the foot of the non-TKA leg back to the ground floor (Figure 12.3). Use the banister as needed for support and/or balance. Complete 3–5 sets of 15–25 repetitions each.

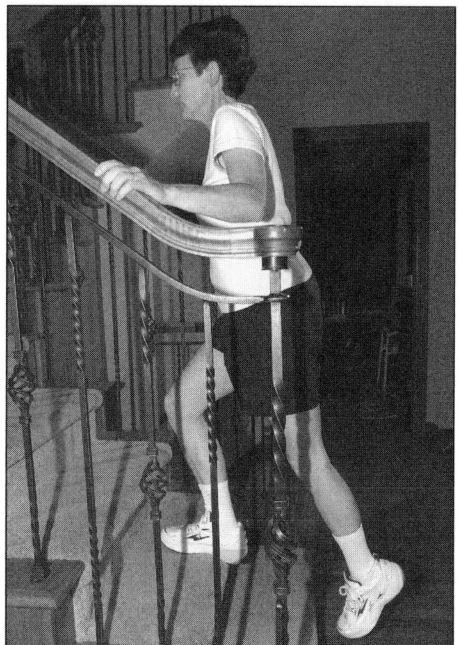

Figure 12.3. Step-strengthening exercise: lifting body weight up two steps

Exercise 129

Lowering Body Weight Two Steps at a Time

Stand on the second step, facing down. Keep the foot of the TKA leg on the second step, and slowly lower the foot of the non-TKA leg toward the ground floor (Figure 12.4). Do not let the non-TKA foot touch the floor. After you have lowered the non-TKA foot as low as possible, slowly straighten your TKA leg once again. Use the banister as necessary. Complete 3–5 sets of 15–25 repetitions each.

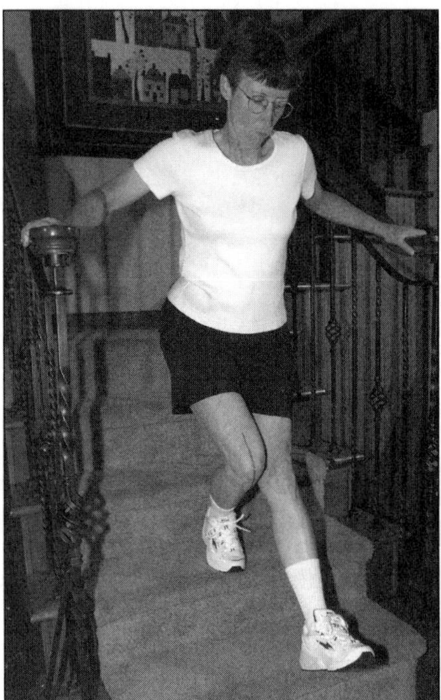

Figure 12.4. Step-strengthening exercise: lowering body weight down two steps

Exercise 130

Lowering Body Weight Sideways on Stairs

Stand sideways on the first step, facing the wall, with the TKA foot closest to the second step. Slowly lower the non-TKA foot toward the ground, but do not let it touch the ground (Figure 12.5). Then straighten the TKA leg until the non-TKA foot is at the level of the step. Complete 3–5 sets of 15–25 repetitions each. Once this exercise becomes easy, try doing it while standing on the second step, lowering the non-TKA foot as close as possible to the ground floor (Figure 12.6).

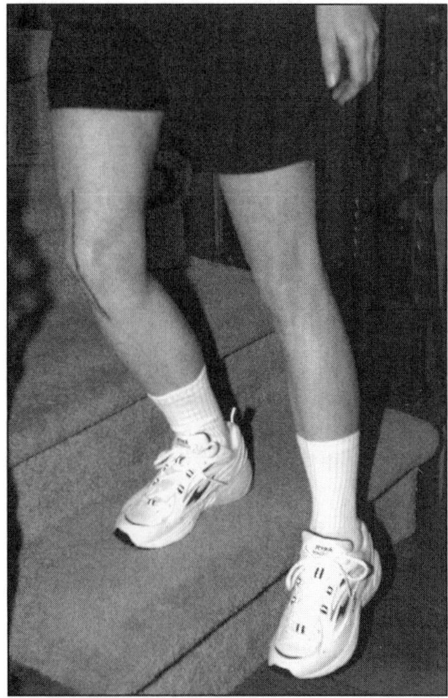

Figure 12.5. Step-strengthening exercise: lifting body weight sideways up steps

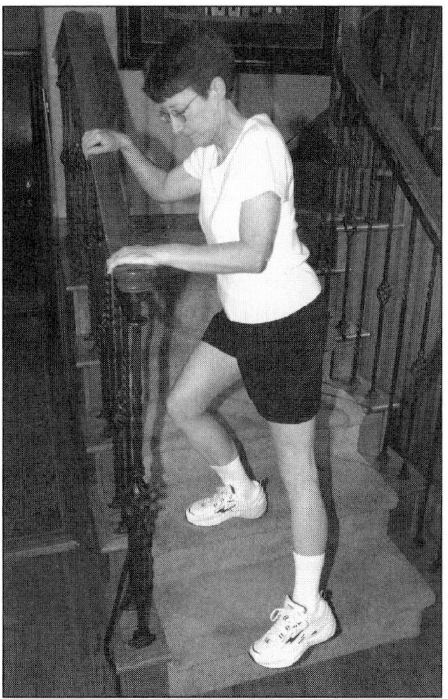

Figure 12.6. Step-strengthening exercise: lifting body weight up two steps (sideways)

Losing the Cane

By this point in your rehabilitation there have probably been many times when you started walking and realized that you had forgotten your cane. Good! If you don't absolutely, positively need the cane to walk, then you are ready to walk without it. But don't give the cane away or sell it at a garage sale. There may be times in the future when you need it for balance, stability, and security, given a particular type of terrain. You may want to use it while walking on uneven surfaces, such as grass, gravel, or hiking trails. Many patients who return to hiking on trails for exercise use their cane whenever they go out. Some purchase an adjustable walking stick (similar to a ski pole) that provides all the stability they need for whatever surface they encounter. As we've suggested before, keep your cane in the back of your vehicle, just in case.

During months three to six post-op, really focus on walking without a limp. Concentrate on the walking exercises we discussed in Chapter 11: spending the same amount of time on each foot, using similar step lengths and swing-phase lengths, keeping the arms moving with the legs, and keeping the head still. By this time, patients can start to feel when they are walking normally and when they are not. If you are still having difficulty with this sensation, have a friend or family member walk with you whenever possible to guide you in the improvement of your walking pattern (see Chapter 11).

Walking is an excellent form of exercise and should be utilized as much as possible. Park the car farther away from the store than usual, and walk. Walk to get the mail at the post office rather than driving the car. Get to the mall early, and walk for twenty to thirty minutes before starting your shopping. As a general guideline, walking for twenty to thirty minutes a day is beneficial not only for your TKA, but also for weight control and cardiovascular fitness. If you want to walk more, try to walk for forty-five minutes. This is the optimal length of time you should walk every day for weight control and cardiovascular health.

What about water walking? If you enjoy pool therapy, and if it is convenient for you to continue with it, the same guidelines apply to walking in the water: Aim for thirty to forty-five minutes per session. Water walking offers the additional benefit of providing more resistance against your body and limbs, causing you to burn more calories and providing a greater challenge to your cardiovascular system. We have several patients who use water walking as their primary means of exercise for their TKA and overall fitness, and they have never felt better!

Balance Training

For a significant number of patients, the one thing that has not returned to normal by now is their balance. Dr. Falkel did not feel that his balance was back to normal for almost eighteen months postoperatively. Balance is influenced by many different types of inputs to the body, and therefore it takes a long time to improve. However, with practice and repetition, balance can indeed be developed, and doing so will significantly enhance your daily activities.

In addition to the balance exercises described in Chapters 10 and 11, try the exercises on the following pages to help gain better balance.

While doing any of the balance exercises in this book it is OK, and actually recommended, for you to use the support of a sink or countertop for stability. As your balance improves, the need for this additional support will decrease, and you should eventually be able to complete the balance exercises without any hand support.

Exercise 131

Balance Exercise on Stairs

Stand on the bottom step of a staircase, facing the floor. Now stand on the TKA foot and, bending the TKA knee, move the other foot forward and down below the level of the step (Figure 12.7). Hold this position for 15–30 seconds, then rest by placing the non-TKA foot back on the step. Repeat 3–5 times.

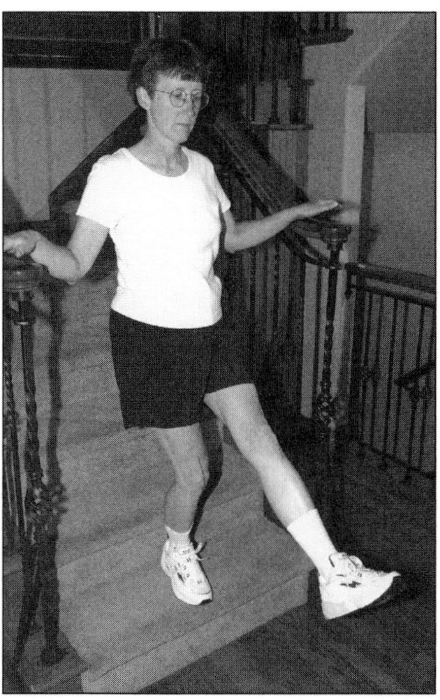

Figure 12.7. Balance exercise, standing on stair step

Exercise 132

Balance Exercise on Two-by-Four

Stand with your TKA foot on the four-inch side of a two-by-four board that is approximately two feet long. Lift the other foot several inches in the air, and try to balance (Figure 12.8). Hold this position for 15–30 seconds, and repeat 5–10 times.

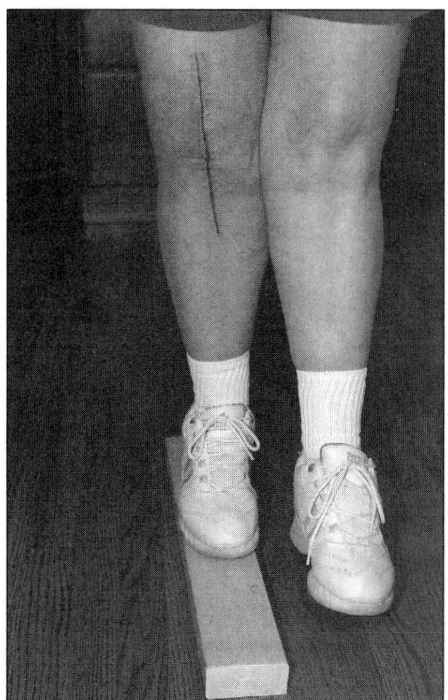

Figure 12.8. Balance exercise, standing on two-by-four

Exercise 133

Foot-Swing Balance Exercise on Two-by-Four

Stand with your TKA foot on the four-inch side of a two-by-four board that is approximately two feet long. Lift the other foot several inches in the air, and while balancing on the TKA foot, swing the other foot forward and backward as far as possible (Figure 12.9). Repeat for 30–60 seconds, 5–10 times.

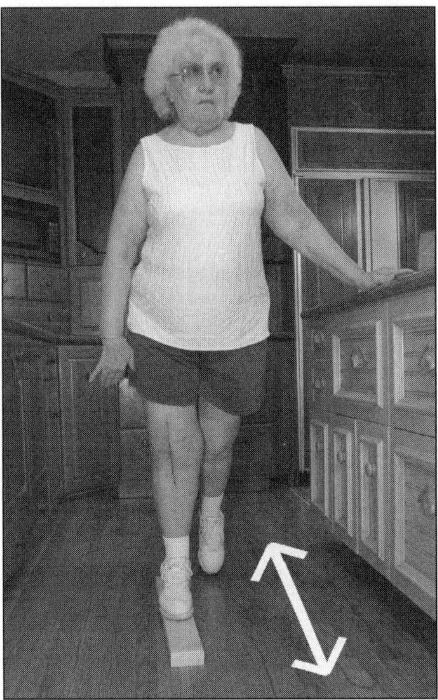

Figure 12.9. Dynamic single-leg-stance balance exercise, standing on two-by-four

As Exercise 133 becomes easier, try the following variations:

Exercise 134

Fast Foot-Swing Balance Exercise on Two-by-Four

Swing the non-TKA foot as fast as possible.

Exercise 135

Slow Foot-Swing Balance Exercise on Two-by-Four

Swing the non-TKA foot as slowly as possible.

Exercise 136

Side-to-Side Swing Balance Exercise in Front of TKA on Two-by-Four

Swing the non-TKA foot out to the side and then across and in front of the TKA foot (Figure 12.10).

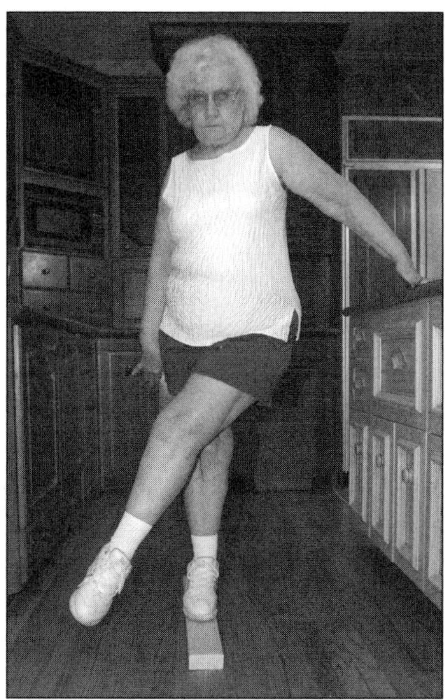

Figure 12.10. Dynamic single-leg-stance balance exercise, swinging leg across and in front of standing leg

Exercise 137

Side-to-Side Swing Balance Exercise Behind TKA on Two-by-Four

Swing the non-TKA foot out to the side and then across and behind the TKA foot (Figure 12.11).

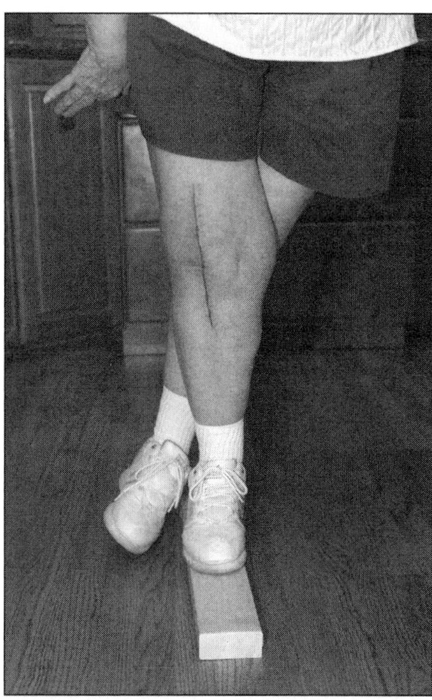

Figure 12.11. Dynamic single-leg-stance balance exercise, swinging leg behind standing leg

Exercise 138

Balancing on TKA While Playing Catch

Stand with your TKA foot on the ground. Lift the other foot several inches in the air, and then have someone throw a ball for you to catch while trying to balance on the TKA foot (Figure 12.12). Avoid letting the other foot touch the ground. Repeat 15–25 times.

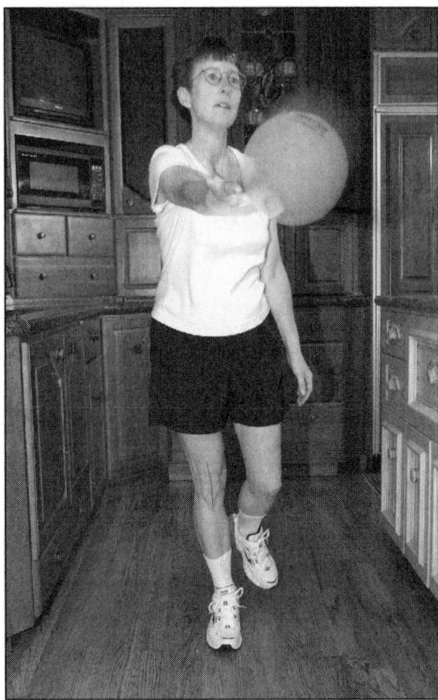

Figure 12.12. Dynamic single-leg-stance balance exercise, playing catch

Exercise 139

Balancing on TKA on Two-by-Four While Playing Catch

Stand with your TKA foot on the four-inch side of a two-by-four board that is approximately two feet long. Lift the other foot several inches in the air, and have someone throw a ball for you to catch while trying to balance on the TKA foot (Figure 12.13). Repeat 15–25 times.

Improving balance takes a lot of practice and dedication. It can be very frustrating while you are first learning how to balance on your TKA leg. Keep at it, because the benefits of good balance are enormous for every aspect of your daily activities.

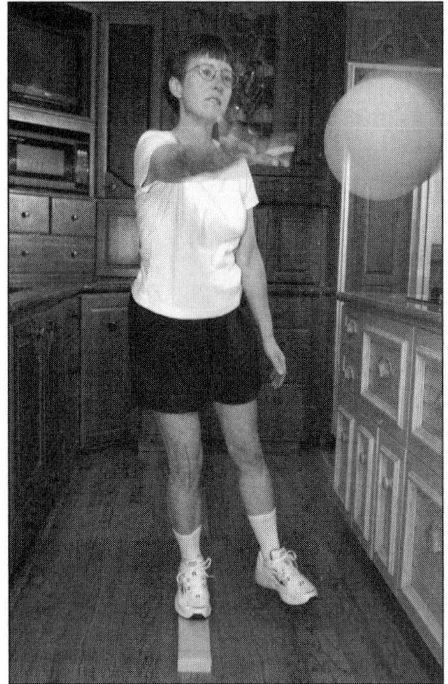

Figure 12.13. Dynamic single-leg stance balance on two-by-four, playing catch

■ ■ ■

If you have read this chapter in anticipation of a TKA, some of these exercises may seem elementary. However, if you have read this chapter after undergoing TKA surgery, you will have a better understanding of our approach to rehabilitation. It is necessary to break down and isolate the mechanics of the simplest things we do in order to better appreciate how to get back to normal. Isolating individual mechanical functions and working to improve them allow us to eventually return to more complicated activities.

Common Questions and Some Answers

Why do my knees feel different before a storm?

There are receptors in the joint that are sensitive to changes in barometric pressure. An approaching storm is accompanied by alterations in the barometric pressure. Our joint receptors sense this, causing pain in the joint. Although it is a poorly understood phenomenon, it is not an "old wives' tale." The sensation is real. For some TKA patients, the sensation is pressure, or tightness. Other individuals actually feel pain.

How long do I have to continue my rehabilitation exercises?

On the average, most patients will find they benefit from doing their rehabilitation exercises for approximately six months. However, this does not mean that you should stop exercising after six months. It is important to continue a regular exercise program that is fun and beneficial for your overall health as well as for your new knee (such as cycling, swimming, walking, doubles tennis, or golf). Even after several months, some patients occasionally find it necessary to do rehab exercises for range of motion when their knee gets stiff or tight.

When should I have my other knee replaced?

Although a significant number of people have arthritis in both knees, they may only require TKA surgery on one knee. The life of the nonoperated knee may be extended, even in the face of severe arthritic disease, because you now have a pain-free knee that can carry its share of weight during activities of daily living. Some of the conservative treatments discussed in Chapter 2 may be more effective since there is less stress and strain on the nonoperated knee. The general guidelines for having the second knee replaced are the same as they are for the first, a topic also discussed in Chapter 2. However, there may come a time when getting the other knee replaced becomes the only option. We recommend that patients wait a minimum of three months between the first and second total-knee-replacement surgeries. This will allow the first TKA to adequately heal and develop enough strength to be designated as the "good leg."

However, having already been through the procedure and rehabilitation once, you are the best judge about when to get the other knee replaced. See more about this topic in the next chapter.

Will I set off the metal detector in an airport?

Most of the TKA prosthetic components are made of metal, either titanium, stainless steel, or cobalt chromium. These implants may set off the alarm in the security screening at major airports. We recommend that before you go through the metal detector you tell the security agent that you have an artificial knee. Some surgeons will offer you a card to carry that explains the metal hardware in your body. Some cards show a picture of your knee X ray with the TKA. If the metal-detector alarm sounds, you will be subjected to the "wand" search, which usually takes only minutes to complete.

When can I start flying again?

After the third postoperative month, most patients can sit comfortably for two hours waiting for a plane or during the flight itself. We recommend that every two hours the TKA patient get up and walk around, even for just a few minutes, so that the TKA knee does not get stiff from being in one position for too long. The same holds true for taking a long road trip in a car: Every two hours, stop and walk for a few minutes to prevent stiffness and keep your TKA knee comfortable.

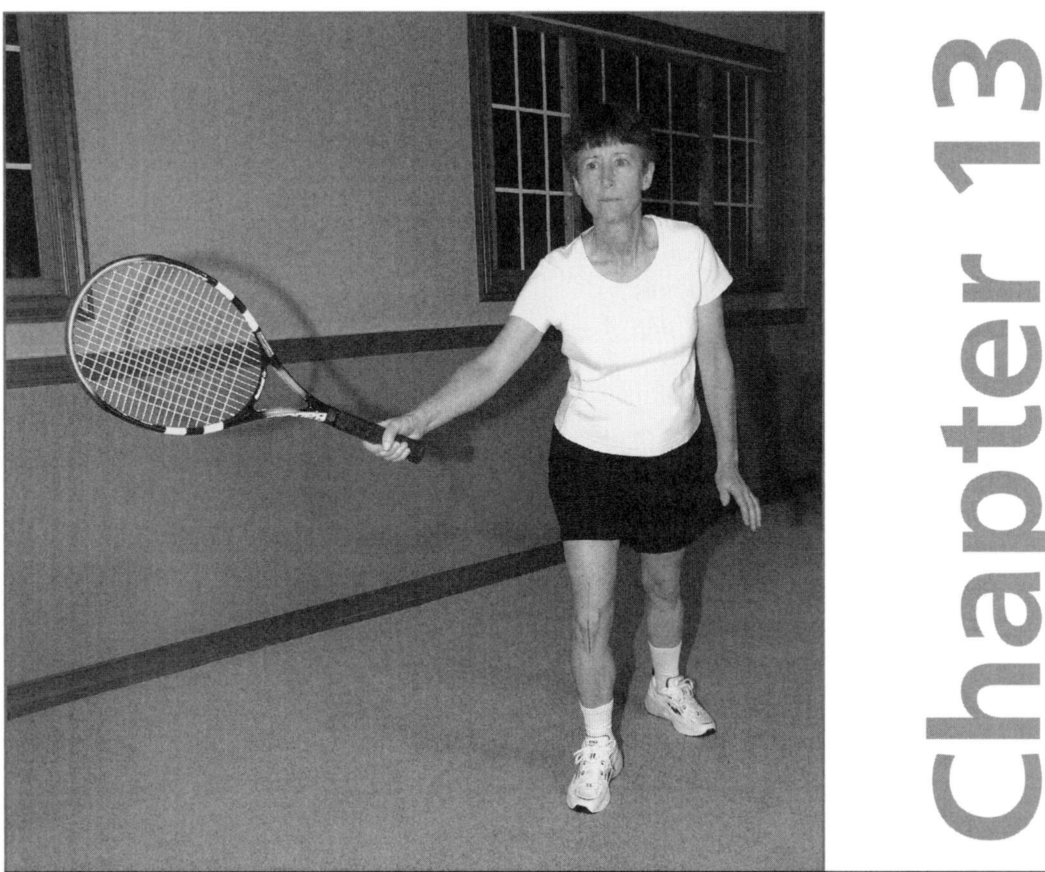

Chapter 13

Six Months to One Year

I Should Have Done This Years Ago!

One of the best things that can happen to someone who has had a knee replaced is the reaction of a friend or family member who has not seen them since before the surgery. Many people have heard "horror stories" about how terrible TKA surgery is and how limiting the artificial knee can be. Then these skeptics see their friend walking without a limp, moving effortlessly, wearing a smile, and they are shocked. That look on people's faces is priceless! After six months of rehabilitation, most patients are finally (or nearly) back to the type of life they had only dreamed about before their surgery. Family members notice that one of the biggest changes in the TKA patient is that they seem to smile a whole lot more. Living without pain is indeed wonderful!

Is It Time to Have the Other Knee Replaced?

What is next for the TKA patient? For many who suffered arthritis in both knees, it is time to start thinking about getting the other knee replaced. Several months ago you probably swore you would never get the other knee replaced, but now the TKA knee is your *good* knee. Your daily activities now may be limited more by the nonoperated knee than by the TKA knee. Some people had a preoperative discussion with their surgeon concerning the pros and cons of having bilateral TKA done simultaneously. Often, the surgeon and/or patient concludes that waiting until the first TKA is healed and rehabilitated is the best option before having the other knee replaced. If the other knee needs to be replaced, there are several considerations about the timing between surgeries:

1. How severe is the arthritis in the other knee? Many times the nonoperated knee is put under less stress after the TKA knee has recovered, and this may delay the need for a second TKA. The TKA is able to handle more of the load, thus relieving the stress on the nonoperated arthritic knee. Relieving this stress may make the conservative treatments for arthritis (discussed in Chapter 2) more effective.

2. What type of family support is available? By now, each patient knows how much they relied on family and friends during the recovery and rehabilitation of the first TKA. Some patients wait until they can arrange to have the necessary family support before getting the other knee replaced.

3. How much time can be taken off from work? Some patients decide to wait until seasonal variations in their workload are low before undergoing a second TKA surgery. One of the main reasons Dr. Falkel had his knees replaced simultaneously was because he had only five weeks of paid time off accrued and knew that the nonoperated knee would not last until he had saved up enough time for an additional rehabilitation.

4. The time of year often influences the decision to have the second surgery. Some patients would rather do their rehabilitation in the fall or winter, while others would rather have their surgery in the spring or summer, when there is less chance of bad weather.
5. Insurance coverage can also play a role in deciding when to have the second knee replaced. It may be necessary to proceed with TKA surgery before or after a change in insurance coverage.
6. The bottom line for most patients considering another knee replacement is that they will usually go to their surgeon when they are ready. Being ready is probably the best reason and time to have the second surgery.

It is worth pointing out once again that just as no two people are the same, no two TKAs are the same. Just about every bilateral knee patient we have treated is of the opinion that while there were many aspects of the recovery and rehabilitation that were similar for both knees, the second TKA was different from the first. One knee may not be better or worse than the other, just different. Dr. Falkel's TKAs are different. The right TKA is tighter, but he has better balance in that leg. The left TKA has more range of motion and is stronger. Were it not for the incision scar, he would never know he had a TKA on the left.

If you are a candidate for eventual bilateral TKAs, it is advantageous to prepare the second leg as well as you can prior to surgery. You already know what demands will be placed on your next TKA with regard to recovery and rehabilitation, so if you are able to keep that leg in the best possible shape, it will make rehabilitation that much easier. The simplest and best way to do this is to perform all the exercises we have described throughout this book with *both* legs, not just the TKA leg. Doing the exercises with the nonoperated leg will not only keep that leg strong and mobile, but it can also provide the TKA leg with a consistent rest interval between sets of different exercises. You may find that you are unable to perform all the exercises with the nonoperated leg because the arthritis in your knee is too severe. In that case, do the exercises that are possible without excessive pain. For this situation, pool therapy is again highly recommended, because the benefits of water are the same for the nonoperated, arthritic knee as for the TKA knee.

Getting Stronger

For a subset of patients, the strength developed during the first six months of rehabilitation has proven to be all they need in order to perform all the activities they want. However, others feel as though they still lack the strength they desire. For such patients, we offer the following suggestions for increasing strength, conditioning, and endurance during the six to twelve months following surgery.

1. If you are using a Total Gym, you can dramatically increase your strength by incorporating the following modifications:

    a. Perform the exercises described in Chapters 3 and 10 using a higher setting for the glideboard.

    b. Perform the exercises with added resistance on the weight bar. (The manufacturer states that six hundred pounds of resistance can be used safely with the Total Gym.)

    c. Perform the exercises using only one leg at a time. This was probably the most effective means by which Dr. Falkel gained strength during this phase of his rehabilitation.

    d. Perform the exercises with additional repetitions and sets.

2. If you are going to a health club or recreation center, you can increase your strength significantly by doing the following:

    a. Perform the exercises with more resistance.

    b. Complete more sets and more repetitions of each exercise.

    c. Do the exercises with only one leg at a time.

3. If you are using a stationary cycle or rowing machine for strength and endurance training, you can increase your level of conditioning a great deal by following these suggestions:

    a. Add more resistance.

    b. Exercise for longer periods at a time (e.g., up to forty-five minutes per session).

    c. Add strength-training sessions on either a Total Gym or other resistance-training device to your workouts on the stationary cycle or rowing machine.

These are just a few suggestions that can dramatically improve your strength and endurance. As we've stated previously, any time you increase the intensity or duration of your training program, do so *gradually.*

Balance Training

The most difficult challenge for Dr. Falkel was recovering his balance. He had been an athlete for many years and had relied on good balance to help him be competitive. But after bilateral TKA surgery, it seemed to take forever for him to regain his balance. Because he had both knees operated on at the same time, it may have taken him longer to regain his balance than it would have following a single TKA surgery. For whatever reason, he was unable to resume playing golf or skiing until after one year postoperatively, primarily because he felt his lack of balance would prevent him from participating in those activities safely.

Balance is such an integral part of almost every daily activity that it should be practiced for many months or even years after TKA surgery. So far in this book we have discussed a number of balance exercises and activities. Now, during this phase of the rehabilitation process, we will shift our focus to a more dynamic type of balance training. Working consistently on these activities will eventually allow patients to safely resume the sports and other activities they enjoyed before they became hindered by knee arthritis.

Balance-Board Exercises

A balance board can easily be constructed out of a 3/4-inch piece of plywood cut to approximately 18 inches by 24 inches. Using screws, attach a piece of wood measuring 24 inches by 3 inches by 3/4 inches along the center of the plywood (Figure 13.1a). Then affix a nonskid surface to the other side of the plywood, and you have a balance board (Figure 13.1b). The following balance exercises are intended for patients who want to return to activities and sports that require more acute balance skills, such as skiing.

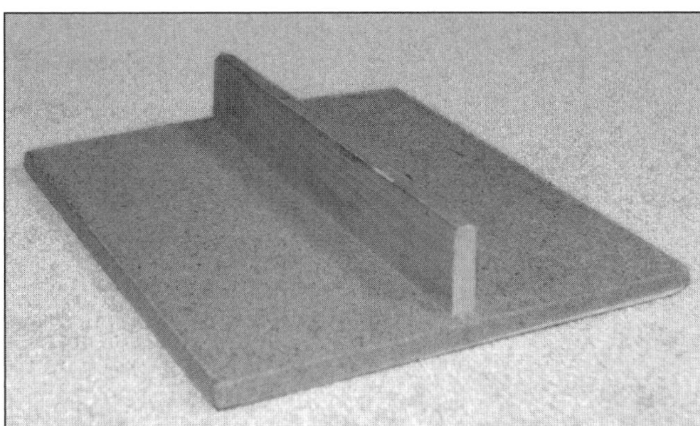

Figure 13.1 a/b. Balance boards

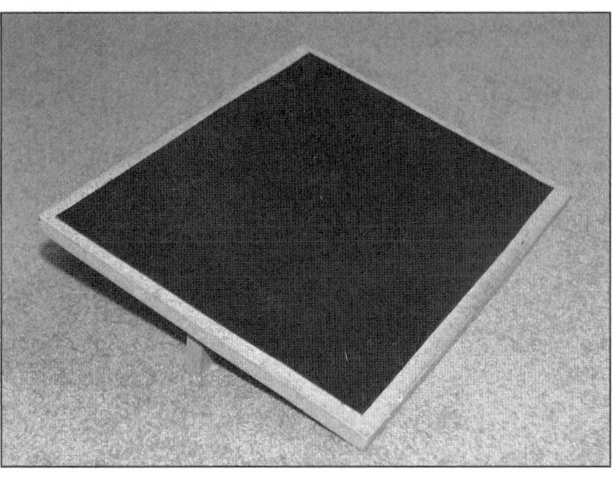

Exercise 140

Feet Parallel to Fulcrum on Balance Board

Practice balancing on the board with your feet parallel to the fulcrum on the bottom (Figure 13.2).

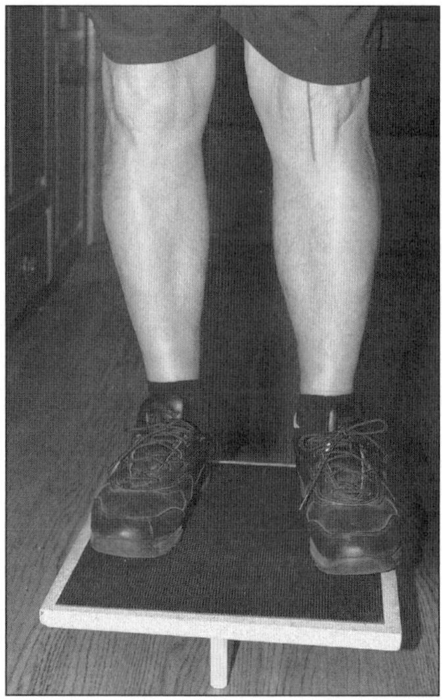

Figure 13.2. Balance-board training: feet parallel to fulcrum

Exercise 141

Feet Perpendicular to Fulcrum on Balance Board

Practice balancing on the board with your feet perpendicular to the fulcrum on the bottom (Figure 13.3).

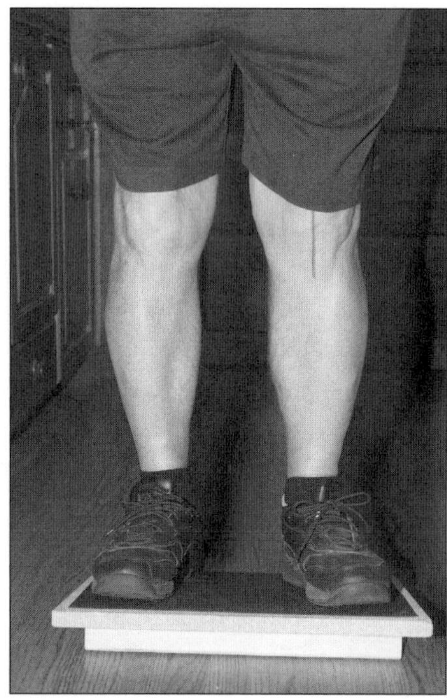

Figure 13.3. Balance-board training: feet perpendicular to fulcrum

Exercise 142

Playing Catch While on Balance Board

Practice balancing on the board while playing catch with someone (Figure 13.4).

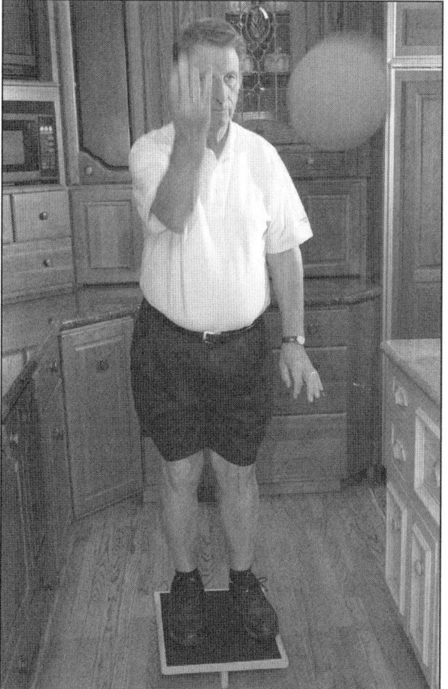

Figure 13.4. Balance-board training: playing catch

Exercise 143

Watching TV While on Balance Board

Practice balancing on the board while watching TV (Figure 13.5).

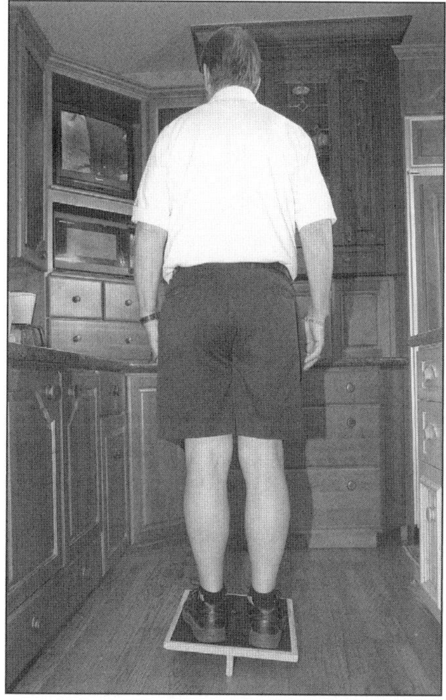

Figure 13.5. Balance-board training: balancing while watching TV

Exercise 144

Keeping Balance Board from Touching Ground

Try to prevent the board from touching the ground for as long as possible.

Exercise 145

One Foot in Front of the Other on Balance Board

Practice balancing on the board with one foot in front of the other (Figure 13.6).

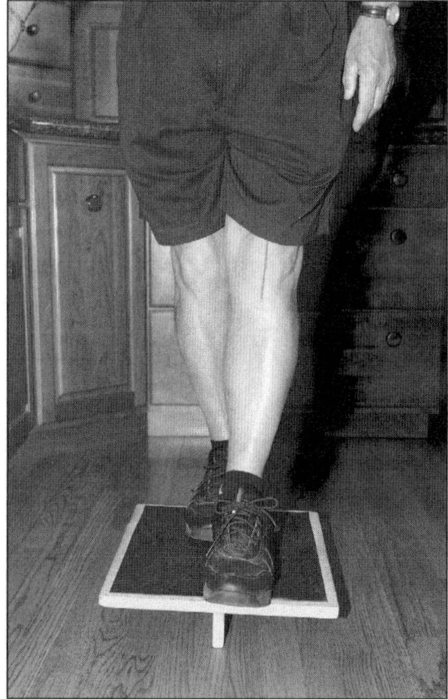

Figure 13.6. Balance-board training: one foot in front of the other

When Can I Start Doing ___________ Again? (Fill in the Blank)

By now, many patients can't wait to start golfing, bowling, or dancing again. They have been unable to participate in a host of activities for years due to their knee arthritis. Beginning about six months after surgery, if you feel ready to try these activities, you probably *are* ready. This section offers some guidelines about when to start various activities and how to participate in them safely.

Golf

In all likelihood, it has been many years since you were able to play golf without pain. Here are some suggestions for getting back into it now:

1. Begin at the driving range. Proceed slowly. Practice hitting iron shots for several sessions before taking out the driver and hitting as hard as you can.
2. Have a golf professional work with you on your swing. If you played golf right up to your surgery, you may have developed some bad habits in your swing because of your knee pain. If you have avoided golf for several years because of your arthritis pain, you may need help with your swing now that you have a new TKA. Dr. Falkel found that moving his right foot back about two inches and turning his left foot slightly out-

ward made all the difference in his golf swing and overall ability. He needed the advice of a golf professional to work out this change in his swing.

3. Once you are ready to start playing, start with an executive or par-three course the first few times. Then progress to nine holes on a regular course, preferably using a golf cart to reduce the amount of walking.
4. Don't be afraid to improve your lie if you are in an awkward place in the rough. Many TKA patients find that with a downhill lie it is very difficult to maintain adequate balance to hit a reasonable shot. When in doubt, pick up your ball and move it to a place where you will have more confidence in your shot.
5. After your swing returns and your endurance improves, if you want to walk while golfing, use a pull cart or similar device to carry your golf bag. Carrying your golf bag on your shoulders for eighteen holes is exhausting and will dramatically alter your gait.

Bowling

Bowling is a great activity for many patients, and it is one that can be safely performed after TKA surgery.

1. Before starting to bowl again be sure you have good single-foot balance on the TKA leg, particularly if the TKA leg is the lead leg on release. Practice sliding the lead foot on the kitchen floor where you have the counter for support if you lose your balance.
2. Before starting to bowl again, practice swinging your bowling ball while in a single-leg stance on the TKA leg (Figure 13.7).
3. Start by bowling only a few frames as part of a game between partners or friends. Eventually work up to bowling a full ten frames. This may take several outings, so be patient.

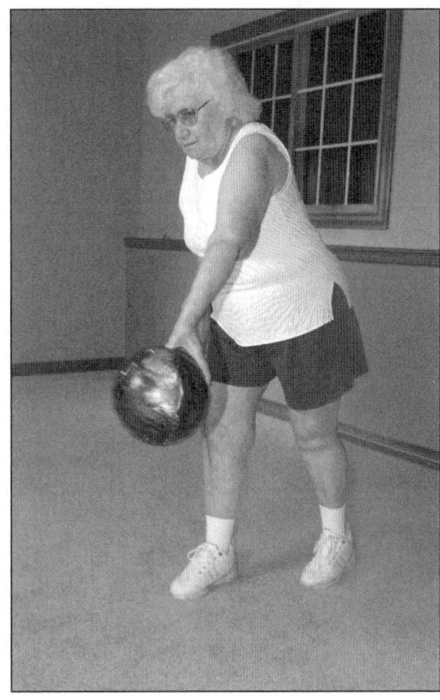

Figure 13.7. Bowling practice at home

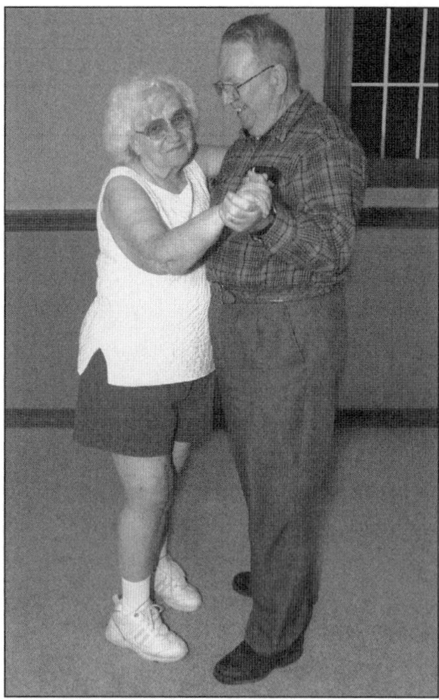

Figure 13.8. Dance practice at home

Dancing

It is surprising how many patients consider a return to dancing a major goal after having had their knee replaced. Dancing is a great form of exercise, and it offers tremendous social benefits as well.

1. As with bowling, be sure to have good single-leg balance in the TKA leg before trying to dance. An exercise to improve single-leg balance is to stand on the TKA foot, swing the other leg forward and backward, and then pivot around on the TKA foot. Be sure to practice this where you have adequate support, such as in the kitchen near the countertop.
2. Practice using an exaggerated motion to step forward, backward, and sideways in both directions with the TKA leg in a single-leg stance and then again with the nonoperated leg in a single-leg stance. Part of dancing is the ability to land on one foot and then move in a different direction off that foot—and that foot may happen to belong to the TKA leg.
3. Begin dancing slowly, practicing with your partner on a surface that will not cause you to trip or slide accidentally (Figure 13.8). You can gradually progress to dancing on different surfaces, but again, be sure to have good footing, and hang on for dear life!

Gardening

For some patients, working in their garden is a dream come true after having undergone TKA surgery.

1. Discuss with your surgeon about kneeling on the TKA knee.
2. Patients who can't kneel often use a small bench on wheels that they can sit on close to the ground. These are available at many garden-supply stores and through mail-order catalogs. Be careful to find a stool that is the proper height so you avoid developing back pain while trying to save your TKA. It may require trial and error to find the proper height.

3. Avoid heavy lifting until your strength and balance are nearly normal.

Skiing

A return to skiing is possible for most patients following TKA as long as they were reasonably competent skiers before surgery.

1. It is a must to have adequate strength, endurance, and (most importantly) balance before attempting to start skiing again. For this reason, we recommend waiting at least one year after TKA surgery before trying to ski.
2. Try the new "shaped" or parabolic skis. They are shaped like an hour glass and are much easier to turn. In addition, you turn the parabolic skis at the same time, as opposed to turning with just the downhill ski, as you do on traditional snow skis.
3. Stay on groomed runs, and *don't even think about skiing the bumps*! Mogul skiing puts tremendous stress on the TKA.
4. Stay away from skiing the deep powder. When skiing in deep powder, the majority of skiers tend to sit back on their skis, which would put excessive stress on the TKA. The other difficulty with powder skiing is that it is very demanding on the thigh muscles in a way that most TKA patients are unprepared for. It is difficult to train the quadriceps muscles adequately to ski in extreme conditions.

Tennis

1. As we mentioned in Chapter 12, discuss playing tennis with your surgeon. Many surgeons will let their TKA patients play doubles tennis because playing doubles involves less running to cover the court.
2. Practice swinging the tennis racquet, both forehand and backhand, while in a single-leg stance on the TKA leg before going to the court.
3. Work on forward, backward, and lateral movements similar to those used in tennis (Figure 13.9 and 13.10). We recommend practicing these movements for several weeks prior to getting on the tennis court.

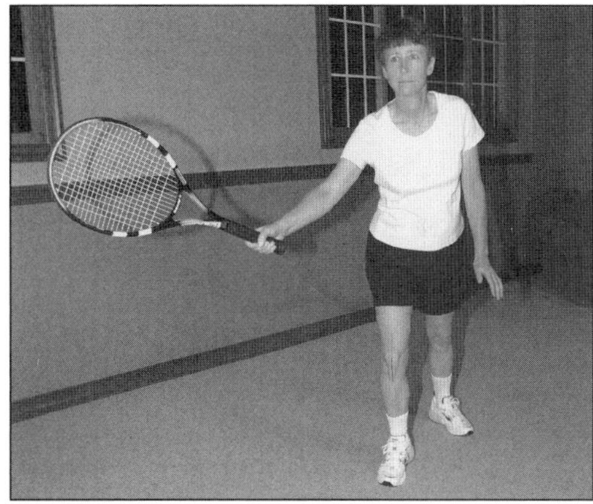

Figure 13.9. Tennis practice at home

4. Begin by hitting or volleying a tennis ball against a wall to see how your new knee reacts to the lateral movements involved.

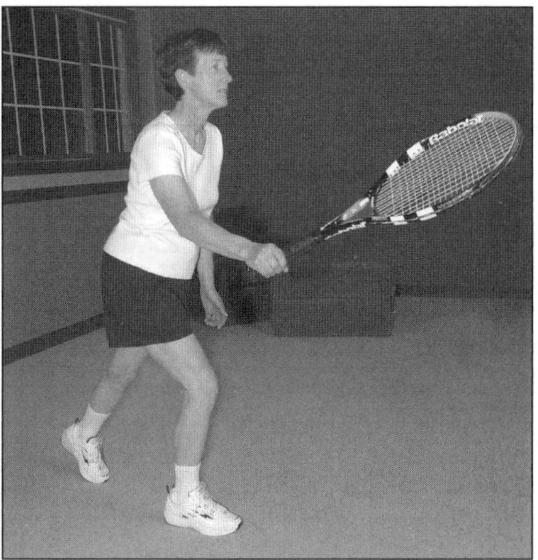

Figure 13.100. Tennis practice at home

5. When you are ready to start playing doubles again, consider having an extra partner available so that you can play for a few minutes and then rest while the substitute plays for a few minutes. By alternating players you avoid getting too tired, and your playing partners can still have a good match.

Other Sports

Other sports can be enjoyed with an artificial knee, such as hiking, cross-country skiing, snowshoeing, biking, hunting, fishing, racquetball, and squash, to name a few. The key in preparing for a return to these sports is to start slowly. Try to simulate some of the movements of the sport with a "dry run" in the kitchen. Don't be discouraged at your initial efforts; it will take time to get back to an acceptable level of performance.

Common Questions and Some Answers

Why does my knee hurt at times?

It is normal for your new knee joint to hurt occasionally. The anatomy of the knee has been surgically altered, and scar tissue has formed in and around the joint that can potentially be a source of some discomfort. In addition, the synovium (the lining of the inside of the joint) can become pinched between the prosthetic parts, resulting in localized pain. And as discussed in Chapter 12, changes in weather can cause pain, stiffness, or tightness in the knee joint. Although pain from various causes can occur without apparent reason, it usually lasts less than twenty-four hours. If knee pain persists for three to four days, contact your surgeon.

Will I hurt something if I try to kneel on my TKA, or will I ever be able to kneel on my TKA?

Kneeling on your TKA will not do any harm to the joint or its artificial components. However, kneeling may be uncomfortable for some time after surgery. For some patients the discomfort is only temporary, but other patients will always experience pain while kneeling on their TKA. The factors that determine pain while kneeling are poorly understood. Therefore, it is difficult to predict who will experience pain while kneeling and who will be able to kneel without any difficulty.

Why does my TKA get "cold" in the winter?

The majority of patients may experience their TKA as being "cold" during the first winter after surgery. The knee and surrounding tissue are probably still healing, and the circulation may be compromised due to swelling and scarring. As the knee heals and the circulation returns to normal, the cold sensation typically subsides. We are of the opinion that the cold sensation is not due to the metal in the knee, because it is well insulated by the surrounding soft tissue.

Why is recovery after my second TKA different from recovery after my first TKA?

Good question! We have discussed this issue quite a bit with colleagues and patients, and no one seems to have a good answer. All patients should be aware that even if they have the same total-knee procedure performed on each knee—at the same time and by the same surgeon—the recovery for each knee will be different.

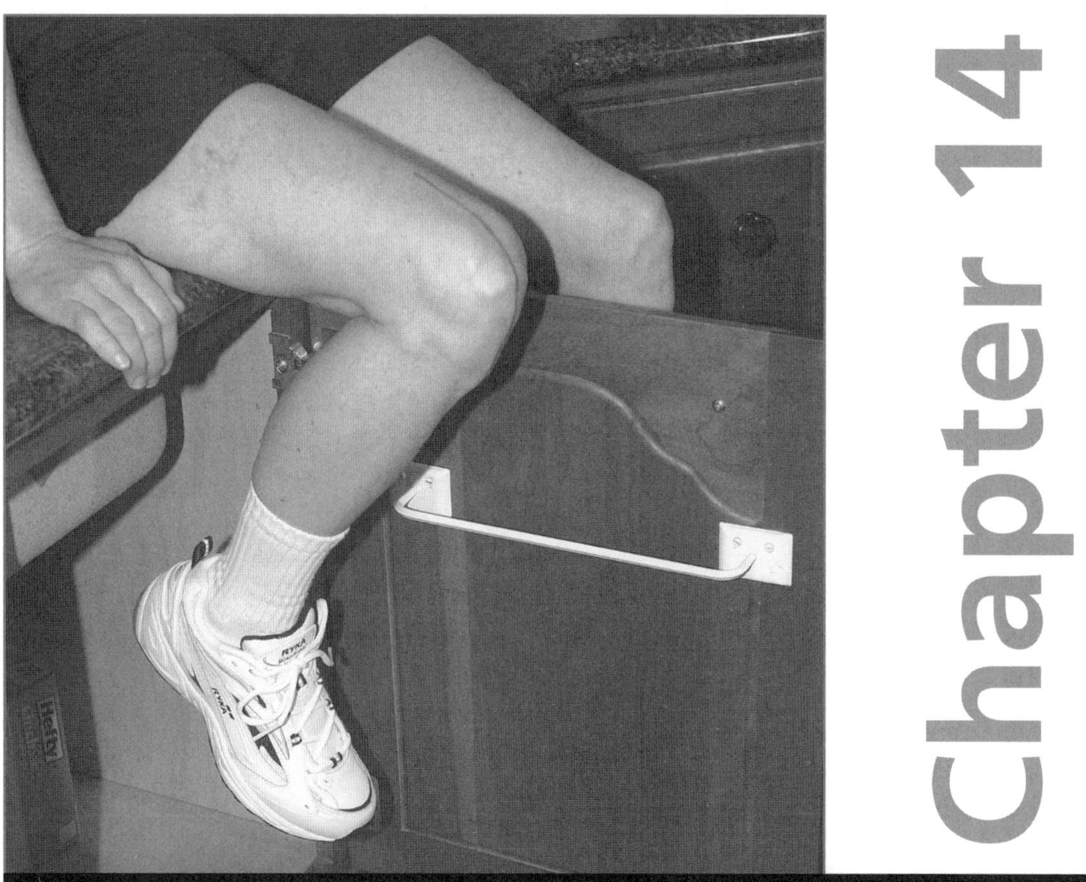

Chapter 14

One Year to Life

My Knee Is My Best Joint

A former patient of ours once said that when he had pants on and could not see his incision, he didn't know he had a TKA. This is our wish for all patients. Living with a TKA has its major emphasis on "living." Ninety to 95 percent of the patients with a new knee joint state that the TKA has indeed given them a new lease on life.

After the one-year postoperative anniversary, the vast majority of TKA patients can do almost anything they desire. There may even be times when they "forget" they have an artificial joint and try something they previously never would have attempted. The first time this happened to Dr. Falkel, he had gone to a patient's home and found the only place for him to sit was on an ottoman in the living room. He didn't even think twice about sitting down on the low footstool and had no difficulty sitting there talking with his patient. However, when he tried to get up he couldn't, because the ottoman was too low. What did he do? He could not ask the patient to help pull him up, but after a few tense moments he realized he could slide down to the floor and get up from there. Because he cannot kneel, getting up off the floor is somewhat challenging—but not impossible. The situation made him realize that he hadn't paid attention to how low the ottoman was, whereas several months earlier he would never even have considered sitting on something that close to the ground!

As we discussed in Chapter 12, if you think you are ready to try something, you are probably right. Most patients tell us that they can sense when it is safe to attempt a certain activity or exercise. Dr. Falkel just "knew" that he was not ready to start skiing one year after surgery, even though his surgeons both gave him the green light. He needed to do more work on his balance and on his skiing-specific strength training before he felt confident and comfortable trying to ski again. But once he had developed his balance and strength, he skied all winter long wearing a big smile on his face!

There will still be some long-term concerns for TKA patients. Some individuals may have trouble standing still for long periods even a year or more after TKA surgery. Unfortunately, there are no easy answers for this problem. Although you can "practice" your standing tolerance, when faced with the actual task of standing your TKA may get stiff, depending on the floor surface, temperature, atmospheric pressure, and length of time you have to stand. Dr. Falkel has no problems standing during an entire soccer match or practice that lasts longer than two hours, but he still does not like to stand in a store checkout line for very long.

Another possible—but rare—experience is a pinching sensation along the joint line of the TKA. Sometimes the prosthetic components will actually pinch a small piece of the joint lining (synovium) or capsule that surrounds the knee. Because the joint lining contains nerve endings, the pinching can be quite painful. It usually subsides with cessation of the activity or exercise and may require some ice and/or treatment with an anti-inflammatory medication for a day or so. However, the first time it happens, it may cause panic, as it feels very similar to some of the pain experienced in the old days prior to TKA surgery.

Sometimes patients continue to feel or hear their TKA "click" even a year after surgery. This is normal, and as long as there is no pain involved it should be of no concern. The only time Dr. Falkel's TKAs regularly click is when he is doing abdominal exercises. If a click becomes consistently painful, it is a good reason to be promptly evaluated by your surgeon. And if your TKA clicks excessively but is *not* painful, be sure to discuss it with your surgeon at your next visit. Many surgeons like to see their TKA patients once a year after surgery, and your annual visit would be a good time to discuss this concern. (For a discussion of other potential complications following knee surgery, see Appendix A.)

Probably the most common question we get asked at this point in the recovery process is "How much longer will I have to do exercises for my TKA?" This is not an easy question to answer. We recommend that all TKA patients perform daily exercise to keep their new knee's motion, strength, and endurance at an optimal level and their own cardiovascular fitness up to par. Daily exercise will also assist in weight control, which is another issue we stress with all patients. However, if a patient is able to return to a job that is physically demanding and allows them to maintain good knee motion, strength, and endurance, this amount of activity in a day may be sufficient. We had a patient who had bilateral TKAs done in November and went back to work as a farmer in April. When we talked to him a year later, he was still working every day on the farm and had not ridden his stationary cycle or been to pool therapy since April. He told us that he probably walked two or three miles every day, climbed on and off farm vehicles fifty or more times each day, and was still able to perform the routine maintenance on his farm vehicles. Even though he was no longer doing his "rehabilitation exercises," he was exercising every day while working.

As a rule of good overall health, as well as good TKA health, we recommend that all TKA patients engage in some exercise every day. It does not have to take as long as your early rehabilitation sessions, and it may be as varied as playing golf one day, exercising on the stationary cycle the next, participating in pool therapy or swimming the day after, and doing strength training the following day. Some patients are content to simply take the dog for a thirty-minute walk every day, and that, too, can be enough. Patients are overjoyed to realize that they now actually look forward to exercise and other daily activities that were nearly impossible before surgery.

While we encourage our readers who have undergone TKA surgery to try to follow our exercise and rehabilitative progressions, we know firsthand that some patients respond faster—and likewise some slower—to the exercises suggested in this book.

Don't use this book as the last word on TKA rehabilitation; rather, use it as a reference. Discuss every step of your recovery and rehabilitation with your surgeon and physical therapist. Consider sharing with them what you have learned from this book. But remember, your surgeon and physical therapist can only do so much. Most of your success in the rehabilitation process is up to *you!*

We wish each person who is reading this book the best of luck with their TKA surgery and with rehabilitation after surgery. It is a potentially life-changing procedure, and for the vast majority of patients the change is for the better. We have enjoyed sharing our knowledge and experience with you. Enjoy your TKA!

Common Questions and Some Answers

What can I do to make my TKA last as long as possible?

Protect your TKA by exercising common sense. Keep in mind the tire analogy: The less stress you place on the tire, the more miles you will get out of it. Likewise, the less stress you place on your new knee, the longer it will last. Low-impact aerobic exercises provide the least stress to the TKA. Striving for optimal weight control will also prolong the life of the TKA (if the tire has to carry less freight, it will last longer). We urge patients to be cautious in their everyday activities, even when doing something as simple as stepping over a puddle. Be careful! Most people want to wait as long as possible before undergoing surgery again. You and only you remember how much "fun" you had after your TKA surgery!

What types of sports can I play in the future with my TKA?

The goal is to have your TKA last as long as possible. Therefore, your sports and recreational activities should be chosen with that in mind. We recommend low-impact, aerobic types of exercises, including cycling, swimming, walking, doubles tennis, golf, and weight lifting, to name a few. Any sport that requires excessive lateral movement or involves quick stops, starts, and turns should be avoided due to the excessive stress those actions place on the knee joint.

Appendix A: Potential Complications of Total Knee Arthroplasty

Overall, the total-knee procedure is a good operation with reliable and reproducible results. Ninety to 95 percent of the time, patients are very satisfied with their new knee(s). Unfortunately, as with any surgical procedure, complications do occur. The following is an overview of some of the potential problems that may arise following TKA surgery. This is not to dissuade patients from having the operation, but rather to make them aware of the possible problems. The potential complications certainly did not deter Dr. Falkel, nor do they deter the hundreds of thousands of patients who undergo successful TKA surgeries each year. An awareness of the potential complications provides an understanding of why certain precautionary measures are needed.

Medical Complications

Since the majority of surgical candidates for TKA are elderly, they frequently have other medical conditions, such as varying degrees of cardiovascular (heart) disease, diabetes mellitus, renal (kidney) disease, and pulmonary (lung) problems. A thorough general medical evaluation preoperatively will allow correction of some of these problems before surgery. Anticipating obstacles that may arise during the surgery allows the surgical team to make adjustments to enable the patient to withstand the rigors of anesthesia and surgery. For patients with multiple and complex medical problems, a doctor who specializes in internal medicine will provide invaluable assistance in the preoperative and postoperative management of any complications. Unfortunately, despite all of the preventive measures, some patients will unavoidably sustain heart attack, stroke, gastrointestinal problems, lung problems, or other medical complications following anesthesia and surgery.

In the immediate postoperative period, care should be taken to prevent problems with the patient's body positioning in bed. Because of the pain experienced with movement and the sedation from pain medications, patients tend to be immobile in bed for the first few days after TKA surgery. Frequent movement and proper positioning can prevent a number of problems. It is necessary to avoid positioning the knees in a flexed position with pillows under the back of the knees for prolonged periods, as doing so can cause joint flexion contractures. Patients and nursing staff must observe the details of positioning to prevent bed sores from developing on the buttocks and heels. Arms and elbows should be moved frequently to prevent nerve injuries. Prophylactic (preventive) antibiotics should be continued as long as invasive IV lines or urinary catheters are in place. Postoperative urinary retention is a common problem. Frequent movement in and out of bed with decreasing amounts of pain medications can minimize this complication. If urinary retention occurs, it typically responds to intermittent catheterization or an indwelling Foley catheter. Further difficulty with urinary retention may require consultation with a urologist.

Sometimes a preexisting medical condition may be worsened after any major surgical procedure. For example, a normally well-controlled diabetic patient may find it difficult to keep his blood sugar regulated after total-knee-replacement surgery. Or someone with high blood pressure may require changes to her medication to keep blood pressure under control postoperatively. Patients with pulmonary problems may need additional respiratory treatments to allow them to breathe more normally. These phenomena occur because of the overall stresses resulting from the TKA surgery and anesthesia. Patients with preexisting medical conditions are more likely to have medical problems postoperatively. If you have a preexisting medical condition, it is very important that you consult with your primary-care doctors prior to TKA surgery in an effort to minimize any potential medical complications after surgery.

Surgical Complications

Infection

Infection is an infrequent complication following TKA. Fortunately, the overall occurrence remains small, in the range of 1–2 percent of all knee replacements performed by competent surgeons.[22] This complication is not entirely preventable, as several factors influence the incidence of infection.

The overall health of the patient may affect the incidence of infection. Factors such as diabetes mellitus, poor nutrition, rheumatoid arthritis, extreme old age, obesity, smoking, and certain prescription medications (e.g., steroids) may all serve to suppress the immune system and increase the chance of infection. Local factors that affect the skin and other soft tissue may also be a factor. These include previous surgery on the knee, prior history of septic arthritis (joint infection), and previous extensive trauma to the knee. All of these factors serve to impair the local blood supply around the joint due to scarring in the soft tissue, thus making the knee more susceptible to infection. A majority of the health issues such as those listed above cannot be controlled.

Surgical technique is an important factor influencing postoperative infection, and it can be controlled by the surgeon and the operating-room staff. Meticulous detail to surgical technique and strict adherence to surgery protocols are critical. Prolonged operating time should be avoided as it theoretically offers a greater chance for bacteria to infect the open surgical site. Careful surgical technique to minimize excessive bleeding and soft-tissue damage will reduce the potential locations where bacteria can thrive. A reputable surgeon will exercise the utmost care to follow these and other standard safety measures.

If infection does occur, it is often diagnosed by physical examination and a blood test. Superficial wound infections are usually easily diagnosed. However, deeper infections may be much more subtle and sometimes require an arthrocentesis. *Arthrocentesis* is a procedure that places a needle in the knee joint to obtain a sample of the knee fluid for a culture. In some cases, a bone scan, gallium scan, indium scan, or MRI scan may be useful in helping to make the diagnosis of infection.

Treatment of the infected knee following TKA can be complicated, depending on the amount, depth, and type of infection. Mild wound cellulitis (i.e., superficial infection of soft tissues) may be treated simply with antibiotics, whereas more involved wound infections may require several surgical wound debridements (washing and cleaning) as well as antibiotic therapy. Infections involving the joint are treated with IV antibiotics and surgical debridement. Deep infections, especially bone infections (osteomyelitis), typically require IV antibiotics, removal of the original prosthesis, and multiple surgical debridements before another prosthesis can be replaced six to eight weeks later.

Since an infection following TKA can have potentially devastating consequences, prevention of infection is taken very seriously. That is why it is so very important to follow the postoperative instructions outlined by your doctor and nurses. Let us reemphasize that although serious, postsurgical infection following TKA surgery is also quite rare, occurring in only 1–2 percent of cases.

Infrequently, a total-knee joint can become infected several months or even years after the surgery. This is due to hematogenous spread (carried by the blood) of bacteria from a source anywhere on the body. A common scenario involves infection following dental work or oral surgery, because manipulation of the gums can allow the normal bacteria of the mouth to enter the bloodstream. The bacteria can then travel through the circulatory system and attach to any foreign object in the body, including the metal and/or plastic components of the TKA. Other sources of infection can include kidney or bladder infections, skin boils or lesions, pneumonia, and the like. In order to reduce the risks of infection even long after TKA surgery, talk with your surgeon about taking preventive antibiotics prior to any type of dental work, even teeth cleaning. In addition, antibiotic treatments should be given prior to any type of surgery in the future. *With any infection, TKA patients are advised to seek early treatment with antibiotics to minimize the possibility of late infection of the total-knee prosthesis. If you have any questions about a remote possibility of infection, see your surgeon or other qualified health-care professional immediately.*

Joint Stiffness

Stiffness in the knee after TKA surgery happens to everyone. The degree and duration of stiffness is influenced by multiple factors. Obesity, infection, excessive bleeding, poor pain control, poor pain tolerance, tight ligaments, and old scars around the joint will contribute to stiffness. Sometimes the knee joint can become stiff for no obvious reason. Most likely this is due to the physical laws of soft-tissue biology, which are currently poorly understood. Regardless of the cause, the initial treatment for stiffness is the CPM machine and aggressive physical therapy. If these measures prove insufficient, a closed manipulation of the joint under general anesthesia may be necessary. Knowing when a closed manipulation is necessary is part of the art of medicine and is usually a joint decision made by the patient, surgeon, and physical therapist.

A closed manipulation is a day-surgery procedure that involves a return trip to the operating room. While there is no incision made on the knee, a general or regional anesthetic is used for the procedure. The surgeon will slowly force the knee through a greater range of motion. This is done so scar tissue that has formed around the TKA can be broken down, allowing the patient to achieve a greater range of motion than could be obtained prior to the manipulation. The procedure is usually followed up with aggressive physical therapy as well as a CPM machine for home use. Very rarely is an arthroscopy or open incision needed to release scar tissue.

Problems with Wound Healing

When it occurs, failure or delay in wound healing after TKA is a serious problem. Any time there is a failure of the wound to heal, the natural barrier to infection is compromised and the risk of infection is increased. Clinical conditions associated with poor wound healing include infection, obesity, rheumatoid arthritis, diabetes mellitus, peripheral vascular disease, and smoking. Scarring around the knee from previous surgery or trauma may impede the blood supply to the area, thus delaying healing of the wound. Treatment ranges from temporarily stopping the CPM machine and rehabilitation program to allow the wound to heal without excessive stress on the surrounding tissue, to multiple surgical debridements and wound closure. These complications are extremely rare, and your surgeon and physical therapist will do all they can to assist you in preventing them.

Neurovascular Complications

Fortunately, serious neurovascular injury (nerve damage) is rare following TKA surgery. Local nerves in the skin are severed during the surgical incision, which commonly results in some "patchy" areas of decreased sensation or complete numbness on the front or sides of the knee. It is particularly common over the lateral (outer) side of the knee. Although the numbness can cause a strange sensation, patients quickly adapt, and it does not impair the overall function of the TKA. Treatment is not needed, and for most patients sensation returns to normal or close to normal within six months to one year postsurgery.

Local skin neuromas (scar tissue around a nerve) near the incision are rare, but they can be troublesome when they occur. The majority improve with time, but nonsteroidal anti-inflammatory medications or injections of local anesthetic and steroids are often necessary. Rarely is surgery needed to remove a neuroma.

The most frequent neurological problem after TKA is peroneal nerve palsy, damage to the nerve that runs along the outer shinbone. Even so, peroneal nerve palsy occurs in less than 1 percent of all total-knee surgeries.[23] Alignment deformities of the knee prior to TKA, surgical technique, and obesity all predispose a patient to this problem. The potential causes of peroneal nerve palsy include injury at the time of surgery, excessive pressure on the nerve from prolonged immobility in bed, or direct pressure from constrictive dressings causing ischemia (lack of local blood supply).

The best treatment for peroneal nerve palsy is prevention. Attention to the details of surgical technique and proper positioning in bed are critically important. Common treatment of a postoperative peroneal nerve palsy requires removal of any tight dressing over the nerve and, if a significant motor deficit exists, an ankle-foot orthosis (brace). The prognosis for healing and return of the nerve function depends on the severity of the original injury.

Thromboembolism

Deep vein thrombosis (DVT) and/or pulmonary embolism (PE) may occur following TKA. The exact incidence of these blood clots and their clinical significance remain controversial. Most doctors agree that asymptomatic DVT and PE occur relatively frequently after this type of surgery. Fortunately, the incidence of potentially symptomatic PE is probably less than 1 percent.[24]

We discussed prevention of blood clots in Chapter 4. A prevention regimen includes using certain medications, such as oral warfarin (Coumadin) or injectable low-molecular-weight heparin (Lovenox, Fragmin), surgical stockings (T.E.D. hose), mechanical foot or leg pumps, and getting the patient up and moving soon after surgery. If a patient develops a postoperative blood clot, a doctor of internal medicine usually supervises the treatment. Treatment typically involves IV heparin and oral warfarin (Coumadin). The IV heparin is continued until the warfarin is adjusted to a therapeutic level. Warfarin may be continued for six months or longer. In addition, the rehabilitation program is temporarily put on hold until the clot is stabilized and the blood is adequately thinned. This is to minimize the possibility of the clot moving. A blood clot that moves to the lungs can be fatal. Usually, the treatment for a blood clot is uneventful and there is no significant effect on the overall surgical result. However, because of the potentially fatal nature of DVT or PE, these complications are taken very seriously.

Other infrequent complications following TKA can include fat embolization, fracture of the bone around the prosthesis, and breakage of the prosthetic knee components. These happen very rarely (usually less than 1 percent of the time), but if you're concerned about them, discuss them with your surgeon.

Revision of the TKA

As the saying goes, "All good things must come to an end." The same holds true for some total knee replacements. The average knee replacement lasts for approximately ten to fifteen years.[25] The longer a patient lives, or the greater the demands that are placed on the artificial knee, the more likely it is that knee-replacement revision may be necessary.

The most common reason for a total knee revision arthroplasty is due to loosening of one of components of the TKA. Depending on the type of fixation (cemented or cementless), either the prosthesis loosens from the bone, the prosthesis loosens from the cement, or the cement loosens from the bone. In any event, it is a painful situation and will require replacement of the TKA. Loosening can be attributed to one of several possible causes: infection, trauma, osteoporosis, misalignment of the joint, or simple wearing down of the prosthetic components. Other reasons for total knee revision include breakage of a component and ligament tears or failure.

The results of a total knee revision vary more than they do with a primary knee replacement, but overall the functional outcome is less satisfactory. After the initial TKA, the bone quality is often compromised, making it more difficult to fit the revision components. Scar tissue can limit motion more. Because the results of most revisions are not as good as they are with the first TKA surgery, most surgeons will encourage a patient to wait as long as is possible or practical before undergoing a replacement.

Rehabilitation after a TKA revision is similar to rehab after the first surgery; however, it tends to take longer to regain range of motion, strength, and function. The main advantage is that the patient has already been through the rehabilitation program once and therefore knows what to expect. The rehabilitation exercises outlined in this book apply to both primary and revision TKAs.

■ ■ ■

We have included this Appendix to discuss some of the more common complications that can occur after TKA surgery. Fortunately, they happen only rarely. Again, this information is not intended to scare patients away from having the operation. We believe—and the statistics confirm—that TKA is a reliable procedure with good, reproducible results. We just want you to have an understanding of the potential complications so that you have the best information available, because the patients with the best information generally get the best results!

Common Questions and Some Answers

How do I know if something is wrong with my TKA?

Unexpected and unexplained pain is usually the first sign that something is wrong with the TKA. The other primary symptom is an unexplained decrease in the range of motion of the TKA. "Clicks" or other noises in the knee that are associated with pain may be an indication of a problem with the TKA. Call your surgeon to discuss any symptom if you feel there is a problem.

How do I know if my TKA is infected?

The cardinal signs of infection are increased pain, swelling, redness, excessive warmth in the skin, and increased body temperature. The first and most consistent sign of infection is usually pain. While some of these symptoms are expected following surgery, it is important to pay attention to any sudden increases in pain, swelling, redness, or warmth around the knee joint. A low-grade fever for the first week following surgery is not unusual, but a persistent high fever requires evaluation and treatment. A reduction in the knee's motion will also accompany infection. In general, be wary of any unexplained increase in pain or swelling of the TKA.

Why is the front of my knee numb?

During surgery, the tiny nerves that supply the skin with sensation are cut. It is necessary to cut through the skin—and consequently cut through these nerves—to gain exposure to the knee. Usually the sensation in the skin around the knee returns during the healing process, but it may take six to twelve months to do so. Sometimes there is an altered sensation (paresthesia) in the skin that may feel strange, but it does not affect the function of the TKA. Two years after surgery, Dr. Falkel still has a numb spot on his knee about the size of a silver dollar, but it has not affected his function in any way.

Why is a blood clot so dangerous?

Blood clots in the extremities (deep vein thrombosis or DVT) can impede the blood flow in the area around the clot. These clots are most dangerous if they dislodge and move in the bloodstream, ending up in the lungs (pulmonary embolism or PE). A blood clot in the lungs, whether it started there primarily or came from another location, has the potential to impede blood flow to a large amount of lung tissue. If a significant amount of lung tissue is affected, it can cause serious respiratory conditions or sudden death.

For how long after my TKA surgery am I at risk for infection?

The most vulnerable time for infection is during the perioperative period (the time around the surgery). The perioperative period lasts from the start of the operation until the incision is completely sealed to the outside world (usually about three to seven days). During that time, bacteria have a chance to get underneath the skin and cause an infection. An infection that starts in the perioperative period usually manifests itself within two or three weeks. That is why so many precautions are taken to prevent infection during the surgery and shortly thereafter. Theoretically, and as discussed earlier in the book, any patient with a TKA is at greater risk of developing an infection in the artificial joint for an indefinite period of time. With time, the probability of infection continues to decrease. Maintaining good health will also lower the lifelong chance of infection. Because of the indefinite risk, even though it is very small, patients who have a TKA are asked to take preventive antibiotics before undergoing any surgery or dental work (see Chapter 11).

Can I get an MRI or CT scan without "hurting" my TKA?

An MRI machine has a large magnet that could theoretically put a stress on your TKA, although we have never seen this to be a problem. A cemented (glued) TKA has immediately stable fixation and will not be affected by an MRI scan. A cementless TKA that relies on bone ingrowth for fixation will not achieve stable fixation for approximately six weeks postoperatively. Unless the MRI is needed for an urgent reason, we recommend waiting for three months after surgery before undergoing an MRI scan. A CT scan will not have any affect on the TKA. An MRI or CT scan of a knee with a TKA in place will not provide good images because the metal components distort the picture. However, computer software is improving to minimize this distortion. The TKA will not affect the images from a scan done on any other part of the body.

Will the sun affect my scar?

For the best possible cosmetic results we recommend using a complete sun-block on your incision for at least 12 months after surgery. The scar tissue of the incision takes at least a year to fully mature and is therefore more susceptible to sunburning for the first year after surgery. The sun will not harm the scar. However, it can make the scar look more noticeable if it is not cared for properly.

Appendix B: Index of Exercises

As a quick reference guide, each exercise in the book is listed here, organized by type of exercise.

RANGE-OF-MOTION EXERCISES

RANGE-OF-MOTION EXERCISES (CONT'D.)

STRENGTHENING EXERCISES

STRENGTHENING EXERCISES (CONT'D.)

STRENGTHENING EXERCISES (CONT'D.)

EXERCISE	DESCRIPTION	PAGE
126	Stair-Walking Variation	217
127	Home Stair Training	217
128	Lifting Body Weight Two Steps at a Time	217
129	Lowering Body Weight Two Steps at a Time	218
130	Lowering Body Weight Sideways on Stairs	218

BALANCE EXERCISES

EXERCISE	DESCRIPTION	PAGE
50	Balancing with Feet Together	139
51	Balancing with Feet Together and Eyes Closed	139
52	Balancing with One Foot in Front of the Other	140
53	Balancing with One Foot in Front of the Other and Eyes Closed	140
54	Balancing on the TKA Leg	140
131	Balance Exercise on Stairs	221
132	Balance Exercise on Two-by-Four	221
133	Foot-Swing Balance Exercise on Two-by-Four	222
134	Fast Foot-Swing Balance Exercise on Two-by-Four	222
135	Slow Foot-Swing Balance Exercise on Two-by-Four	222
136	Side-to-Side Swing Balance Exercise in Front of TKA on Two-by-Four	223
137	Side-to-Side Swing Balance Exercise Behind TKA on Two-by-Four	223
138	Balancing on TKA While Playing Catch	224
139	Balancing on TKA on Two-by-Four While Playing Catch	224

BALANCE EXERCISES (CONT'D.)

HOT-TUB AND POOL EXERCISES

HOT-TUB AND POOL EXERCISES (CONT'D.)

Appendix B: Index of Exercises

FUTEBOL EXERCISES

THERA-BAND EXERCISES

WALKING EXERCISES

Notes

1. Rogers, C. *American Academy of Orthopaedic Surgeons Bulletin* February 2002, 50 (1): 13.

2. Ibid.

3. Buckwalter, J. A., Martin, J., and Mankin, H. J. "Instructional Course Lectures," ed. Price, C.T. In *American Academy of Orthopaedic Surgeons* 49 (2002): 481–89; Felson, D. T. "Epidemiology of Osteoarthritis." In *Osteoarthritis*, ed. Brandt, K. D., Doherty, M., and Lohmander, L. S. Oxford, England: Oxford University Press, 1998. 13–22; Felson, D. T. "The Epidemiology of Osteoarthritis: Prevalence and Risk Factors." In *Osteoarthritic Disorders*, ed. Kuettner, K. E., and Goldber, V. M. Rosemont, IL: American Academy of Orthopaedic Surgeons, 1995. 13–24.

4. Buckwalter, J. A., Martin, J., and Mankin, H. J. 481–89.

5. Buckwalter, J. A., Martin, J., and Mankin, H. J. 481–89; Felson, D. T. "Epidemiology of Osteoarthritis." 13–22; Felson, D. T. "The Epidemiology of Osteoarthritis: Prevalence and Risk Factors." 13–24; Praemer, A., Funter, S., and Rice, D. P., ed. *Musculoskeletal Conditions in the United States.* Rosemont, IL: American Academy of Orthopaedic Surgeons, 1992.

6. Gabriel, S. E., Crowson, C. S., and O'Fallon, W. M. "Costs of Osteoarthritis: Estimates from a Geographically Defined Population." *J Rheumatology* 22 (1995), suppl. 43: 23–25; Yelin, E. "The Economics of Osteoarthritis." In *Osteoarthritis*, ed. Brandt, K. D., Doherty, M., and Lohmander, L. S. Oxford, England: Oxford University Press, 1998. 23–30.

7. Buckwalter, J. A., Martin, J., and Mankin, H. J. 481–89.

8. Buckwalter, J. A., and Lane, N. E. "Aging, Sports and Osteoarthritis." *Sports Med Arthroscopic Rev* 4 (1996): 276–87.

9. Buckwalter, J. A., Lane, N. E., and Gordon, S. L. "Exercise as a Cause of Osteoarthritis." In *Osteoarthritic Disorders*, ed. Kuettner, K. E., and Goldber, V. M. Rosemont, IL: American Academy of Orthopaedic Surgeons, 1995. 405–17; Martin, J. A., and Buckwalter J. A. "Articular Cartilage Aging and Degeneration." *Sports Med Arthroscopic Rev* 4 (1996): 263–75.

10. *Primer on the Rheumatologic Diseases.* 9th ed. Atlanta: Arthritis Foundation, 1998. 83–96.

11. Buckwalter, J. A., Martin, J., and Mankin, H. J. 481–89.

12. Price, C. T., ed. "Instructional Course Lectures." In *American Academy of Orthopaedic Surgeons* 49 (2000): 491–94.

13. Theodosakis, J., Adderly, B., and Fox, B., ed. *The Arthritis Cure.* New York: St. Martin's Press, 1997.

14. Price, C. T., ed. "Instructional Course Lectures." 491–94; Tapadinhas, M. J., Rivera, I. C., and Bignamini, A. A. "Oral Glucosamine Sulphate in the Management of Arthritis: Report on a Multicenter Open Investigation in Portugal." *Pharmatherapeutics* 3 (1982): 157–68.

15. Price, C. T., ed. "Instructional Course Lectures." 491–94; McCarty, M. F. "The Neglect of Glucosamine as a Treatment for Osteoarthritis: A Personal Perspective." *Med Hypothesis* 43 (1994): 323–27.

16. Price, C. T., ed. "Instructional Course Lectures." In *American Academy of Orthopaedic Surgeons* 49 (2000): 495–502.

17. Ibid.

18. Lussier, A., Cividino, A. A., McFarlane, C. A., et al. "Viscosupplementation with Hylan for the Treatment of Osteoarthritis: Findings from Clinical Practice in Canada." *J Rheumatology* 23 (1996): 1579–85.

19. Peterson, L. "Articular Cartilage Injuries Treated with Autologous Chondrocyte Transplantation in the Human Knee." *Acta Orthop Belgium* 62 (1996), suppl.: 196–200; Peterson, L. "Current Approaches and Results of Chondrocyte Transplantation." Proceedings of the American Academy of Orthopaedic Surgeons 64th Annual Meeting. Rosemont, IL: American Academy of Orthopaedic Surgeons, 1997. 183.

20. Friel, J. P., ed. *Dorland's Illustrated Medical Dictionary.* Philadelphia: WB Saunders, 1974.

21. Insall, J. N., Hood, R. W., Flawn, L. B., and Sullivan, D. J. "The Total Condylar Knee Prothesis in Arthritis: A Five- to Nine-Year Follow-Up of the First Hundred Consecutive Replacements." *J Bone Joint Surg* 65A (1983): 619.

22. Bernard, F., and Rand, J. A. "Infection." In Morrey, B. F., ed. *Joint Replacement Arthroplasty.* New York: Churchill Livingston, Mayo Foundation Publishers, 1991. 1067–80.

23. Asp, J., and Rand, J. A. "Peroneal Nerve Palsy Following Total Knee Arthroplasty." *Orthop Trans* 12 (1988): 717.

24. Rand, J. A. "Complications of Total Knee Arthroplasty." In Morrey, B. F., ed. *Joint Replacement Arthroplasty.* New York: Churchill Livingston, Mayo Foundation Publishers, 1991. 1085–92.

25. Rand, J. A. "Revision of the Total Knee Arthroplasty: Techniques and Results." In Morrey, B. F., ed. *Joint Replacement Arthroplasty.* New York: Churchill Livingston, Mayo Foundation Publishers, 1991. 1093–1104.

Index

A

B

E

F

G

H

L

M

N

O

P

Q

R

S

T

U

V

W

X

Y

More Hunter House books on TAKING CARE OF YOUR BODY

TREAT YOUR OWN KNEES

by Jim Johnson, P.T. ... Foreword by James R. Roberson, M.D.

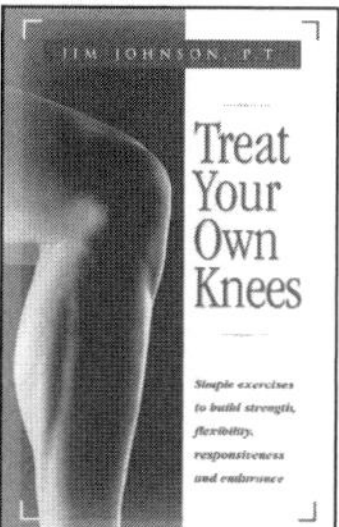

An inexpensive, compact, useful book. The author, a physical therapist, reviewed hundreds of scientific journal articles to find the most simple and effective do-it-yourself treatments for knee pain. Simple illustrations depict the muscles responsible for knee pain and the correct way to perform exercises that can enhance the four crucial abilities every knee must have: muscular strength, flexibility, responsiveness (proprioception), and endurance. The last chapter combines the concepts and exercises in a time-efficient exercise program.

128 pages ... 21 illus. ... Paperback $10.95

TREAT YOUR BACK WITHOUT SURGERY: The Best Nonsurgical Alternatives for Eliminating Back and Neck Pain

by Stephen Hochschuler, M.D., and Bob Reznik

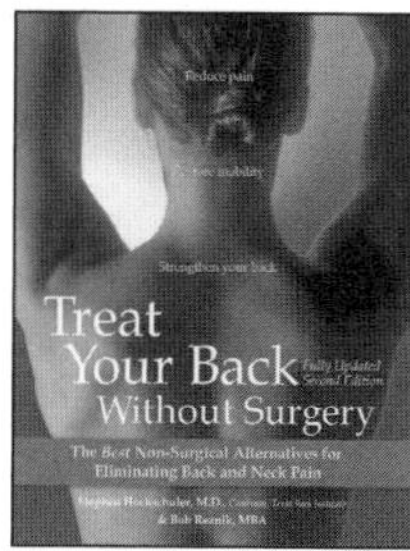

Eighty percent of back pain sufferers can get well without surgery. Be one of them! From the authors of *Back in Shape,* this new guide discusses a range of nonsurgical techniques — from tai chi and massage therapy to chiropractic treatment and acupuncture — as well as exercise plans, diet and stress management techniques, and tips to ease everyday pain. Because surgery is sometimes necessary, you'll also get advice on how to find the best surgeon and what questions to ask.

224 pages ... 58 b/w photos ... 6 illus. ... Paperback $15.95

THE CHIROPRACTOR'S SELF-HELP BACK AND BODY BOOK: How You Can Relieve Common Aches and Pains at Home and on the Job

by Samuel Homola, D.C.

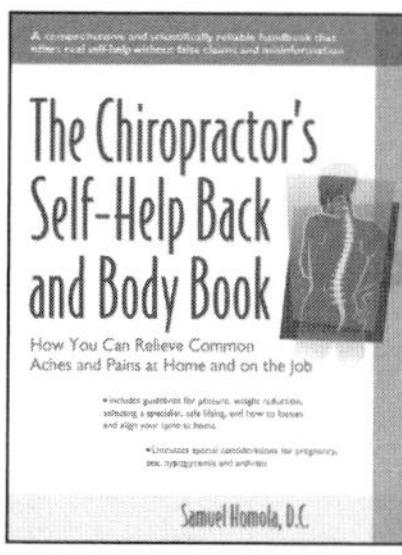

Written by a chiropractor with over 40 years experience, this book is for people with chronic head, neck, arm, wrist, back, hip, leg, and shoulder pain as well as sufferers from osteoporosis, a weak back, sciatica, arthritis, and hypoglycemia. It includes information on how to handle arthritis, how to protect a weak back during sex and pregnancy, and how to tell sense from nonsense in the chiropractic care of your back pain. The book is illustrated with 42 line drawings prepared by a professional artist.

320 pages ... 42 illus. ... Paperback $17.95

To order or for our FREE catalog call (800) 266-5592

More Hunter House books on BODY HEALTH & FITNESS

THE GOOD FOOT BOOK: A Guide for Men, Women, Children, Athletes, Seniors — Everyone ... *by Glenn Copeland, DMP, with Stan Solomon*

As baby-boomers reach the wear-and-tear stage of life they can find foot problems seriously impeding their mobility. Glenn Copeland, a leading podiatrist, provides the latest information and advice on preventing and curing foot problems.

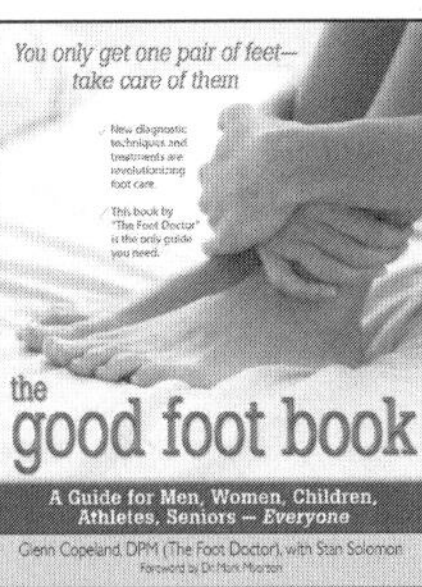

His book covers common foot problems — bunions, hammer toes, corns, calluses and warts — and the problems faced by diabetics, seniors, and athletes. It discusses diagnostic and treatment procedures including ankle replacement surgery and explains orthotic foot therapy and what it can do for the feet and the whole body.

256 pages ... 47 illus. ... Paperback 16.95 ... SEPTEMBER 2004

GET FIT WHILE YOU SIT: Easy Workouts from Your Chair
by Charlene Torkelson

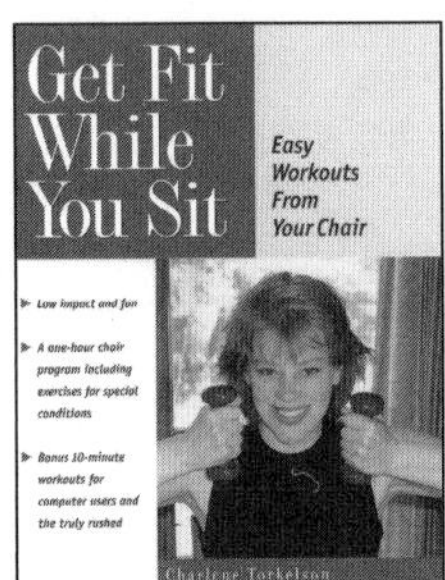

Here is a total-body workout that can be done right from your chair, anywhere. It is perfect for office workers, travelers, and those with age-related movement limitations or special conditions. This book offers three programs. The One-Hour Chair Program is a full-body, low-impact workout that includes light aerobics and exercises to be done with or without weights. The 5-Day Short Program features five compact workouts for those short on time. Finally, the Ten-Minute Miracles is a group of easy-to-do exercises perfect for anyone on the go.

160 pages ... 210 photos ... Paperback $14.95

SHAPEWALKING: Six Easy Steps to Your Best Body
by Marilyn Bach, Ph.D., and Lorie Schleck, M.A., P.T.

Millions of Americans want an easy, low-cost fitness program. *ShapeWalking* is the answer. It includes aerobic exercise, strength training, and flexibility stretching and is ideal for exercisers of all levels who want to control weight; develop muscle definition; prevent or reverse loss of bone density; and spot-shape the stomach, buttocks, arms, and thighs. The second edition includes over 70 photographs as well as updated exercises and resources.

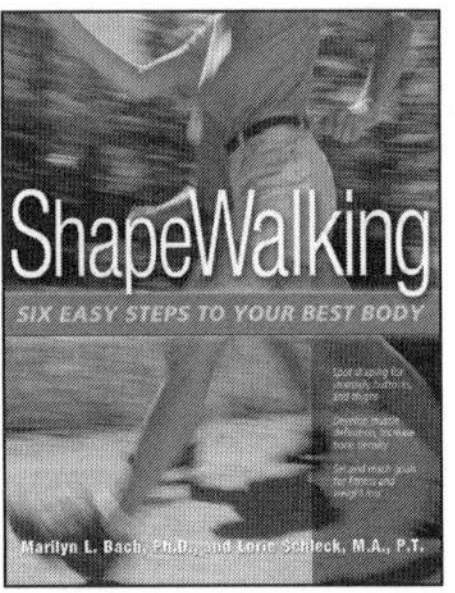

144 pages ... 73 photos ... Paperback $14.95

Prices subject to change without notice